Advances and Technical Standards in Neurosurgery

Volume 47

This series, which has earned a reputation over the years and is considered a classic in the neurosurgical field, is now relaunched under the editorship of Professor Di Rocco, which relies on the collaboration of a renewed editorial board.

Both volumes focused on recent advances in neurosurgery and on technical standards, and monographs devoted to more specific subjects in the neurosurgical field will implement it. Written by key opinion leaders, the series volumes will be useful for young neurosurgeons in their postgraduate training but also for more experienced clinicians.

Dachling Pang • Kyu-Chang Wang

Editors

Spinal Dysraphic Malformations

Science and Surgery - Volume 47

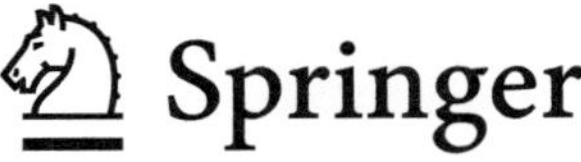 Springer

Editors
Dachling Pang
NHS Trust
Great Ormond Street Hospital
LONDON, UK

Kyu-Chang Wang
Center for Rare Cancers
National Cancer Center
Goyang, Korea (Republic of)

ISSN 0095-4829 ISSN 1869-9189 (electronic)
Advances and Technical Standards in Neurosurgery
ISBN 978-3-031-34983-6 ISBN 978-3-031-34981-2 (eBook)
https://doi.org/10.1007/978-3-031-34981-2

This Springer imprint is published by the registered company Springer Nature Switzerland AG
The registered company address is: Gewerbestrasse 11, 6330 Cham, Switzerland

Preface

Advances and Technical Standards in Neurosurgery (ATSN) represents the successful achievement of the wish of Jean Brihaye, Bernard Pertuised, Fritz Loew, and Hugo Krayenbuhl to provide the European neurosurgeons in training with a high-level publication to accompany the teaching provided by the European post-graduate course. The project was conceived during the joint meeting of the German and Italian Neurosurgical Societies in Taormina in 1972, and the first volume was published in 1974. The English language was chosen to facilitate the international exchange of information and the circulation of scientific progress. Since then, the ATSN has hosted chapters by eminent European neurosurgeons and has become one of the most renowned educational tools on the continent for both young and experienced neurosurgeons. The successive editorial boards have maintained the ATSN's high scientific quality and ensured a good balance between contributions dealing with advances in neurosciences over the years and detailed descriptions of surgical techniques as well as analyses of clinical experiences. Additional appeal has been added by freedom granted by the Editor and Publisher in the length, style, and organization of the published papers.

The current series aims to preserve the original spirit of the publication and its high-level didactic function but intends to present itself not only as a historic European publication but as a truly international forum for most advanced clinical research and modern operating standards.

Hannover, Germany   Concezio Di Rocco

Contents

Gastrulation and Split Cord Malformation

Zubair Tahir and Claudia Craven

Definition

Split cord malformation (SCM) is a form of closed spinal dysraphism, in which two hemi-cords are present, instead of a single spinal cord. SCM is categorised into type 1 and type 2 [1]. SCM type 1 and type 2 are always distinct but can occur as composite SCMs in the same individual at different vertebral levels.

1. Type 1 SCM is defined by the presence of a bony or osseocartilaginous spur between the hemi-cords (Fig. 1a). The hemi-cords are contained within separate dural tubes. Type 1 was previously referred to as diastematomyelia (diasterma = cleft, myelos = marrow or spinal cord, in Greek).
2. Type 2 SCM has no bony spur, and the two hemi-cords are contained within a single dura, with minimal or no fibrous tissue between (Fig. 1b). Type 2 was previously referred to as diplomyelia.

Nomenclature

The term diastematomyelia was first described by pathologist Ollivier d'Angers in 1837 [2]. At one point, three terms were being used to describe split cord malformations: diastematomyelia, hemidydemia and diplomyelia [3]. Not only were these considered by many to have very different embryological origins, but the nomenclature usage was inconsistent and, at times, confusing [2].

Z. Tahir (✉) · C. Craven
Great Ormond Street Children Hospital, London, UK
e-mail: zubair.tahir@gosh.nhs.uk

© The Author(s), under exclusive license to Springer Nature Switzerland AG 2023
D. Pang, K.-C. Wang (eds.), *Spinal Dysraphic Malformations*, Advances and Technical Standards in Neurosurgery 47,
https://doi.org/10.1007/978-3-031-34981-2_1

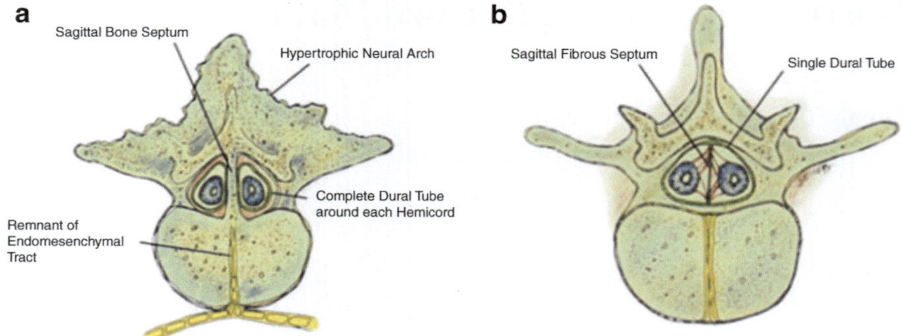

Fig. 1 (**a**) Type 1 SCM is defined by the presence of a bony spur between the hemi-cords. (**b**) Type 2 SCM with no bony spur and the two hemi-cords are contained within a single dura (Figure adapted from Pang 2020 [6])

Diastematomyelia and diplomyelia have since been replaced with SCM type 1 and type 2 respectively, in 1992, after Pang proposed a unified theory for the pathophysiology [1]. This also reduced use of diastematomyelia and diplomyelia, although you will still see these terms in the literature.

In addition to type 1 and type 2 SCM, Mahapatra et al. have proposed four type 1 subtypes a–d, based upon the location of the bony spur (being superior, inferior, or straddling the bifurcation) [4]. This additional nomenclature is rarely used in day-to-day clinical practice. In 2020, Meena and colleagues proposed a type 1.5 SCM, to explain the rare cases with mixed features of type 1 and type 2, where an extradural partial bony septum is present (like type 1) but the hemi-cords were found to be a single dural sac (like type 2) [5]. However, this phenomenon is rare, and few use the type 1.5 SCM terminology, owing to controversy over whether it is a variation of type 1 [6].

Epidemiology

SCM has affected humans for centuries, with the oldest known specimen dating back to AD 100, in a skeleton recovered from a burial site in the Israeli desert [7, 8]. SCMs have an estimated prevalence of 0.02%, with a slight female preponderance (1.3:1) [1, 9]. SCMs are rare and represent less than 5% of all congenital spinal abnormalities [1]. Type 1 occurs more commonly than type 2 [1, 9]. Although rare, SCM is important to understand and recognise, given the potential for neurological deterioration.

Pathology

Macroscopic: Type 1 SCM will always have the presence of a midline bony spur (best identified with computed tomography) between the hemi-cords, whereas type 2 will lack this. The most common locations for SCM are thoracic region (38%), followed by lumbar (38%), thoraco-lumbar (24%), cervicothoracic (6%) and lumbosacral (4%). Type 1 SCM occurs more commonly in the thoraco-lumbar region whereas type 2 occurs in the cervicothoracic region [1]. In 5–10% of type 1 SCMs, the bony septum is oblique. The majority of hemi-cords (91%) reunite caudally [10]. The spinous process and lamina at the level of bony septum are usually hypertrophic. Anomalies of the adjacent vertebrae, including anomalous segmentation and defects of the posterior arch, are common and may result in progressive scoliosis.

Microscopic: Dorsal and ventral septae are often associated with blood vessels, fat, and muscle, visible macroscopically and also demonstrable on histopathology slides [6]. Paramedian nerve roots often adhere to the septum (Fig. 2a) and can occur in 75–90% in both SCM 1 and 2, and therefore cannot be used to differentiate the two entities as previously thought [1, 6]. Nerve roots can also adhere to the dura or adjacent fat, forming a meningocele manqué (Fig. 2b) [6, 10].

Aetiology

SCM appears to be a sporadically occurring phenomenon. Unlike for open neural tube defects, folate plays no known role in SCM formation [11]. The underlying cause of SCM appears to be partly epigenetic, and partly environmental, with no known responsible genes [11].

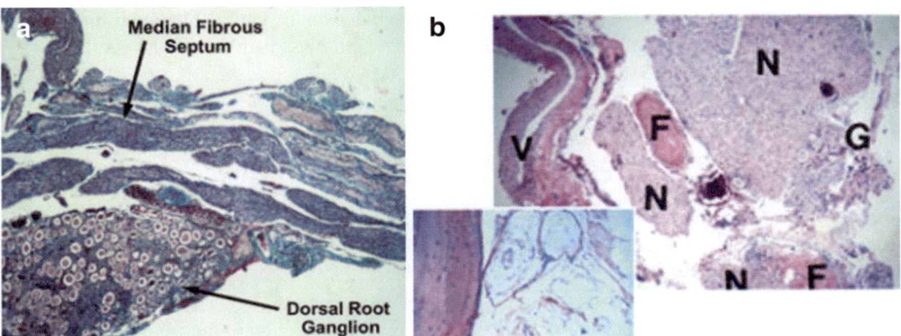

Fig. 2 (**a**) Paramedian dorsal root inside the median fibrous septum (with a dorsal root ganglion attached). (**b**) Histological slide of the extradural 'meningocele manqué' containing vessels (V), nerves (N) (paramedian dorsal roots), fibrous bands (F) and ganglion cells (G). The inset shows a Pacinian corpuscle developing also. (Figure adapted from Pang 2020 [6])

SCM has been hypothesised to originate during the embryological phase of gastrulation [1]. Whilst there are animal models for open neural tube defects, this is not the case for SCM [11–14], and embryological explanations are largely theoretical and knowledge gleaned from animal studies should be interpreted with caution. Gastrulation differs widely between species and may not be directly extrapolated to humans.

Before detailing putative embryological mechanisms leading to SCM, it is prudent to revise the processes that underpin early embryonic development, gastrulation, and notochord formation.

Embryology: Germinal Phase

Table 1 summarises the key stages that occur from fertilisation, the germinal phase (the 10 days of division of the zygote to implantation) and the resulting bilaminar disc consisting of a hypoblast and an epiblast layer. At this early stage, cell destiny

Table 1 Early stages of embryogenesis prior to gastrulation

Fertilisation (day 0)	Fertilisation of the egg occurs. The resulting single cell is called a zygote, and is within a zona, with a polar body in the zona, and has pronuclei
Cleavage (day 2)	Soon after fertilisation, cells divide into a sphere of identical cells (blastomeres) referred to as the 'morula'. Stochastic (or random) gene expression starts to alter the interactions between cells
Compaction (day 3)	Compaction of the cells starts to occur, and the cells interact with one another via tight cell junctions. The most peripheral cells of the sphere have reduced cell–cell interaction and altered physical forces [11]
Differentiation (day 4)	Due to the different forces on the outer cells, a different cascade of intracellular events results in the outer cells forming a distinct layer of trophoblasts called 'trophoectoderm'
Cavitation (day 5)	The trophoectoderm (which will become placental membranes) secretes fluid resulting in a fluid cavity called the blastocoelic cavity. The remaining cells become the 'inner cell mass'. The overall mass inside the zona is now a blastocyst
Zona hatching (day 6)	The blastocyst hatches from the zona
Implantation (day 7)	The blastocyst implants into the uterine epithelium
Differentiation (day 9)	Again, owing to reduced cell–cell interactions and forces, the peripheral cells of the inner cell mass differentiate into the 'hypoblast' layer. The remaining cells of the inner cell mass form the epiblast
Bilaminar disc formation (day 12)	The outer cells of the hypoblast become the yolk sac. The epiblasts separate from the surrounding layer creating an adjacent amniotic cavity. At this stage, the embryo consists of a bilaminar disc, consisting of a hypoblast layer (facing the yolk sac), and an epiblast layer (facing the amniotic cavity). The epiblast will eventually differentiate to become the three primitive germ layers, in the next phase (gastrulation)

is determined by location in physical space, the forces applied to the cells and the cell–cell interactions [11].

Embryology: Gastrulation

Gastrulation is a critical embryological stage occurring in third week of life, in which the bilaminar disc becomes trilaminar, producing three primitive germ layers: the ectoderm, mesoderm, and endoderm (layers destined to form organs) (Fig. 3) and a notochord (Fig. 4). It is also during gastrulation that three-dimensional polarity to the cell is established. Therefore, errors at this stage can result in major anatomical defects. Indeed, the embryologist Lewis Wolpert once said, 'It is not birth, marriage or death but gastrulation which is truly the most important time of your life' [15]. Tables 2 and 3 outline the key stages observed in various animal models and studies for gastrulation and notochord formation, respectively.

Dysraphism and Embryology

Split cord malformation has been hypothesised to be an error occurring during the embryological phase of gastrulation [1, 21]. Many other dysraphic states have been attributed to errors in various stages of embryogenesis. Table 4 shows the classification of spinal dysraphism according to putative stages in embryogenesis [6]. Table 5 shows the various congenital abnormalities attributed to events occurring in gastrulation [11].

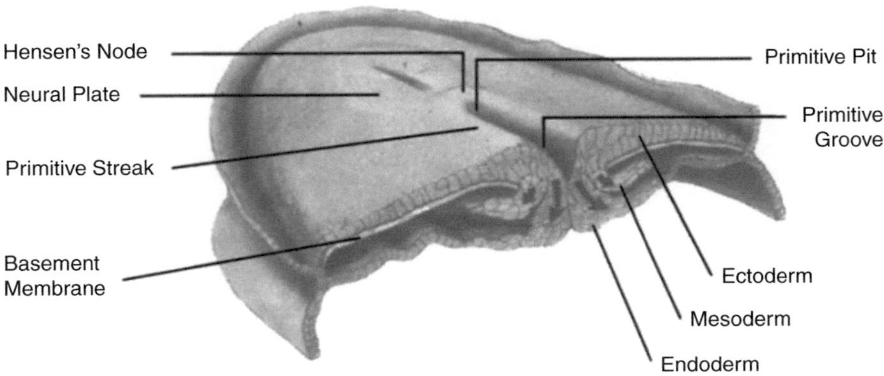

Fig. 3 Gastrulation. Epiblast cells move from the dorsal surface (indicated by arrow) to form deeper layers (mesoderm and endoderm), via the primitive streak. (Adapted from Pang 2020 [6])

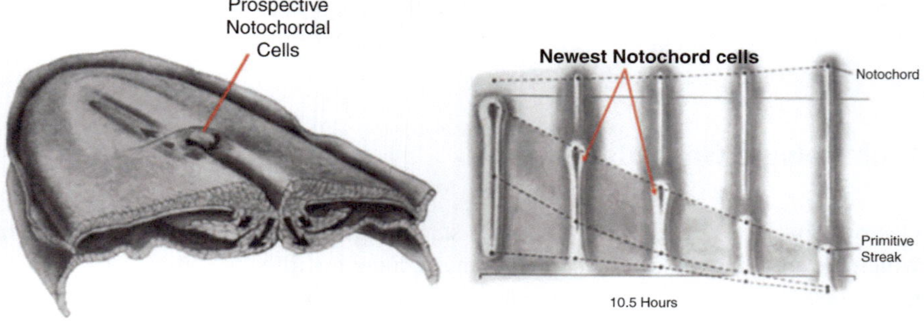

Fig. 4 Formation of the notochord. (**a**) Epiblasts move through the primitive pit and lie between ectoderm and endoderm, forming a tube-like structure called the notochord. (**b**) The notochord adds cells to the caudal end, then elongates cranially (Adapted from Pang 2020 [6])

Table 2 Key stages of gastrulation

AVE formation	Gastrulation starts on day 18 post ovulation. The hypoblast cell–cell interactions and position within the disc result in further gene activations differentiating cells from their neighbours. These cells migrate to the edge of the hypoblast, forming the 'anterior visceral endoderm' (AVE) [11]
Epiblast inhibition	The AVE sends inhibitory signals to epiblasts, preventing them from maturing and migrating too early
Primitive streak formation	The inhibitory signals do not reach all epiblast cells. The few epiblast cells that are uninhibited respond to signalling proteins causing them to migrate to the centre, thus forming the dorsal primitive streak
Cranio-caudal polarity	The primitive streak initially forms at the 'caudal' end of the embryo, thus starting embryonal polarity. The primitive node (also known as Hensen's node), a mass of epiblasts, forms at the 'cranial' end
Epiblast intercalation	As epiblasts continue to evade the inhibitory signals, more cells 'intercalate' into the primitive streak, causing it to elongate
Epiblast internalisation (Emboly)	The primitive node releases signalling proteins. These proteins mobilise epiblast cells from adjacent cells and activate motility proteins in the cytoskeleton, causing the cells to migrate towards and into the primitive streak via the primitive pit [16] (Fig. 1). Those closest to the node will migrate first, due to the higher concentration gradient
Epithelial to mesenchymal transition (EMT)	The cells that first migrated through the primitive streak displace hypoblast cells laterally and transform to become the endoderm. The cells that migrated later through the primitive streak transform to the mesoderm, the layer between endoderm and the epiblast [17]. The dorsal epiblast cells then become the ectoderm. EMT is a self-amplifying positive feedback process [18]
Epiboly	These sheets of similar cells then extend by spreading out and thinning. The direction of the sheet growth is controlled by signalling pathways
Convergence and extension	The Wnt and planar cell polarity (PCP) signalling pathways encourage cranio-caudal lengthening and transverse narrowing [19]. This is achieved through downregulation of adhesion molecules, thus enabling movement and shape changes. At the end of gastrulation, the embryo is an elongated shape with three-dimensional polarity

Table 3 Key stages of notochord formation and relevant latter stages

Notochord formation	
Early notochord formation	Cells from the primitive node (below the epiblast) move through the primitive pit and lie between ectoderm and endoderm, forming the tube called the notochord under the direction of signalling proteins Wnt, VegT and BMP [20] (Fig. 2a)
Notochord elongation	Around day 16, the primitive streak starts to regress caudally, and the notochord starts to form and grow cranially (Fig. 2b)
Neurenteric canal intercalation	Around day 18, the tubular notochord (the notochordal canal) briefly intercalates with the endoderm, dorsally communicating with the amniotic cavity and ventrally with the yolk sac, forming the neurenteric canal
Neurenteric canal extracalation	Around day 20–26, the canal then separates (extracalates) away from the endoderm
True notochord formation	The tubular canal forms a solid cord (the true notochord) running cranio-caudally
Relevant later embryological stages	
Primary neurulation	This process is not part of gastrulation but is summarised to demonstrate the big picture and future role of the notochord. During primary neurulation, the notochord signals via sonic hedgehog (SHH) to ectoderm to fold into the neural tube, which caudally will become the spinal cord. The closure of the neural tube starts at distinct points referred to as neuropores. The cranial neuropore closes on day 23–25 and the caudal on days 25–27
Meninx primitiva	On day 29, meninx primitiva cells (bipotential cells for bone and dura) appear between the notochord and neural tube. They migrate around the neural tube to form dura and bony arches

Split Cord Malformation and Embryology

The embryological basis of SCMs remains unknown. There have however been numerous attempts to explain the phenomenon of SCM from a developmental perspective from the earliest by Dareste in 1839, through the most widely accepted unified theory from Pang in 1992 [1, 22]. All of these are embryological and morphological hypotheses, most of which apply the rule of Ockham's razor. To better contextualise the 'unified' theory, we describe historical and more recent developments in the theory of SCM development in Table 6.

In 1940, Herren and Edwards suggested the 'twinning' model, a phenomenon where the neural folds fuse with the neural plate in the midline, resulting in two hemi-cords [26]. Since then, most theories have focused on errors during gastrulation. Lichtenstein (who had coined the term 'spinal dysraphism' in 1940) first proposed that gastrulation was in fact the more likely embryological stage of error [27]. He suggested that the bony septum was due to a defect in mesoderm formation resulting in a midline malformation and a split neural plate. Rokos in 1975 postulated that, if SCM and spina bifida can coexist, a destructive phenomenon directly to the neural tube or its precursor must occur [3].

Bremmer hypothesised that, in SCM, the previous ectodermal-endodermal interface can persist as an adhesion in the midline [21]. This adhesion disrupts the

Table 4 Classification of spinal dysraphism by putative embryonic stages (Table adapted from Pang et al. [6])

Gastrulation
Split cord malformation (type 1 and type 2)
Neural tube defects: primary neurulation
Open neural tube defects
Neural tube defects: premature disjunction
Dorsal lipoma
Neural tube defects: delayed disjunction
Limited dorsal myeloschisis
Dermal sinus and cyst
Secondary neurulation
Fatty filum
Terminal lipoma
Caudal agenesis
Retained medullary cord
Terminal myelocystocele [cavitation of the caudal cell mass]
Mixed primary and secondary neurulation
Transitional lipoma
Chaotic lipoma

Table adapted from Pang et al. [6]

Table 5 Stages of gastrulation and examples of congenital abnormalities (Table adapted from Thompson [11])

Stage	Anomaly	Congenital abnormality
Primitive streak	Duplication	Conjoined twins
Notochord	Notochord rests	Chordoma
Notochord	Notochord splitting	Split cord malformation
Neurenteric canal	Accessory neurenteric canal	Neurenteric cyst
Caudal mesoderm	Impaired migration	Caudal agenesis and sirenomyelia
Caudal mesoderm	MNX1 mutation	Currarino syndrome

midline integration notochord progenitor cells, resulting in a 'split' or duplicated notochord (Fig. 5a) [1]. This subsequently results in separate neurulation of the two hemi-neural plates, and ultimately two hemi-cords developing (Fig. 5b) [1].

Building upon this theory, Pang and colleagues proposed that primitive mesenchyme cells (destined to become bone) and meningeal progenitor cells (destined to become dura, respectively) are invested around the adhesion, forming an endomesenchymal tract (Fig. 5c) [1]. These cells then form between the hemi-cord and hemi-neural tube (Fig. 5d) [1].

Table 6 The evolution of embryological hypothesis for SCM development

Year	Authors	Embryo stage	Hypothesised error
1839	Dareste [3, 22]	Germinal phase	Proposed amniotic adhesions to explain the double cord (a duplication event)
1881 1938	Koch [23] Schiderling [24]	Neurulation	Each half of the neural plate closed separately
1881 1889	Koch [3] Pick [3, 25]	Neurulation	After neurulation, a medio-sagittal septum forms to divide the cord
1940	Herren and Edwards [26]	Neurulation	'Twinning' model. The neural folds are exaggerated and fuse with the neural plate in the midline, resulting in two hemi-cords. They also stated that the SCM could not be due to arrested development
1940	Lichtenstein [27]	Gastrulation	An error of mesoderm formation, resulting in a malformed midline and split neural plate
1958	Beardmore and Wigglesworth [3, 28]	Gastrulation	Notochordal splitting and endomesenchymal tract formation consequent on endodermal–ectodermal adhesion
1973	Gardner [29]	Neurulation	Hydromyelia distends the neural tube, and it ruptures into two cords, with subsequent fibrous tissue (mesenchymal cell) repair in the midline to form the bony spur
1975	Rokos [3]	Notochord formation	SCM and spina bifida can coexist even at the same level suggests a possible common pathogenesis that destructive phenomenon occurs to the neural tube or its precursor
1952	Bremmer [21]	Gastrulation	Ectodermal–endodermal interface can persist as an adhesion in the midline, disrupting the midline integration of notochord progenitor cells, resulting in a 'split' or duplicated notochord
1992	Dias and Walker [30]	Gastrulation	SCMs were associated with skin lesions, and intestinal malformations, affecting organs derived from all germ layers. They therefore hypothesised that simultaneous disruption of cells during gastrulation resulted in SCM
1992	Pang [1]	Gastrulation	Built upon Bremmer's hypothesis. The unified theory includes both SCM 1 and SCM 2 under the same gastrulation error, with a final difference owing to the presence or absence of the meninx cells in the median cleft
2022	Sun [31]	Gastrulation	Built upon Bremmer's hypothesis but is alternative to the unified theory, both SCM 1 and 2 start with a bony septum, however type 1.5 and type 2 occur due to regression of the bony septum. The amount of condensing of meninx primitive might determine if the septum extends to the opposite dura

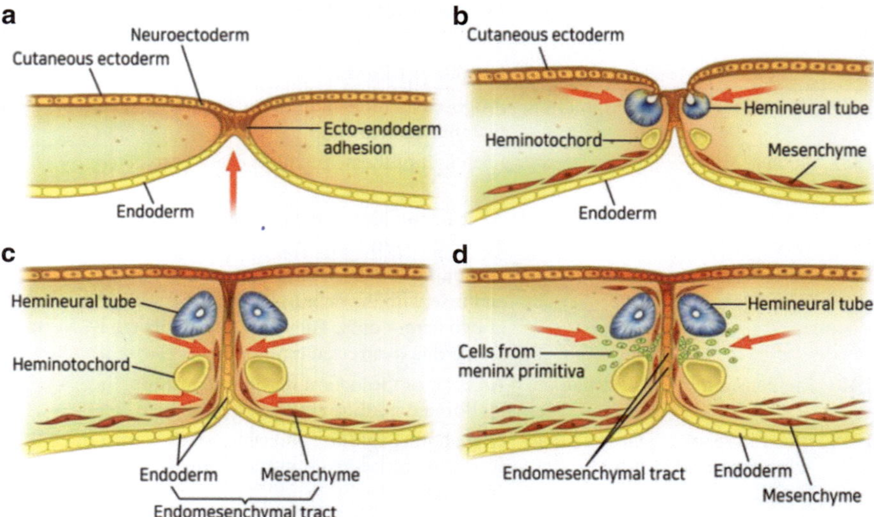

Fig. 5 (**a**) An accessory neurenteric canal may begin as an ecto-endodermal adhesion, bisecting the midline neuroectoderm to give two hemi-plates. (**b**) Each hemi-neural plate neurulates independently. (**c**) Mesenchyme condenses around the fistula to form endomesenchymal tract. (**d**) Cells from meninx primitiva appear between the hemi-neural tube and hemi notochord. (Text and Figure adapted from Pang et al. 2020 [6])

The presence of the meninx cells in the median cleft (Fig. 6a) results in the bony spur seen in type 1 SCM (Fig. 6b). In type 2 SCM, the endomesenchymal tract does entrap the meninx cells. The absence of the cells in the median cleft (Fig. 6c) results in no dural layer, no bone and no cartilage, just a thin fibrous septum between the hemi-cords of type 2 SCM (Fig. 6d) [1, 6]. It is unclear why some endomesenchymal tracts trap the meninx cells while other tracts exclude them [6]. The cervical spine undergoes early neurulation so the meninx cells are too late to be incorporated into the endomesenchymal tract, hence the cervical spine has typically type 2 SCM [6].

Combined dysraphic pathology with SCM is common and can support or refute the unified theory [32–35]. These include cases of SCM with a dorsal bony spur [36, 37], or a cervical type 1 SCM (something which should not occur in unified theory [38] or intermediate appearing types with a midline ventral bony spur (as seen in SCM type 1) but with a single dural sac encasing both the hemi-cords (consistent with SCM type 2) [5, 39]. To explain the latter, Sun and colleagues have proposed an alternative theory, whereby both SCM 1 and 2 start with a bony septum; however, type 1.5 and type 2 occur due to regression of the bony septum [30]. They hypothesise that the amount of condensing of meninx primitive might determine if the septum extends to the opposite dura [31].

To date, there are no confirmatory studies for any of the aforementioned embryological hypotheses. The unified theory is the most widely accepted to date, owing to the large series and elegance of the hypothesis.

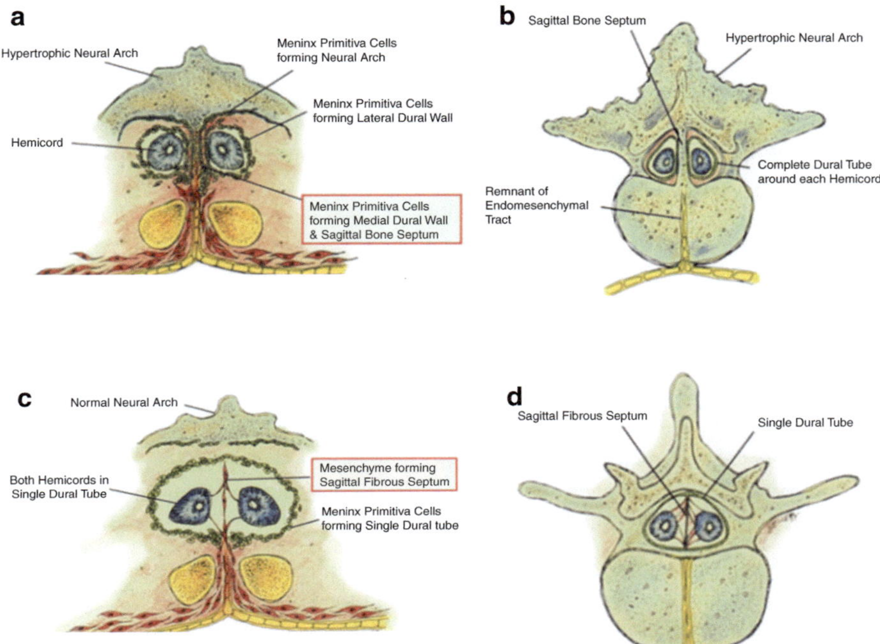

Fig. 6 (**a**) Formation of type 1 SCM, with meninx primitive cells forming medial dural wall and sagittal bony septum. (**b**) Type 1 SCM with a typical hypertrophic neural arch and bony septum, with the remnant of endomesenchymal tract. (**c**) Formation of type 2 SCM, with meninx primitive cells forming a single dural tube. (**d**) Type 2 SCM with a thin sagittal fibrous septum. (Text and Figure adapted from Pang et al. 2020 [6])

Split Cord Malformation and Experimental Evidence

Few replicable animal models for SCM exist. Experimental evidence to support the unified theory is limited. In the newt model *Cynops pyrrhogaster*, a fistula was made across the neural plate during gastrulation, to attempt to replicate the above adhesion processes. A splitting of the spinal cord reminiscent of SCM resulted [40, 41]. One early model of ethanol-induced spinal cord duplications have been reported in the Zebra fish embryo *Brachydanio rerio* [42]. Other avian models also support the SCM is likely to be an error of gastrulation, and that atopic mesoderm has a role to play in bony septum formation [43, 44].

However, there are few experimental studies strongly supporting any of the embryological hypotheses. Neural tube closure is known to be carefully genetically regulated, through activation of some identified individuals or clusters of genes [12–14]. In future, genetic explanations will be able to further elucidate the pathophysiology of SCM also, which in term will further explain the mechanisms in which SCM occurs [32].

Signs and Symptoms

Cutaneous changes, sympathetic dystrophy, neurological symptoms (including urinary symptoms) and neuro-orthopaedic signs are the predominant presenting features of SCM. Table 7 summarises the presenting signs and symptoms in SCM.

Cutaneous stigmata of SCM are most common, occurring in 90% of patients, with hypertrichosis occurring in around 60% of cases (Fig. 7) [45, 46]. Neurological symptoms and signs are often non-specific but progressive sequelae of spinal cord tethering, including back pain, radiating leg pain and lower extremity paraesthesia (44%), leg weakness (73%), and urinary incontinence (in at least 33%) are well recognised [46, 47]. Unlike other dysraphic tethering lesions, SCM carries a higher likelihood of left-right discrepancy in neurological function, relating to the difference in size of hemi-cords. Baseline urodynamics are advised, particularly prior to surgical intervention [48].

Both types of SCM are tethering lesions; however, type 1 has higher incidence of getting symptomatic. The clinical picture is similar between type 1 and type 2 patients, with following noted exceptions:

1. Type 1 patients are more prone to have prominent pain of both dysaesthetic type in legs and perineum and the localised pain at the split cord site.
2. The incidence of progressive scoliosis is significantly higher in type 1.
3. Signs of chronic sympathetic dystrophy such as a nonhealing ulcer, thin shiny skin, hairlessness, and anhidrosis are much more common in type 1.

The timing of the clinical presentation varies. Naturally patients with cutaneous stigmata in infancy would undergo a subsequent screening MRI scan and, as a result, the majority of presentations will be in infancy. Patients with SCM can also be initially asymptomatic but may present later in life with tethering or scoliosis [45, 49]. Some patients will present with an associated condition such as syringomyelia (see associated conditions section). Finally a small proportion of patients will present acutely with spinal cord injury after trauma (as they are more predisposed to injury with tethering and bony spur), or after spinal surgery for scoliosis (if undiagnosed) [49].

Table 7 Presenting signs and symptoms in SCM

Cutaneous stigmata	Hypertrichosis, haemangiomas, lumbar dimples, or lumbar subcutaneous masses
Chronic sympathetic dystrophy	Nonhealing ulcers, thin shiny skin, hairlessness, anhidrosis
Tethering with neurological symptoms	Back pain, radiating leg pain, lower extremity paraesthesia, leg weakness, and urinary incontinence. Left-right discrepancy in neurological function
Neuro-orthopaedic	Scoliosis, torticollis, leg length discrepancy and talipes equinovarus

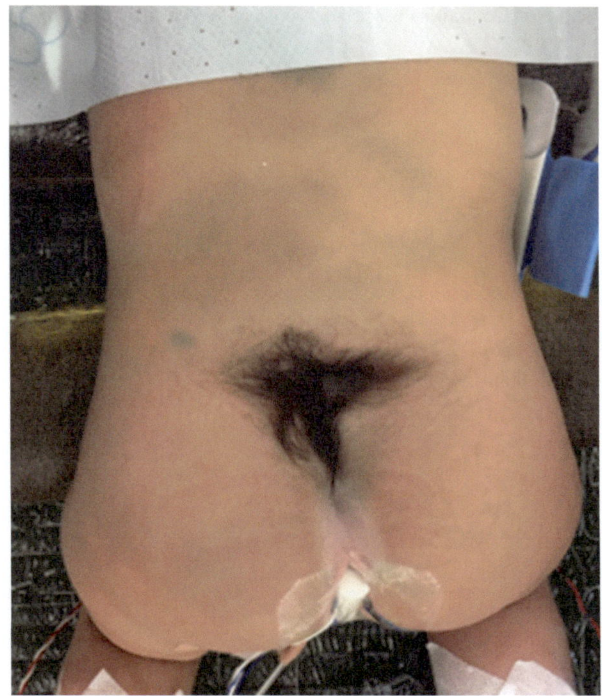

Fig. 7 Lumbar hypertrichosis is a common skin stigmata of SCM

Associated Conditions

Associated congenital spinal deformity occurs in 85% of patients with SCM type 1 [10]. This can include:

1. Composite split cord malformations (e.g. a SCM type 1 occurring at L2–L3 and SCM type 2 occurring at L5, in the same patient) [50, 51].
2. Other dysraphic conditions, including those occurring in gastrulation (neurenteric cysts) [10], primary neurulation (myelomeningocele) [10, 52] and secondary neurulation (terminal myelocystocele or terminal lipoma) [32].
3. Other developmental anomalies such as segmentation anomalies of spinal vertebrae [10, 32, 53].
4. Conditions that are likely to be a consequence of the SCM (tethered cord and syringomyelia) [45].

Some of these coexisting pathologies affect both hemi-cords (e.g. a twin dorsal lipoma) whilst others just one hemi-cord [54, 55]. Table 8 lists some of these pathologies, from commonly occurring (such as scoliosis) to the rarely coexisting conditions. One particularly rare mixed malformation is the SCM and hemi-limited dorsal myeloschisis (LDM) [54]. Pang et al. reported only one hemi-LDM in SCM 1 and one hemi-LDM in SCM 2 in a series of 255 cases SCM [54]. Interestingly, in

Table 8 Conditions associated with split cord malformation (organised from common to rarely coexisting)

Associated conditions	Frequency	References
Scoliosis	79%	[10, 45, 58]
Radiological tethered cord	75%	[6, 10]
Segmentation and fusion anomalies	60%	[10, 32, 53, 59]
Composite SCM 1 and SCM 2 (at different levels)	Common	[50]
Thickened filum terminale	40–90%	[10, 60]
Syringohydromyelia	50%	[10]
Myelocele (or hemi-myelocele) and myelomeningocele	15–39%	[10, 52]
Dorsal lipoma	26%	[10, 55, 61]
Chiari malformation	15–20%	[10, 62]
Dermoid cysts	13%	[10, 63–65]
Neurenteric cysts	Rare	[10]
Lipomyelocele and lipomyelomeningocele	Rare	[61]
Dorsal myelocystocele	Rare	[66]
Terminal myelocystocele	Rare	[32, 67]
Terminal lipoma	Rare	[54]
Limited dorsal myeloschisis (LDM) and hemi-LDM	Rare (0.8%)	[54, 60]
Caudal regression	Rare	[67]
Sacral agenesis	Rare	[68]

one of these cases, the patient also had a terminal lipoma. Therefore, potentially this individual had disruption to the three major stages of neural tube development: gastrulation (resulting in SCM), primary neurulation (non-dysfunction stage of the hemi-cord, resulting in the LDM) and secondary neurulation (resulting in the terminal lipoma).

As previously mentioned, combined pathologies with SCM can either support previous hypotheses, such as unified theory or introduce new etiological questions [32–35, 51, 56, 57].

Neuroimaging

The main radiological investigations for SCM include

1. On antenatal ultrasound. The hyperechogenic focus in the midline can suggest SCM [69].
2. A plain radiograph (X-ray). An X-ray can enable a diagnosis of scoliosis (if standing whole spine views), can identify posterior defects, and associated congenital abnormalities such as hemivertebrae.

3. Computed tomography (CT). CT can demonstrate the bony spur seen in type 1 SCM and is often required for surgical planning.
4. Magnetic resonance imaging (MRI) will identify the hemi-cords, any fibrous septum, tethering, associated conditions such as hydro or syringomyelia and myelomalacia. It should be noted that in some series, only 40% ventral tethering was picked on preoperative MRI (so it should not be ruled out on imaging alone) [6, 70]. On MRI, conus is found lower than L2 level in 75% of type 1 SCM patients along with fatty filum [6] (Fig. 8a–d).
5. A CT myelogram can be used in patients who cannot undergo MRI.

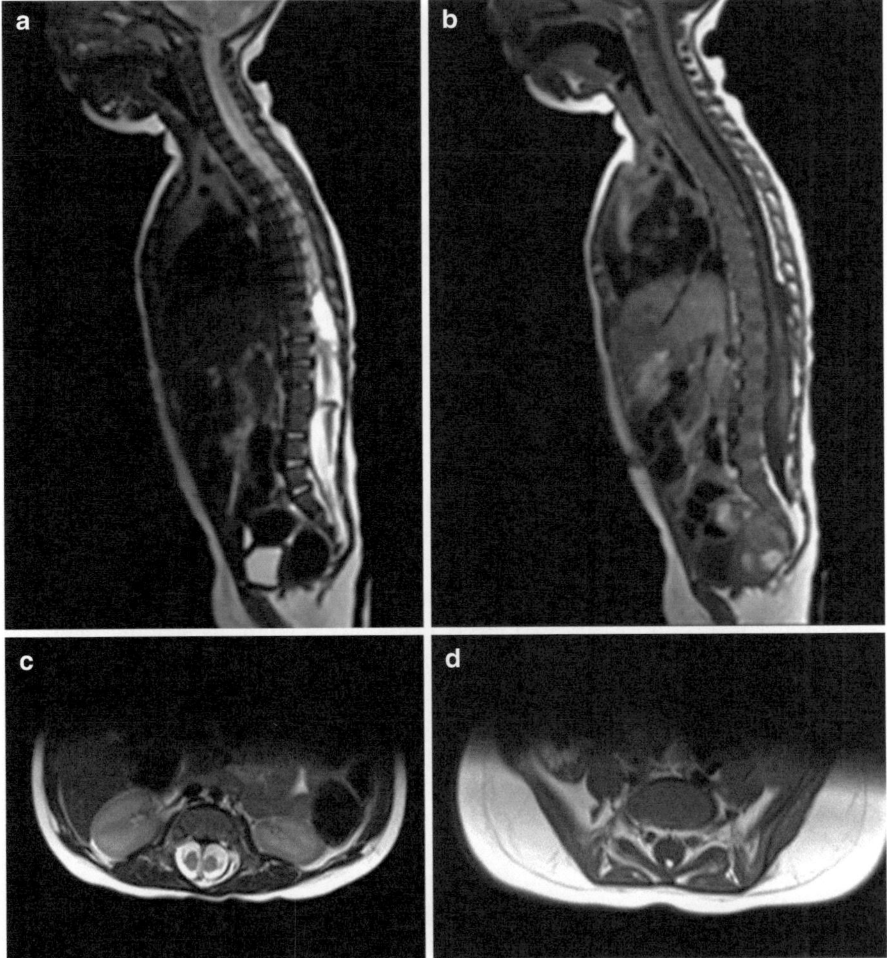

Fig. 8 Case of type 1 SCM. (**a**) T2 and (**b**) T1 sagittal MRI scan showing bony spur at L2/L3 level along with low-lying conus and fatty filum. (**d**) T2 and (**c**) T1 axial MRI scans showing bony spur, two hemi-cords and fatty filum

Management

Management options include (1) observation (for asymptomatic or minimally symptomatic patients) or (2) surgery (either prophylactically or in response to symptoms).

Type 1 SCM is often managed with surgery prophylactically, given the risk of both tethering and spinal cord injury from the bony spur. Type 1 SCM should also be treated prior to any scoliosis surgery, as deformity correction could result in severe spinal cord injury [71, 72]. Type 2 SCM can be managed with observation if asymptomatic or incidental, or with surgery if symptomatic.

Surgery for Type 1 SCM

Surgery involves decompression of the neural elements, careful excision of bony spur and reconstruction of the duplicated dural sac (to prevent re-tethering). Additionally, some patients have low-lying conus and fatty filum, which requires division. The filum should be divided after the bony spur has been removed, as injury to the spinal cord can occur at the level of the crotch due to retraction of cord.

Adjuvants: Intraoperative neuro-monitoring (IONM) can alert the surgeon to inadvertent spinal cord injury during surgical manipulation and should be used where available. Hence, total intravenous anaesthesia (TIVA) is used, and muscle relaxants are avoided. Foley catheter is placed to keep bladder empty and avoid venous hypertension.

Positioning: Patient is positioned prone on gel rolls making sure the abdomen is not compressed and pressure points are well padded. Level is confirmed with X-rays and incision is marked. Planning the skin incision requires knowledge of the exact vertebral level of the median septum.

Approach and exposure: A linear midline skin incision is made to span at least two laminar levels above and two levels below the septum. Depending upon the level of the bony spur and its distance from the filum, either single or two separate incisions are used. Subperiosteal elevation of para-vertebral muscles are carried out to expose the posterior bony elements. The spinal canal is characteristically widened in SCM and so the surgeon needs to be prepared for a wider exposure than usual.

Laminectomy and excision of extradural bony septum: Usually, the spinous process and lamina at the level of the bony septum are hypertrophic. The bony septum is attached to the inner aspect of the lamina. The extent of the laminectomy should be at least one level rostral and one level caudal to the septum bearing laminae. During removal of lamina, attention should be paid to avoid excessive movement of lamina as it can lead to injury of hemi-cords from bony septum. Therefore, laminae are removed under microscopic magnification by carefully drilling and using Kerrison punches in piecemeal fashion, leaving an island of bone in the midline where bony septum is attached. After exposing dura on each side of bony septum, further extradural removal of bony septum is carried out with diamond burr, taking precaution not to cause dural tear (Fig. 9a).

Intradural resection of bony septum: Once maximum bony removal has been achieved, dura should be opened from cranial to caudal direction, making an elliptical incision around midline split (Fig. 9b). Both hemi-cords can be visualised at this stage. Aberrant nerves and fibrous bands are stretched from the dorsomedial aspects of the hemi-cords to end blindly within the median dural sleeve. These can be directly stimulated by a probe and divided.

Further drilling of bony septum may be required until this is flush with the posterior wall of the vertebral body. Afterwards the empty dural sleeve is removed. It requires coagulation of central vessels close to ventral attachment of sleeve and cutting it flush with the ventral dural wall. The ventral dural defect does not require suturing as dura is adherent to surrounding bone which precludes CSF leakage. Careful inspection to ensure removal of any ventral adhesions should also be performed [70].

Division of filum: Attention is then paid to divide the filum. For lumbar SCM, this can be achieved through the same dural opening. Fatty filum is separated from surrounding nerves, confirmed with direct stimulation, coagulated, and divided (Fig. 9c). For thoracic lesions, an additional dural exposure and opening is required to expose conus and filum (Fig. 10).

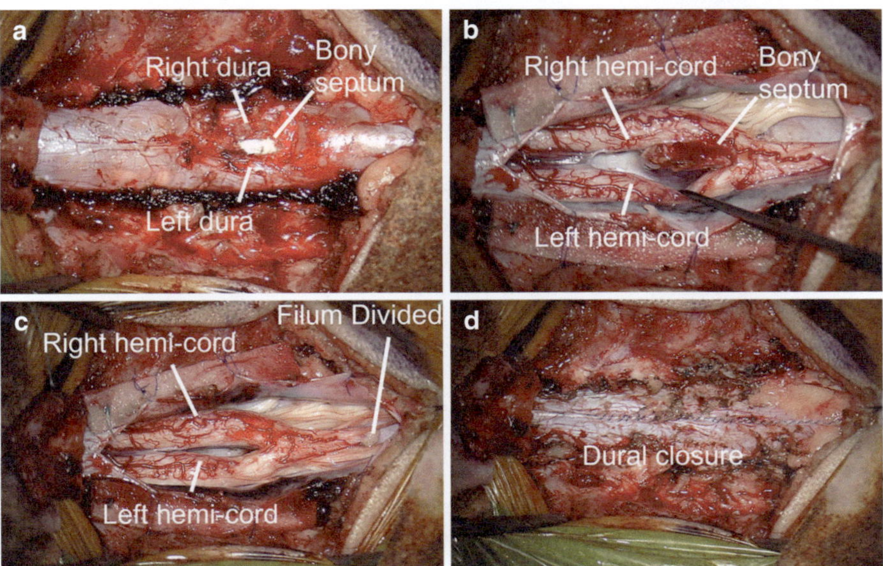

Fig. 9 (a) Intraoperative photograph after removal of posterior neural arch. Two dural sleeves and midline bony septum are visible. (b) Left hemi-cord is retracted to show dural sleeve and bony septum. (c) View at the end of removal of bony septum and division of filum to achieve complete untethering. (d) Watertight dural closure

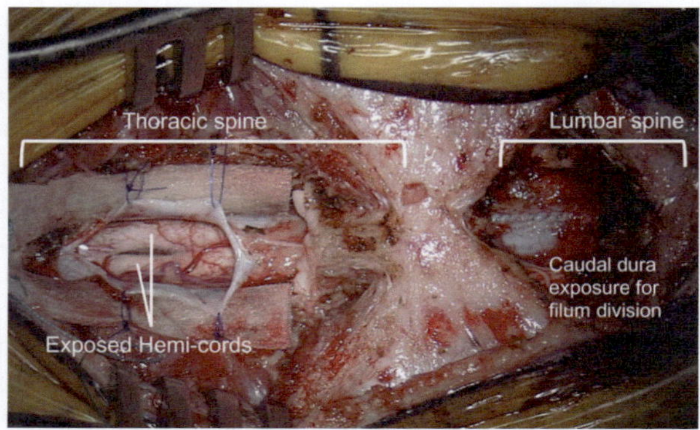

Fig. 10 Intraoperative photo of a different patient, showing the two different dural exposures to achieve (1) removal of bony spur and (2) division of filum

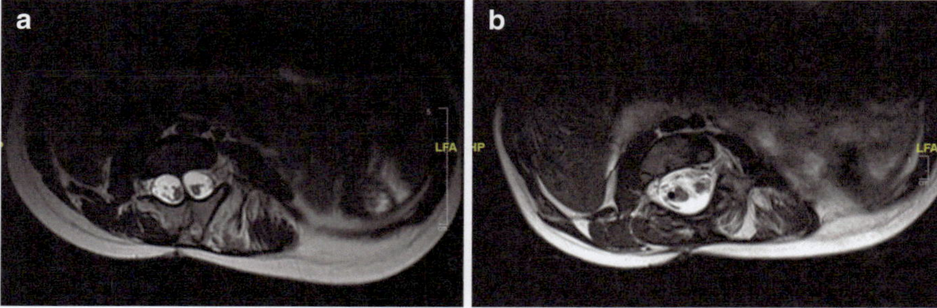

Fig. 11 A T2-weighted MRI of SCM type 1 showing (**a**) preoperative image with bony septum and (**b**) postoperative type 1 SCM showing posterior decompression the removal of the bony septum

Cutting the filum terminale is very important in SCM and is a stage that should not be missed [73]. Histological evidence of loss of elasticity of the filum terminale (increased hyalinization and loss of elastic fibres) has been found in patients with SCM, even in patients with a normal level of the conus medullaris on MRI [73]. This suggests that cord is under tension in SCM and can be damaged from traction, and therefore cutting of the filum terminale is advised as part of the surgical procedure of SCM.

Closure: At the end of procedure, both hemi-cords reside in a single dural sac and dura is closed primarily in a watertight fashion (Fig. 9d). Continuous intraoperative neuro-monitoring (including at the least Somatosensory Evoked Potentials (SEEP) and Motor Evoked Potentials (MEP)) are vital. Figure 11 shows the typical preoperative and postoperative MRI for a type 1 SCM.

Caution: In 5–10% of type 1 SCMs, the bony septum is oblique. The major hemi-cord contained within the larger compartment is much larger than the hemi-cord in the smaller compartment. In these cases, the exposure of the minor hemi-cord is hampered because it is partly sheltered by the overhanging oblique bone spur as well as being ventrally rotated away from the surgeon's view. The delicate smaller hemi-cord is at risk of inadvertent injury, and this pattern of asymmetric splitting must be recognized on preoperative imaging to avoid any complications.

Surgery for Type 2 SCM

In contrast to type 1 SCM, natural history of type 2 SCM is usually benign. The incidental finding of type 2 SCM in an asymptomatic child is managed conservatively. Sometimes type 2 SCM is associated with fatty filum or limited dorsal myeloschisis (LDM) tract [54]. In this subgroup, the chances of getting tethered cord symptoms are high and surgery may be indicated [54].

The basic surgical principles are the same as type 1 SCM like use of IONM and TIVA to achieve complete untethering. However, the solid bony spur is absent, and both hemi-cords have a single dural sleeve. Hypertrophic and fused laminae, common in type 1 lesions, are seldom found in type 2 SCMs. In fact, the neural arches of type 2 lesions are often attenuated or even bifid.

Like type 1 bony septa, type 2 fibrous septa are found near the caudal end of the split. Once dura is opened and both hemi-cords are exposed, un-tethering is achieved by removal of fibrous bands around the split. Intra-cleft exploration is not recommended. The excessive width of the spinal canal should allow the hemi-cords to be rolled gently to one side for ventral inspection. Additional steps such as division of the filum or removal of LDM tract are performed based on individual cases and careful preoperative assessment of imaging.

Complications

Particular attention should be paid to these three risk categories: (1) neurological deficits, (2) CSF leaks or wound complications and (3) future tethering.

1. Worsening of neurological functions occurs in less than 3% of patients following surgery of SCM [6]. Permanent bladder function deterioration occurs in around 3% of children [70]. Neurological complications can be minimised by using IONM, and extra careful during piecemeal removal of bony spur, especially with oblique orientation [74]. Wide laminectomy at the site of septum provides better exposure of both dural sacs.
2. Wound complications are rare, provided meticulous attention is given during layered closure. Watertight dural closure should be confirmed with Valsalva manoeuvre. Additionally, these children should rest fully flat for 2–3 days after surgery.
3. Re-tethering is uncommon in type 2 SCM. The recurrence rate for type 1 SCM is less than 5%. Possible causes include ventral tethering after inadequate resection of bone spur [70]. Closure of the ventral dural defect can lead to dense adhesions and is not recommended [70]. Patients presenting with symptoms of re-tethering require re-exploration.

Prognosis

Both types of SCM have potential to cause tethering. Of those with symptoms, 72% were SCM type 1 and 64% SCM type 2 [6, 45]. Type 1 SCM is at higher risk of deterioration because of the differential growth of the bony spine in relation to the hemi-cords. Patients with ventral tethering are significantly more likely to deteriorate than patients with dorsal tethering [70].

If operated, the prognosis for type 1 SCM is excellent, with less than 3% of patients deteriorating [74]. In one large series of over 200 patients, 40% had improvement in motor power, 31% regained continence [46]. Of the few who do deteriorate postoperative, the main reason is re-tethering [75]. The prognosis for type 2 SCM (with or without surgery) is better than type 1, owing to less tethering and much lower rates of spinal cord injury.

Pang and colleagues found that increasing age was correlated with a strong likelihood of deterioration in SCM type 1 (R^2 value of 0.76) and in SCM type 2 to a lesser degree (R^2 value of 0.61) [6]. Adults with SCM have been reported to deteriorate after trauma or strenuous exercise, but the current data does not support prophylactic surgery [49].

Conclusion

Split cord malformations (SCM) are hemi-cords divided either by a bony septum (type 1 SCM) or by a fibrous septum and within a common dura (type 2 SCM). SCM often coexists with other developmental anomalies. Years of exploration into embryological hypothesis suggests that the aetiology lies within the embryological stage of gastrulation. Genetic research will further this knowledge of the aetiology of SCM and its coexisting developmental anomalies. Although SCMs are rare but they are important to identify and manage, given the progressive tethering and neurological deterioration that can ensue. When managed promptly, outcomes are excellent.

References

1. Pang D, Dias MS, Ahab-Barmada M. Split cord malformation: part I: a unified theory of embryogenesis for double spinal cord malformations. Neurosurgery. 1992;31:451–80.
2. Kerr J, Nelson SL. Split cord malformation. In: Johnston M, editor. Developmental malformations. MedLink Neurology; 1994. p. 1.
3. Rokos J. Pathogenesis of diastematomyelia and spina bifida. J Pathol. 1975;117:155–61.
4. Mahapatra AK, Gupta DK. Split cord malformations: a clinical study of 254 patients and a proposal for a new clinical-imaging classification. J Neurosurg. 2005;103:531–6.
5. Meena RK, Doddamani RS, Gurjar HK, Kumar A, Chandra PS. Type 1.5 split cord malformations: an uncommon entity. World Neurosurg. 2020;133:142–9.

6. Pang D, Hou YJ, Wong ST. Classification of spinal dysraphic malformations according to embryogenesis: gastrulation defects and split cord malformation. In: Di Rocco C, Pang D, Rutka JT, editors. Textbook of pediatric neurosurgery. Cham: Springer International Publishing; 2020. p. 2295–340.

7. Saker E, Loukas M, Fisahn C, Oskouian RJ, Tubbs RS. Historical perspective of split cord malformations: a tale of two cords. Pediatr Neurosurg. 2017;52:1–5.

8. Edelson JG, Nathan H, Arensburg B. Diastematomyelia—the "double-barreled" spine. J Bone Jt Surg Br B. 1987;69:188–9.

9. Bademci G, Saygun M, Batay F, Cakmak A, Basar H, Anbarci H, Unal B. Prevalence of primary tethered cord syndrome associated with occult spinal dysraphism in primary school children in Turkey. Pediatr Neurosurg. 2006;42:4–13.

10. Ross JS, Moore KR. Diastematomyelia. In: Diagnostic imaging: spine. 3rd ed. Philadelphia: Elsevier; 2015. p. 148–51.

11. Thompson DNP. Gastrulation: current concepts and implications for spinal malformations. J Korean Neurosurg Soc. 2021;64:329–39.

12. Copp AJ, Brook FA, Estibeiro JP, Shum AS, Cockroft DL. The embryonic development of mammalian neural tube defects. Prog Neurobiol. 1990;35:363–403.

13. Copp AJ. Genetic models of mammalian neural tube defects. Ciba Found Symp. 1994;181:118–34.

14. Copp A, Cogram P, Fleming A, Gerrelli D, Henderson D, Hynes A, Kolatsi-Joannou M, Murdoch J, Ybot-Gonzalez P. Neurulation and neural tube closure defects. Methods Mol Biol. 2000;136:135–60.

15. Hopwood N. "Not birth, marriage or death, but gastrulation": the life of a quotation in biology. Br J Hist Sci. 2022;55:1–26.

16. Voiculescu O, Bertocchini F, Wolpert L, Keller RE, Stern CD. The amniote primitive streak is defined by epithelial cell intercalation before gastrulation. Nature. 2007;449:1049–52.

17. Ferrer-Vaquer A, Viotti M, Hadjantonakis A-K. Transitions between epithelial and mesenchymal states and the morphogenesis of the early mouse embryo. Cell Adhes Migr. 2010;4:447–57.

18. Voiculescu O, Bodenstein L, Lau I-J, Stern CD. Local cell interactions and self-amplifying individual cell ingression drive amniote gastrulation. elife. 2014;3:e01817.

19. Roszko I, Sawada A, Solnica-Krezel L. Regulation of convergence and extension movements during vertebrate gastrulation by the Wnt/PCP pathway. Semin Cell Dev Biol. 2009;20:986–97.

20. Xanthos JB, Kofron M, Tao Q, Schaible K, Wylie C, Heasman J. The roles of three signaling pathways in the formation and function of the Spemann Organizer. Development. 2002;129:4027–43.

21. Bremer JL. Dorsal intestinal fistula; accessory neurenteric canal; diastematomyelia. AMA Arch Pathol. 1952;54:132–8.

22. Brocklehurst G. The pathogenesis of spina bifida: a study of the relationship between observation, hypothesis, and surgical incentive. Dev Med Child Neurol. 1971;13:147–63.

23. Dominok GW. Zur Frage der Dipbmyelia. Deutschen Zeitschrift Nerven-Heilk. 1962;183:340–50.

24. Schneiderlin W. Unvolkommene dorso-ventrale Verdoppelung des Ruccken-markes. Virchows Arch Pathol Anat Physiol. 1938;301:479–89.

25. Pick A. Beitraege zur Lehre von Hoelenbildungen in meschlichen reuckenmarkes. Arch Psychiatry Nervkrankh. 1899;31:736–69.

26. Herren RY, Edwards JE. Diplomyelia (duplication of the spinal cord). Arch Pathol. 1940;30:1203–14.

27. Lichtenstein BW. Spinal dysraphism: spina bifida and myelodysplasia. Arch NeurPsych. 1940;44:792–810.

28. Beardmore HE, Wigglesworth FW. Vertebral anomalies and alimentary duplication. Pediatr Clin N Am. 1958;5:457–74.

29. Gardner WJ. The dysraphic states, from syringomyelia to anencephaly. Amsterdam: Excerpta Medica; 1973. p. 1–201.
30. Dias MS, Walker ML. The embryogenesis of complex dysraphic malformations: a disorder of gastrulation? Pediatr Neurosurg. 1992;18:229–53.
31. Sun M, Tao B, Luo T, Gao G, Shang A. Type 1.5 split cord malformation: a new theory of pathogenesis. J Korean Neurosurg Soc. 2022;65:138–44.
32. Solanki GA, Evans J, Copp A, Thompson DNP. Multiple coexistent dysraphic pathologies. Childs Nerv Syst. 2003;19:376–9.
33. Sattar MT, Bannister CM, Turnbull IW. Occult spinal dysraphism—the common combination of lesions and the clinical manifestations in 50 patients. Eur J Pediatr Surg. 1996;6(Suppl 1):10–4.
34. Katoh M, Hida K, Iwasaki Y, Koyanagi I, Abe H. A split cord malformation. Childs Nerv Syst. 1998;14:398–400.
35. Borkar SA, Mahapatra AK. Split cord malformations: a 2 years experience at AIIMS. Asian J Neurosurg. 2012;7:56–60.
36. Akay KM, Izci Y, Baysefer A. Dorsal bony septum: a split cord malformation variant. Pediatr Neurosurg. 2002;36:225–8.
37. Chandra PS, Kamal R, Mahapatra AK. An unusual case of dorsally situated bony spur in a lumbar split cord malformation. Pediatr Neurosurg. 1999;31:49–52.
38. Ye DH, Kim DY, Ko EJ. An unusual case of torticollis: split cord malformation with vertebral fusion anomaly: a case report and a review of the literature. Children. 2022;9(7):1085. https://doi.org/10.3390/children9071085.
39. van Aalst J, Beuls EAM, Vles JSH, Cornips EMJ, van Straaten HWM. The intermediate type split cord malformation: hypothesis and case report. Childs Nerv Syst. 2005;21:1020–4.
40. Emura T, Asashima M, Furue M, Hashizume K. Experimental split cord malformations. Pediatr Neurosurg. 2002;36:229–35.
41. Emura T, Asashima M, Hashizume K. An experimental animal model of split cord malformation. Pediatr Neurosurg. 2000;33:283–92.
42. Laale HW. Ethanol induced notochord and spinal cord duplications in the embryo of the zebrafish, *Brachydanio rerio*. J Exp Zool. 1971;177:51–64.
43. Rilliet B, Schowing J, Berney J. Pathogenesis of diastematomyelia: can a surgical model in the chick embryo give some clues about the human malformation? Childs Nerv Syst. 1992;8:310–6.
44. Klessinger S, Christ B. Diastematomyelia and spina bifida can be caused by the intraspinal grafting of somites in early avian embryos. Neurosurgery. 1996;39:1215–23.
45. Pang D. Split cord malformation: part II: clinical syndrome. Neurosurgery. 1992;31:481–500.
46. Sinha S, Agarwal D, Mahapatra AK. Split cord malformations: an experience of 203 cases. Childs Nerv Syst. 2006;22:3–7.
47. Kobets AJ, Oliver J, Cohen A, Jallo GI, Groves ML. Split cord malformation and tethered cord syndrome: case series with long-term follow-up and literature review. Childs Nerv Syst. 2021;37:1301–6.
48. Kearns JT, Esposito D, Dooley B, Frim D, Gundeti MS. Urodynamic studies in spinal cord tethering. Childs Nerv Syst. 2013;29:1589–600.
49. Akay KM, Izci Y, Baysefer A, Timurkaynak E. Split cord malformation in adults. Neurosurg Rev. 2004;27:99–105.
50. Vaishya S, Kumarjain P. Split cord malformation: three unusual cases of composite split cord malformation. Childs Nerv Syst. 2001;17:528–30.
51. Alzhrani GA, Al-Jehani HM, Melançon D. Multi-level split cord malformation: do we need a new classification? J Clin Imaging Sci. 2014;4:32.
52. Kumar R, Bansal KK, Chhabra DK. Occurrence of split cord malformation in meningomyelocele: complex spina bifida. Pediatr Neurosurg. 2002;36:119–27.
53. Moriya J, Kakeda S, Korogi Y, Soejima Y, Urasaki E, Yokota A. An unusual case of split cord malformation. AJNR Am J Neuroradiol. 2006;27:1562–4.

54. Pang D, Devadass A, Thompson D. Limited dorsal myeloschisis involving one hemicord of a split cord malformation—a "hemi-LDM". Childs Nerv Syst. 2022;38(11):2223–30. https://doi.org/10.1007/s00381-022-05599-0.

55. Jamaluddin MA, Nair P, Divakar G, Gohil JA, Abraham M. Split cord malformation type 2 with double dorsal lipoma: a sequela or a chance. J Pediatr Neurosci. 2020;15:135–9.

56. Izci Y, Kural C. Composite type of split cord malformation: rare and difficult to explain. Pediatr Neurosurg. 2011;47:461.

57. Akay KM, Izci Y, Baysefer A, Timurkaynak E. Composite type of split cord malformation: two different types at three different levels: case report. J Neurosurg. 2005;102:436–8.

58. Qureshi MA, Asad A, Pasha IF, Malik AS, Arlet V. Staged corrective surgery for complex congenital scoliosis and split cord malformation. Eur Spine J. 2009;18:1249–54.

59. McMaster MJ. Congenital scoliosis caused by a unilateral failure of vertebral segmentation with contralateral hemivertebrae. Spine. 1998;23:998–1005.

60. Erşahin Y, Demirtaş E, Mutluer S, Tosun AR, Saydam S. Split cord malformations: report of three unusual cases. Pediatr Neurosurg. 1996;24:155–9.

61. Salunke P, Kovai P, Malik V, Sharma M. Mixed split cord malformation: are we missing something? Clin Neurol Neurosurg. 2011;113:774–8.

62. Beals RK, Robbins JR, Rolfe B. Anomalies associated with vertebral malformations. Spine. 1993;18:1329–32.

63. Akhtar S, Azeem A, Shamim MS, Tahir MZ. Composite split cord malformation associated with a dermal sinus tract, dermoid cyst, and epidural abscess: a case report and review of literature. Surg Neurol Int. 2016;7:43.

64. Udayakumaran S, Onyia CU. Split cord malformation associated with congenital dermoid cyst and myeloschisis—case-based literature review on possible embryonic derivation and implications. Br J Neurosurg. 2020;2020:1830947.

65. Mishra A, Nadeem M, Prabhuraj AR, Paul P, Bhat D. Tetrad of split cord malformation I with neurenteric cyst, dermoid cyst, and thickened filum terminale in a 2-year-old child: a case report. Pediatr Neurosurg. 2021;56:448–54.

66. Khandelwal A, Tandon V, Mahapatra AK. An unusual case of 4 level spinal dysraphism: multiple composite type 1 and type 2 split cord malformation, dorsal myelocystocele and hydrocephalous. J Pediatr Neurosci. 2011;6:58–61.

67. Schmitt HP, Kawakami M. Unusual split of the spinal cord in a caudal regression syndrome with myelocystocele. Brain Dev. 1982;4:469–74.

68. Mankotia DS, Satyarthee GD, Sharma BS. A rare case of thoracic myelocystocele associated with type 1 split cord malformation with low lying tethered cord, dorsal syrinx and sacral agenesis: pentad finding. J Neurosci Rural Pract. 2015;6:87–90.

69. Anderson NG, Jordan S, MacFarlane MR, Lovell-Smith M. Diastematomyelia: diagnosis by prenatal sonography. AJR Am J Roentgenol. 1994;163:911–4.

70. Pang D. Ventral tethering in split cord malformation. Neurosurg Focus. 2001;10:e6.

71. Hamzaoglu A, Ozturk C, Tezer M, Aydogan M, Sarier M, Talu U. Simultaneous surgical treatment in congenital scoliosis and/or kyphosis associated with intraspinal abnormalities. Spine. 2007;32:2880–4.

72. von Bazan UKB, Rompe G, Krastel A, Martin K. Diastematomyelia—its importance in the treatment of congenital scoliosis. Z Orthop Ihre Grenzgeb. 1976;114:881–9.

73. Barutcuoglu M, Selcuki M, Selcuki D, Umur S, Mete M, Gurgen SG, Umur. Cutting filum terminale is very important in split cord malformation cases to achieve total release. Childs Nerv Syst. 2015;31:425–32.

74. Pang D. Split cord malformations, theories and practice. In: Batjer HH, Loftus CM, editors. Textbook of neurological surgery. Philadelphia: Lippincott Williams & Wilkins; 2002. p. 916.

75. Proctor MR, Scott RM. Long-term outcome for patients with split cord malformation. Neurosurg Focus. 2001;10:e5.

Fetal Surgery for Myelomeningocele: Neurosurgical Perspectives

Dominic N. P. Thompson, Philippe De Vloo, and Jan Deprest

Introduction and Experimental Background

In the early 1990s, Meuli and colleagues developed a reproducible sheep model of spina bifida. Hysterotomy was performed in a pregnant ewe to expose the back of the fetal lamb. A skin opening was created over the lower spine, followed by paraspinal muscle removal, laminectomy, dual opening and exposure of the spinal cord. The fetal lamb was then returned to the intrauterine environment to complete gestation. At birth, the lambs had a spinal lesion that morphologically resembled myelomeningocele, and had similar functional consequences comprising sensorimotor paraplegia and bladder/bowel incontinence. They went on to perform a second series of experiments in which fetal lambs had a spina bifida lesion created as above, but were then exposed and reoperated 3 weeks later to cover the lesion. Following birth, these "repaired" lambs showed improved neurological and urological function confirmed by clinical and electrophysiological examination, compared with their unrepaired counterparts [1].

There were two important implications of Meuli's experiments. Firstly the authors had demonstrated the feasibility of creating a large animal model of spina bifida that mimicked the human anomaly, and secondly, their results challenged the concept that the deficits associated with spina bifida were a *fixed* consequence of

D. N. P. Thompson (✉)
Department of Pediatric Neurosurgery, Great Ormond Street Hospital for Children NHS Trust, London, UK
e-mail: dominic.thompson@gosh.nhs.uk

P. De Vloo
Department of Neurosurgery, UZ Leuven, Leuven, Belgium

J. Deprest
Department of Obstetrics and Gynaecology, UZ Leuven, Leuven, Belgium

© The Author(s), under exclusive license to Springer Nature Switzerland AG 2023
D. Pang, K.-C. Wang (eds.), *Spinal Dysraphic Malformations*, Advances and Technical Standards in Neurosurgery 47,
https://doi.org/10.1007/978-3-031-34981-2_2

congenital malformation. This led to the emergence of the "two-hit hypothesis" suggesting that, in addition to a primary anomaly of neural tube closure, secondary deleterious changes also occur as a consequence of exposure of viable neural tissue to the intrauterine environment, and moreover that the neurological consequences of these secondary changes might be rescued by fetal surgery.

There have since been other animal studies to support the two-hit hypothesis. In a mutant mouse model in which spina bifida occurs spontaneously, Stiefel et al. showed that neuronal connectivity and spinal cord development proceeds in a relatively normal fashion early in gestation only to deteriorate later with evidence of neurodegeneration and loss of function as the pregnancy proceeds [2].

Whilst animal models have continued to play an essential part in understanding the pathophysiological mechanisms underlying myelomeningocele and in developing and evaluating surgical techniques for fetal repair, the limitations in extrapolating from fetal model to human need to be borne in mind. A systematic review of the fetal lamb model of spina bifida concluded that there was good experimental evidence supporting the safety and efficacy of two-layer closure of experimentally induced spina bifida; however, this review highlighted the lack of standardisation within the fetal lamb model [3]. The timing of the lesion, the incorporation of myelotomy during creation of the lesion and the subsequent mode of repair were among the important variables identified. The lamb model is a lesion *induced* in an otherwise normally developing spinal cord; this of course is a major difference with human myelomeningocele. Furthermore, in order to maintain the defect in the lamb model (and avoid spontaneous healing), the lesion is necessarily large, incorporating five-level laminectomy and removal of paraspinal musculature, resulting in lesions proportionately more severe than typically seen in clinical practice.

Nonetheless, since the innovative experiments of Meuli, there have been subsequent attempts to standardise and validate the fetal lamb model [4]. This model can now reliably reproduce not only the sensorimotor consequences of spina bifida but also the phenomenon of hindbrain herniation akin to the Chiari II malformation. Additionally, the use of quantitative electrophysiological studies-somatosensory and motor evoked potentials (SSEP and MEP) as well as techniques to determine the watertightness of surgical closure and ovine postnatal MRI studies have further endorsed use of the fetal lamb model to develop, test and compare surgical techniques [5, 6].

Clinical Studies

The management of myelomeningocele study (MOMS) remains the only randomised controlled clinical trial of fetal repair versus postnatal repair [7]. The trial, restricted to three study centres, compared the open fetal surgery technique, performed prior to 26 weeks of gestation with conventional postnatal repair. The trial concluded that prenatal surgery reduced the need for ventricular shunting and improved motor outcomes at 30 months. Improvement in hindbrain herniation was also identified. There has since been a proliferation of centres offering prenatal surgery for myelomeningocele and the finding of the MOMS trial have been replicated in subsequent case series and cohort studies [8–10].

In spite of the apparent neurological benefits to the fetus, the MOMS trial identified both maternal and fetal risks. Separation of the placental membranes (which is associated with increased risk of premature membrane rupture) occurred in one quarter of women following prenatal surgery. Thinning of the uterine wall or dehiscence at the hysterotomy site was also seen in more than one third of cases, which is not only a risk for the index pregnancy but increases the risk of uterine scar rupture in future pregnancies, and thus it is mandated that all future pregnancies are delivered by caesarean section. Furthermore, fetuses repaired prenatally were more likely to be born prematurely (only 21% reached 37 weeks gestation) and with reduced birth weight. It is these adverse consequences of fetal surgery that have been motivation behind modifications of surgical technique, in particular mini hysterotomy [11] and fetoscopy [12–14].

Neurosurgery Perspectives

The principles underlying repair of myelomeningocele are the same for both prenatal and postnatal surgery, namely, separation of the exposed neural placode from surrounding skin and meninges, protection of neural tissue from ongoing damage by layered closure, and prevention of cerebrospinal fluid (CSF) leakage at the spinal defect by means of healthy, durable skin closure. The proclaimed benefits of parental repair over conventional repair can be considered under the following headings.

Hydrocephalus

In the MOMS trial, at 12 months follow up, placement of a shunt to treat hydrocephalus was required in 40% of infants who had been repaired prenatally compared with 82% of the postnatal group ($p < 0.001$), and this effect was maintained at 5 years of age. This beneficial effect on shunt placement rates has since been replicated in other large series [8, 15, 16]. In a systematic review, Inversetti et al. concluded that for every two babes treated prenatally there was one fewer who required a shunt [15]. It has also been observed that shunt revision rates are also significantly less following prenatal as compared with postnatal repair [17], although the reasons for this are unclear.

It is often stated that the risk of developing hydrocephalus is related to the level of the MMC; however, in the MOMS trial, the spinal level of the lesion at screening was not correlated with the subsequent need for shunt placement in either the prenatal or postnatal closure groups.

Interestingly, endoscopic third ventriculostomy (ETV), a treatment option previously thought to be less effective in the context of myelomeningocele-associated hydrocephalus seems to yield more beneficial results in myelomeningocele infants who develop hydrocephalus after prenatal repair [18]. These findings raise the possibility that fetal repair of myelomeningocele might modify the underlying pathophysiology of hydrocephalus in this group of patients, and Elbaba et al. suggest that improvement in the hindbrain herniation might be an important factor in this regard. Another observation supporting the hypothesis that the pathophysiology of hydrocephalus might be altered by prenatal surgery is the finding that age at treatment of hydrocephalus (by shunt or ETV) is significantly later for prenatal repair patients compared with postnatal [19].

Whilst the avoidance of shunt placement is a laudable goal of fetal surgery, the "headline" rates of reduced shunt placement need to be critically appraised. Outside a clinical trial, variability in the criteria and thresholds for shunt placement are inevitable. Given the acknowledged burden of shunt-dependent hydrocephalus, even prior to MOMS there had already been a trend toward shunt avoidance in the postnatal closure population with large centres reporting shunt placement rates of between 50 and 65% [20, 21]; rates that are significantly lower than the perceived norm. Increasingly paediatric neurosurgeons have become more influenced by clinical signs of raised intracranial pressure (bulging fontanelle, sutural splaying etc.) than by ventricular dimensions alone to guide their clinical decision-making [17]. It might be argued that this philosophy of "permissive ventriculomegaly" is particularly likely to be resorted to in prenatally treated patients where there is an even greater vested interest in shunt avoidance for the parents as well as for the neurosurgeon.

A second factor that needs to be considered is that the reduction in shunt placement rate is not evenly distributed amongst fetal repair cases. It is now apparent that fetal surgery "halts" rather than "reverses" progression of ventricular dilation [17, 22]. Ventricular size, measured by atrial diameter or front-occipital horn ratio, on USS or MRI at the time of prenatal closure is strongly correlated with the likelihood of shunt placement postnatally [19]. When ventricular size is >15 mm at the time of closure, the rate of shunting is similar to that following postnatal closure. There are of course other benefits of prenatal closure, so ventricular size alone should not preclude the option of fetal surgery, but this needs to be clearly stated during the counselling process. Peralta et al. emphasise the importance of gestational age at the time of closure suggesting that the "shunt avoidance" benefits of fetal surgery become less with advancing gestational age (Fig. 1).

Finally, as concluded in the systematic review by Inversetti et al. neurodevelopmental outcomes are similar between prenatal and postnatal patients [15] and so, on the basis of current evidence at least, parents should not be counselled that the avoidance of shunt as a result of prenatal surgery confers a clear cognitive advantage.

Chiari II Malformation

At 1 year, complete reversal of hindbrain herniation was seen in 36% of prenatal and 4% of postnatal repair cases in the MOMS trial; this difference was maintained at more than 5 years of follow-up. The efficacy of fetal surgery in improving

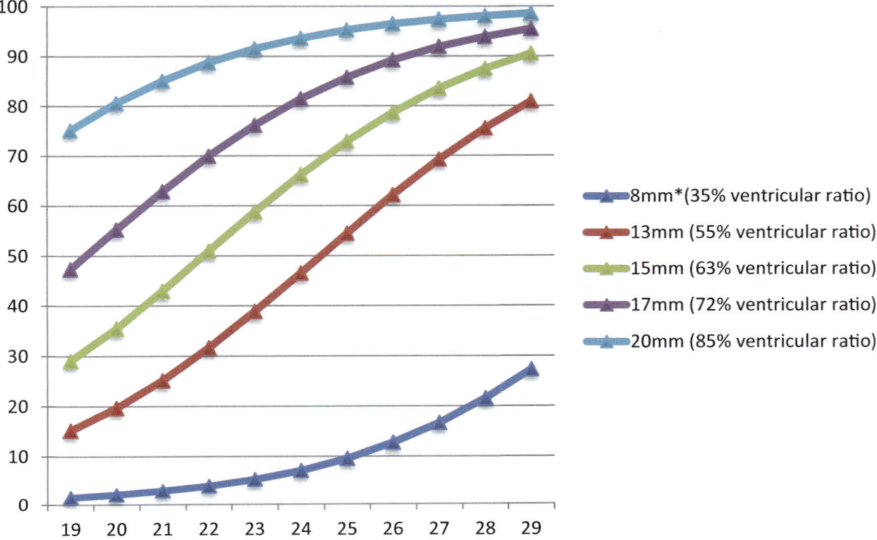

Fig. 1 Change in ventricular size during pregnancy depending on initial ventricular measurement. (From Peralta 2020). There is progressive increase in ventricular dimensions as pregnancy progresses. This is used in support of earlier fetal intervention in an attempt to halt progression of ventriculomegaly

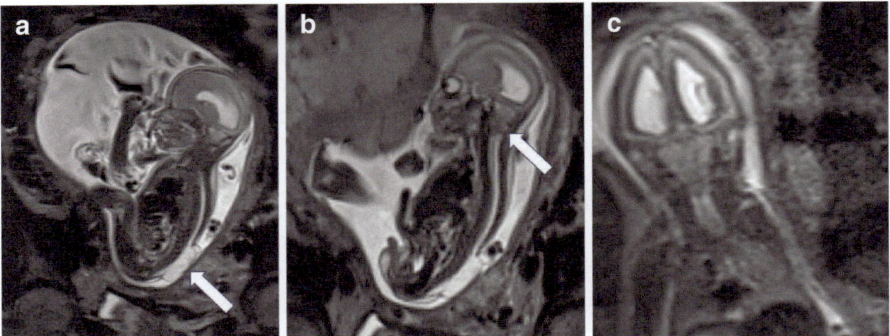

Fig. 2 In utero MRI showing lumbosacral MMC sac (**a**) hindbrain herniation (**b**) and ventriculomegaly (**c**)

hindbrain herniation has been replicated in subsequent surgical series outside the MOMS centres [8, 10, 23] and has become one of the more objective parameters by which the success of fetal surgery is measured (Fig. 2). Radiological confirmation of hindbrain herniation remains one of the inclusion criteria for fetal surgery; the reasons for this are twofold. Firstly, hindbrain herniation is so frequently associated with myelomeningocele that it is considered pathognomonic of the condition and helps distinguish cases of "open" myelomeningocele from "closed" dysraphic

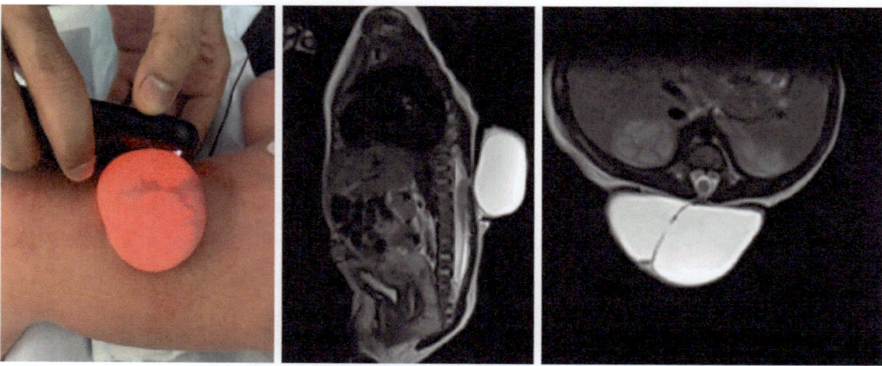

Fig. 3 Limited dorsal myeloschisis. Clinical and MRI appearances of LDM, a lesion that can be confused with MMC

anomalies such as saccular limited dorsal myeloschisis and myelocystocele, which may also appear as cystic spinal malformations but are skin covered and not appropriate for fetal intervention (Fig. 3). Secondly, in cases of myelomeningocele without hindbrain herniation, it is considered that the risk of hydrocephalus is smaller and therefore the benefits of fetal intervention are less compelling. Absence of hindbrain herniation at the time of screening is the single most common fetal reason for exclusion from fetal surgery [24].

In 1989, David McLone proposed a "unifying theory" by which the Chiari II malformation could be explained on the basis of chronic CSF leakage at the myelomeningocele site during early development [25]. On the basis of clinical observations and experiments in the Splotch (Spd/Spd) mouse model of open neural tube defect, he suggested that impaired growth and distension of the primitive brain vesicle and ventricular system precipitated a state of craniocerebral disproportion in which the posterior fossa was too small and insufficient to contain the developing hindbrain structures which were displaced into the cervical spinal canal as a result. Subsequent studies on fetal lambs, in which hindbrain herniation could be induced by surgically creating a myelomeningocele defect provided further evidence to corroborate the McLone theory [26]. Furthermore, these same studies demonstrated that hindbrain herniation did not occur after fetal repair of the defect, suggesting a degree of reversibility of the Chiari II "malformation".

More recently, Joyeux and colleagues have refined and validated the lamb model such that it can be used to assess the efficacy of newer fetal therapies and modifications of surgical technique. In their model, they highlighted the importance of myelotomy in addition to dural opening in reliably reproducing the key features of the Chiari II complex, namely, hindbrain herniation, small posterior fossa, and ventriculomegaly [4]. In an elegant series of experiments, the model was used to demonstrate the importance of "watertightness" at the fetal repair site in ensuring reversal of hindbrain herniation as well as neural protection. Evidence of leakage and the closure site resulted in less favourable outcomes [3].

Are their clinical benefits of reversing hindbrain herniation? Recent decades have seen a trend toward reduced rates of decompression for Chiari II malformation amongst patients treated by conventional postnatal closure [27]. Nonetheless, severe brainstem dysfunction continues to have catastrophic consequences in a minority of cases and hence there would appear to be a clinical advantage to minimising the extent of hindbrain herniation in this population. This notion is supported by a late follow-up study of MOMS patients in which it was found that resolution of hindbrain herniation occurred in 85.1% of fetal repairs compared with 32.6% of postnatal closures and that 6/62 patients in the postnatal repair group required decompression surgery for Chiari II malformation at a mean age of 8.8 months compared with none in the fetal repair group [19]. Additionally, in this study, resolution of hindbrain herniation was significantly associated with absence of clinical hydrocephalus on univariate analysis; a finding in keeping with the observation of others, that persistence of hindbrain herniation following fetal repair was a strong predictor of the need for hydrocephalus treatment [28].

A clear causal association between hindbrain herniation and hydrocephalus is not universally accepted; in a small series of prenatal repair patients Lu et al. reported progressive hydrocephalus in spite of reversal of hindbrain herniation [29]. Overall, however, observations from fetal surgery patients strengthen the argument that disturbed CSF flow in the posterior fossa is likely a contributory factor in the pathophysiology of MMC-associated hydrocephalus.

In summary, improved hindbrain herniation following fetal repair does appear to have measurable clinical benefits and prognostic implications. The presence of hindbrain herniation will continue to be an important component of the selection criteria, not the least because of its sensitivity in excluding cystic closed malformations. Given the inherent problems in objectively diagnosing hydrocephalus and in correlating anatomical and functional motor level, reversal of hindbrain herniation is perhaps the most objective radiological parameter by which the success of fetal surgery can be measured.

Motor Function

Motor outcomes following surgery for myelomeningocele are described by comparing the highest functional myotome on clinical examination with the rostral limit of the spinal defect determined by ultrasound or MRI. In the MOMS trial, at 30 months of age, following prenatal repair, 32% had a functional level that was at least two levels better than anatomical level, compared with 12% following postnatal repair. In approximately 25% of cases, there was no difference between functional and anatomical level for either group. In practical terms, by 2.5 years of age, independent mobility (with or without orthotic support) was achieved in 71% and 57% in the prenatal and postnatal groups, respectively.

On statistical analysis, the benefits to motor function following fetal repair are less significant than for hydrocephalus and hindbrain herniation. Inversetti et al.

calculated that for every two babies treated prenatally, one fewer would require a shunt, expressed as NNT (number needed to treat) = 2. However, for hindbrain herniation NNT = 4 and for motor function, for every five treated prenatally, one extra would walk independently, that is, NNT = 5 [15]. The differing benefits of fetal surgery across various domains of outcome likely reflect differing mechanisms of action of fetal surgery; improvements in hydrocephalus and hindbrain herniation being a hydrodynamic consequence of preventing ongoing spinal CSF losses whereas improvements in motor outcome reflect protection of the neural placode and amelioration of the "second hit" component of the two-hit hypothesis.

Impaired mobility is one of the major disabilities associated with MMC and so it is pertinent to examine the predictors of motor outcome in the light of lessons learned from fetal surgery.

Anatomical Level

It is well established that the anatomical level of the lesion is a major prognostic factor for lower limb function. Prenatal ultrasound and MRI have similar efficacy in determining anatomical level [30, 31]. In a recent study, precise correlation between prenatal ultrasound and postnatal imaging was reported in 22.8% of cases, and in 66.7% of cases the prediction was correct to within one level [32]. However, both modalities (ultrasound and MRI) have a margin of error of up to two levels. This is important to recognise in prenatal counselling as an error of two levels can have significant functional consequences. When the accuracy of prenatal imaging is judged according to postnatal functional level (determined by physical therapist), ultrasound and MRI had a concordance with muscle charting to within one level in 65% and 59% of cases, respectively [31].

MMC Sac vs No Sac

Neurosurgeons have long recognised that the morphology of MMC lesions can vary between a true sac (or "coele") and a flat type, referred to as myeloschisis; however, no prognostic significance has previously been ascribed to these differences. Based on a case of S1 level MMC that was born with severe talipes, Wilson et al. hypothesised that traction on nerve roots due to distension of a MMC sac might be an additional factor worsening lower limb function. They went on to perform a detailed retrospective review of cases and found that leg function at 1 year was better in cases with no sac but this did not reach statistical significance [33]. More recently, evidence has accrued that the presence of a MMC sac (and larger sac volume) does indeed portend a worse neurological outcome, suggesting that nerve root traction within an expanding MMC sac is an additional component of the "second hit" [34, 35].

Gestational Age at the Time of Fetal Repair

In a series of patients operated between 19.7 and 26.9 weeks of gestation using the open technique, but by means of mini-hysterotomy, Peralta et al. found that in addition to the level of the MMC, gestational age at the time of surgery was a significant predictor of the ability to walk, with or without orthoses by 2.5 years [22]. This, and the observation that intact motor function at the time of repair predicts better motor function, further supports the notion that there is a neuroprotective effect of fetal surgery that can mitigate the progressive deterioration of neural placode function that would otherwise occur.

It is important to consider motor outcomes over the longer term. Currently, published motor outcomes following fetal surgery are limited to the first decade of life, and during this period the early benefits appear to be sustained [36]. However, it has been recognised for many years that around a third of MMC patients will have decreased ambulation if followed up beyond 10 years [37]. Spasticity, pain, adolescent weight gain and neuro-orthopaedic factors are among the reasons for this. A recent longitudinal study found that most deterioration in ambulation occurred by the end of the second decade, and that those with low lumbar level MMC were particular at risk [38]. Long-term follow-up will be essential to see how patients that have undergone fetal repair perform by the time they reach the transition to adult care to ensure that the apparent motor benefits are not eroded by time.

Bladder Function

Neuropathic bladder dysfunction in children with MMC not only has major implications for health of the renal tract but also for the associated problems of continence that have profound implications for quality of life. Unsurprisingly, the effects of fetal MMC repair on urological outcome have been eagerly anticipated. Early reports suggested that urodynamic studies and rates of clean intermittent catheterisation (CIC) were not improved by fetal surgery [39–41].[1] In a 30 month follow-up of the MOMS cohort, MOMS 1, whilst rates of CIC were not improved there was less evidence of bladder trabeculation and open bladder neck [43]. In a subsequent analysis of children that had reached school age, the number of children requiring CIC at least three times per day was statistically less in the prenatal group (62% vs 87%), and there was also a higher rate of volitional voiding in the prenatal group [44]. This latter study has however received criticism for its reliance on questionnaire and patient-centred feedback and so further data will be necessary to substantiate these claims.

Urological outcomes are difficult to quantify as continence and bladder function can be variously defined. Thresholds to instigate CIC vary amongst urologists and, as pointed out in a recent review, the conduct and interpretation of urodynamic

---

[1] See table in Clayton [42].

studies is by no means standardised across institutions [42]. As with motor function, early coverage of the neural placode and the release of tension in stretched nerve roots may protect, or indeed improve bladder innervation, but further evidence is required before this can be confirmed. An additional concern is the impact of secondary neurosurgical interventions on bladder function; re-tethering rates and inclusion cyst formation are more common following fetal repair, particularly fetoscopic repair, and surgery to deal with these complications can impart additional neurological injury [45],

Cognitive Function

Teenagers and young adults with spina bifida tend to perform less well in areas of executive functioning and behavioural adaptive skills (a composite of conceptual, social and practical life skills) when compared to the normal population. The detrimental impact of hydrocephalus and shunt history (revisions for blockage and infection) on these domains has been highlighted in many studies. In spite of this the majority of spina bifida patients will have an IQ within the normal range.

In a long-term follow-up of prenatally repaired patients, Danzer et al. found that the majority of children scored within the normal range across a variety of tests of cognitive and behavioural function and that the majority were able to successfully manage everyday tasks both at home and in school. They noted that problems of behavioural adaptive skills were more common than impaired executive function [46]. In the MOMS cohort, at 30 months, Bayley Scales of Infant Development were marginally better in the prenatal group compared with postnatal but this did not reach statistical significance [47].

Any benefits of fetal surgery on cognitive outcome through avoidance of hydrocephalus need to be balanced against the potential detrimental effects of prematurity. Moderate prematurity, around 34 weeks, is a well-documented complication of fetal surgery by any technique, with more that 10% of cases delivering before 30 weeks. In a systematic review, Inversetti et al. sought to address this question. They found that the risk of neurodevelopmental impairment was similar between pre- and postnatal repair in spite of the much higher rates of prematurity (<34 weeks) in the prenatal group [15]. Interestingly, in the prenatal group, the risk of such impairment was similar between shunted and non-shunted patients (comparable data was not available for the postnatal group).

Complications at the Myelomeningocele Repair Site

Ensuring coverage of the neural placode and prevention of ongoing CSF leakage are fundamental requirements of any prenatal myelomeningocele closure technique.

Problems of Wound Healing

Using the fetal lamb model, Joyeux et al. demonstrated that the watertightness of the repair was not only important for reversal of hindbrain herniation and preservation of lower limb function but also appear to result in better preservation of brain histology [48]. Postnatal wound breakdown with CSF leakage therefore not only constitutes a significant infection risk but may compromise the efficacy of fetal surgery. Wound dehiscence, CSF leakage and the need for postnatal surgery at the repair site are significantly more likely to occur following fetoscopic techniques compared with open [49]. Interestingly, Tulipan et al. observed that wound leakage as a criterion for shunt placement was much higher following postnatal repair (25%) compared with open prenatal repair (1.1%) [17].

Inclusion Cysts

Historically, following postnatal closure, inclusion cysts occur in approximately 5% of cases. There is mounting evidence to suggest that this figure is significantly higher following prenatal surgery. Prior to the MOMS trial, the Philadelphia group identified inclusion cysts in 14/54 (26%) prenatal repair patients; cysts occurred in the context of "tethered cord syndrome" in ten cases and as an incidental finding in the remaining four [50]. In a more recent series, inclusion cysts occurred in 30% of cases [45]. The majority of inclusion cysts present within the first 2 years of life, and based on these two series half of cases will require neurosurgery to resect the cyst. It is therefore sobering to note that two thirds of the patients who required surgery for inclusion cyst incurred a new motor deficit as a result of the intervention. This led the authors to suggest that the complication of inclusion cyst constituted a "third hit." Given the high incidence of inclusion cysts (many of which are asymptomatic), and the propensity for these lesions to grow and cause deficits, there is a strong argument to perform surveillance MRI as part of follow-up (Fig. 4).

Re-tethering of Spinal Cord

Symptomatic deterioration due to re-tethering of the spinal cord is well recognised in MMC patients, and surgery for this also incurs an additional threat to long-term function. Re-tethering remains an issue following fetal repair; however, currently there is no evidence that the rates of re-tethering (not associated with inclusion cyst) are any different between pre- and postnatal repair.

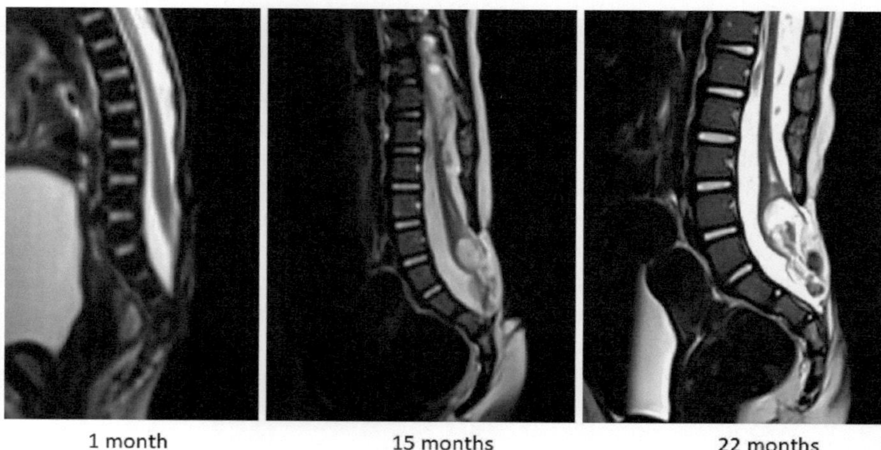

Fig. 4 MRI images showing evolution of an inclusion cyst at the site of previous prenatal repair of MMC

Selection Criteria for Fetal Surgery

For the purposes of the MOMS trial, the maternal and fetal selection criteria were somewhat empirical (Table 1). The time frame for surgery was limited to between 19 + 0 and 26 + 0 weeks. There are technical constraints in operating on the fetus prior to 19 weeks, and there are additional practical limitations imposed by the time from diagnosis to completion of the necessary screening investigations and counselling. An upper limit of 26 weeks ensured that there would be adequate time to derive benefit, acknowledging the progressive natural history of untreated MMC. MMC lesions needed to be between T1 and S1; below S1 the prognosis is generally favourable with postnatal intervention and thus difficult to justify additional risks of prenatal surgery. As already noted, the presence of hindbrain herniation is an important inclusion criterion; not only does this reflect severe myelomeningocele with potential adverse implications for bulbar function and CSF circulation, but also serves to distinguish myelomeningocele from occult dysraphic conditions such as segmental myelocystocele and saccular limited dorsal myeloschisis, lesions that can appear very similar on fetal USS or MRI based on sac morphology alone.

Selection criteria based on the MOMS trial continue to be used in the majority of fetal surgery centres. There have, however, been modifications as experience has grown. A maternal BMI of 35 or more, an initial exclusion has now been extended in many centres after reports that maternal morbidity and fetal outcomes were not compromised if the BMI was greater [51]. More controversial is the suggestion to extend the upper time limit for fetal repair beyond 26 weeks. A recent South American study found that rates of premature rupture of membranes, chorioamnionitis, oligohydramnios, preterm delivery, and maternal complications were no different, and shunt insertion rates were similar if surgery was performed

Table 1 Maternal and fetal inclusion and exclusion criteria for open fetal surgery for spina bifida

Inclusion criteria	
Maternal	Fetal
• Singleton fetal pregnancy • No serious maternal medical complications • Maternal cervix long and closed • Known HIV, Hepatitis B and Hepatitis C status	• Ultrasound confirmation of spinal bifida aperta between T1 and S1 • Gestational age of 19 + 0 to 25 + 6 weeks • Amniocentesis or chorionic villus sampling with karyotype or microarray • Fetal kyphoscoliosis <30° • Fetal MRI confirmation of Chiari II

Exclusion criteria	
Maternal	Fetal
• Multifetal pregnancy • Previous spontaneous singleton delivery prior to 37 weeks as a contra-indication to a safe near-term delivery • Current or planned cervical cerclage (a stitch placed around the cervix to keep it closed during pregnancy) or documented history of cervical insufficiency • Placenta praevia or previous placental abruption • Short cervical length less than 20 mm measured by transvaginal ultrasound • Maternal-fetal Rhesus isoimmunisation, Kell sensitisation or a history of neonatal alloimmune thrombocytopenia • Uterine anomaly such as large or multiple fibroids or Mullerian duct abnormality • A previous hysterotomy in the active segment of the uterus (whether from a previous classical caesarean, uterine anomaly such as arcuate or bicornuate uterus, major myomectomy resection, or previous fetal surgery). A previous uncomplicated caesarean section scar is acceptable • Other maternal medical condition which is a contraindication to surgery or general anaesthesia • Maternal hypertension which increases the risk of preeclampsia or preterm delivery (including, but not limited to: uncontrolled hypertension, chronic hypertension with end organ damage and new onset hypertension in pregnancy)	• Fetal anomaly not related to spina bifida aperta which MDT review considers likely to significantly impact on the fetal surgery or the short or long term outcome for the baby

up to 27 + 6 weeks compared with standard limit of 26 weeks [52]. However, the fetal outcome metrics for this study were limited and the conclusions are somewhat at variance with the notion that MMC is progressive in utero, and the earlier the intervention the better [53].

Operative Technique: Standard Open Fetal Repair of MMC

The procedure of open fetal repair of MMC is carried out under general anaesthesia using a balanced anaesthetic technique with a combination of volatile agents, nitrous oxide, propofol and muscle relaxation. An intravenous infusion of tocolytic drugs (atosiban or magnesium sulphate) is commenced prior to surgery and continued into the immediate post-operative period.

Abdominal Opening

Via a low transverse abdominal incision, the uterus is exposed. When the placenta is anterior, the rectus muscles may have to be divided to permit exteriorisation of the uterus and improve access for a more posterior hysterotomy.

Hysterotomy

Intraoperative ultrasound is used to establish the exact position of the placenta which is mapped out and marked with surgical pen or cautery. The hysterotomy needs to be parallel to, and at least 6 cm from the placental margin. The fetus may have to be repositioned to ensure that the MMC lesion will lie beneath the uterine opening. Under US guidance, two full thickness sutures are placed on either side of the planned uterine incision; this anchors the underlying placental membranes to the uterine wall. The myometrium is then carefully opened using electrocautery to minimise blood loss. The uterus can be entered directly or via initial placement of a cannulated trocar. Through this initial opening, a stapling device is placed which will deploy a line of staples that is both haemostatic and further secures the placental membranes to the uterine wall. Stapling of hysterotomy was used in the MOMS trial though some surgeons have since preferred to place additional sutures instead.

Fetal Monitoring

Once the fetus is exposed an intramuscular injection of fentanyl, atropine and muscle relaxant are given. Throughout the procedure, echocardiography is used to monitor fetal heart rate and contractility. An intrauterine infusion of warmed Ringers lactate is used to help maintain fetal temperature and buoyancy.

Standard Open Repair

The principles of MMC repair are little different to postnatal repair. In view of the small circulating blood volume of the fetus, meticulous haemostasis is essential. In cases where there is a large sac, this is initially incised to release CSF and facilitate mobilisation of the neural placode. Sharp dissection is carried out circumferentially around the neural placode, care being taken to avoid leaving epithelial tissue attached to the placode which may predispose to inclusion cyst formation. The placode and terminal spinal cord are mobilised and separated from any tethering bands of arachnoid membrane. There is no consensus regarding neurulation of the placode; advocates of neurulation claim that this reduces the likelihood of re-tethering in postnatal life and lowers the risk of additional neurological damage during subsequent surgery for dermal inclusion cysts or symptomatic tethering [8], whilst others consider that the placement of sutures into the delicate placode risks damage to potentially viable neural tissue [54].

The dura is identified proximally and then mobilised from the margins of the defect, the dura is often friable, particularly distally and mobilising sufficient dura to create a terminal thecal sac can be difficult. In general, it seems that the dural quality is better in myeloschisis compared with myelomeningocele-type lesions. The dura is closed with 6/0 PDS monofilament suture. It should be noted that neither neurulation nor dural closure are attempted with most fetoscopic closure techniques.

The myofascial layer is then closed, occasionally this is achieved by simple approximation, more usually however, lateral parallel relieving incisions in the lumbodorsal facia are necessary to allow tension-free closure using a 4/0 PDS monofilament suture. Finally, the skin is undermined as extensively as possible using blunt dissection. The skin edges are trimmed to ensure healthy tissue along the suture line. A continuous 4/0 PDS suture is used for skin closure. Fetal skin tears easily and so to facilitate closure full-thickness sutures should be used; these can be kept loose initially and then, using a blunt hook each loop is successively tightened before the final knot is tied.

This is the standard three-layer closure for open fetal MMC repair (Fig. 5b). Not infrequently the technique has to be modified. For example, where the dura is too thin, insufficient, or absent, a collagen patch (e.g. DuraGen® Integra NJ USA) can be placed over the placode, alternatively the rudimentary dura can be left attached to the paraspinal tissues and incorporated into the myofascial closure.

Skin Patch Repair

The MMC lesion is sometimes deemed too wide for primary skin closure, in this scenario lateral relieving skin incisions are best avoided as there is a risk of CSF leakage through the release site and late wound healing problems. A patched repair provides a more immediate and durable closure. The authors preference for skin patch is Integra Dermal Regeneration Template® (Integra NJ USA). This is a bilaminar patch comprising a layer of bovine collagen backed by a thin silicone sheet. The patch is cut to size and sutured into the defect with a continuous 4/0 PDS suture. Within a few days of birth, the silicone layer is gently lifted off leaving the collagen to incorporate into the surrounding skin (Fig. 6). The early and late appearances of the repair site following standard open repair and patched repair are shown in Fig. 7.

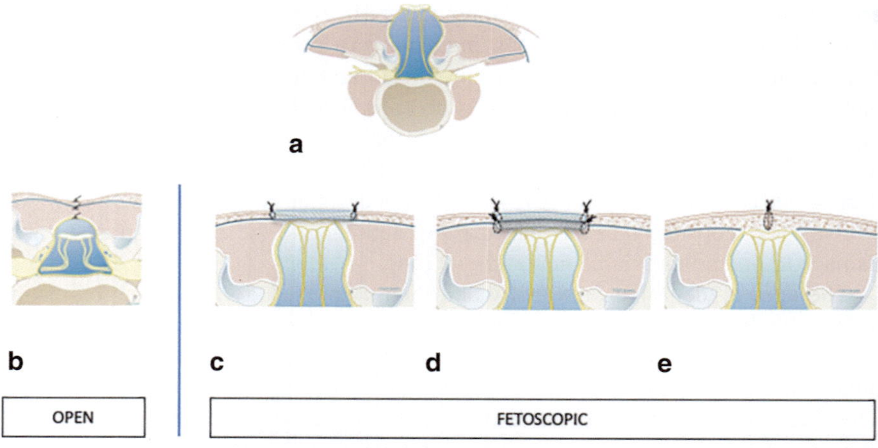

Fig. 5 Diagram to illustrate variations in technique of fetal repair of MMC. (**a**) Anatomy of MMC lesion, (**b**) three-layer open repair (dura/fascia/skin). Neurulation of the placode is sometimes performed in this technique (not shown here), (**c**) fetoscopic repair with skin patch only, (**d**) fetoscopic repair with two-layer patch, (**e**) fetoscopic repair two layer (fascia and skin) without patch. [Illustration with permission Prof. Jan Deprest, UZ Leuven (Χοπψριγητ)]

Fig. 6 Intraoperative illustration of open repair with patch closure

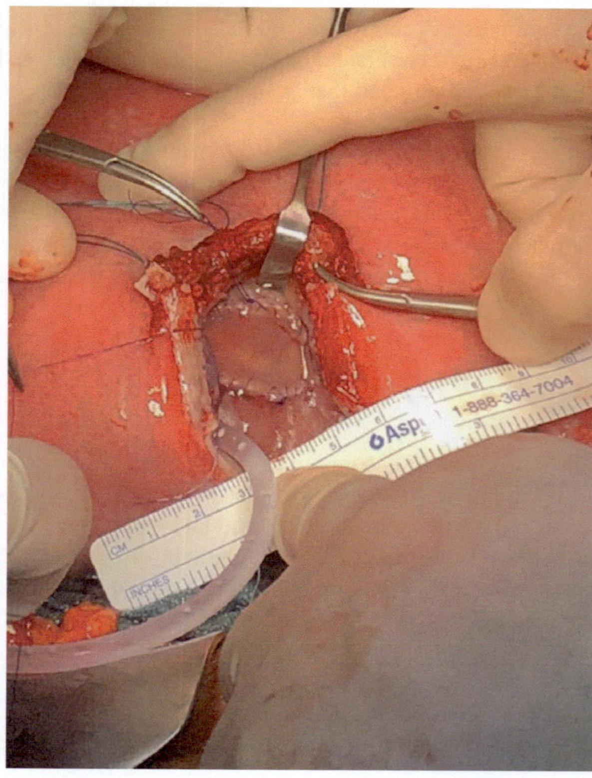

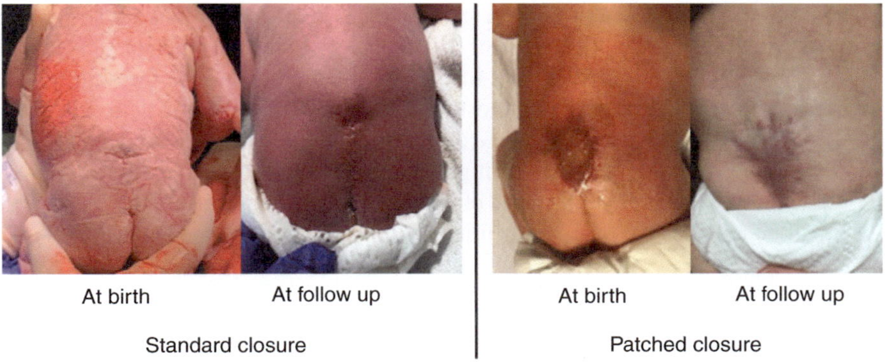

Fig. 7 Clinical appearances of repair site following standard open repair and after patched open repair

Alternative Techniques

Whilst the fetal benefits of prenatal surgery for spina bifida aperta are largely acknowledged, the maternal morbidity, specifically uterine thinning and the implications for mode of delivery for the index and subsequent pregnancies have been the impetus to pursue less invasive techniques. Foremost among these is fetoscopic spina bifida aperta repair (FSBAR).

Fetoscopic Repair (FSBAR)

In contrast with the standardised technique of open repair described above, fetoscopic techniques have evolved in a variety of ways. It is important to recognise that FSBAR techniques vary in two aspects, namely, fetoscopic access to the fetus and mode of repair of the MMC lesion.

1. Uterine access. In FSBAR, the endoscopic ports may be placed percutaneously [55] (CECAM) or following exteriorization of the uterus [56, 57]. In the former, three ports are placed whilst in the latter some groups rely on only two ports. These techniques avoid the need for "formal" hysterotomy and have been shown to have a negligible risk for dehiscence or uterine thinning. Vaginal delivery can be permitted following either technique.
2. Mode of repair. Using current technology, the constraints of fetoscopic operating mean that the surgical technique to close the spina bifida aperta defect has to be modified (Fig. 5c–e). The simplest technique involves dissection of the neural placode from the surrounding skin, followed by suturing a patch into the skin defect (Fig. 5c). This technique was pioneered by Kohl in Germany; however, in

some of their patients a two-patch technique has been used; a biocellulose patch is placed over the dural defect, prior to placement of the skin patch [13]. Pedreira et al. in Brazil also place a patch in the dural defect, and close the skin with a second patch if primary skin closure is not feasible (Fig. 5d). In a further development of FSBAR, the Texas group advocates a two-layer closure (musculofascial and skin) avoiding patches altogether (Fig. 5e). Where the defect is too large for simple skin closure, they use lateral releasing incisions to facilitate tension-free skin apposition.

Given these technical variations in FSBAR and given the differing outcome perspectives (fetal vs maternal) it is an oversimplification to make a binary comparison between open and fetoscopic techniques. In a systematic review, perinatal mortality and shunt rates were comparable between open and fetoscopic techniques. Uterine thinning or dehiscence did not occur following fetoscopy but were reported in over one third of open repair cases [58]. However, FSBAR was associated with higher rate of preterm rupture of membranes (PROM), earlier gestational age at delivery and a tenfold increase in the need for post-delivery surgery at the site of repair, for problems such as wound breakdown, CSF leakage or inclusion cyst. Additionally, operation time is longer for FSBAR and the learning curve to achieve procedural competency is also longer [59].

Some proponents of fetoscopy have extended the gestational age limit for surgery in an attempt to obviate the problems of premature delivery. In the CECAM trial of percutaneous FSBAR, the median age at delivery was 32.4 weeks, and this was in spite of extending the time of intervention to 28 weeks—there was an average of only 5.6 weeks between repair and delivery [55]. The issues of prematurity and PROM seem much improved using the exteriorised uterus technique of FSBAR [57]. Nonetheless, this group still experienced wound-related problems at the closure site (although these improved with increasing experience), and amongst 28 cases, four had to be converted to open and two abandoned.

A recent study using data from an International registry of FSBAR, comprising results from 300 cases, provided further confirmation of the maternal advantages of avoiding hysterotomy; there were no instances of uterine thinning or dehiscence, and vaginal delivery was possible in one third of cases [60]. This study also concluded that postnatal outcomes for the child were similar for FSBAR (in comparison to MOMS); however, the infant outcomes did not report beyond 12 months and were limited to shunt placement rates. Only the motor level at birth was mentioned, and there were no references to ventricular size or hindbrain herniation. A further criticism of this study is that percutaneous and exteriorised uterus techniques were analysed together thus obscuring the increasing evidence that the latter technique is statistically superior.

Whilst FSBAR has clear maternal benefits, important differences in repair technique should not be overlooked. Longer and more rigorous follow-up are required in order to confirm that the advantages to the fetus of prenatal repair are not compromised.

Mini-Hysterotomy

In an attempt to maintain the advantages of open microsurgical repair whilst improving maternal morbidity, Peralta and colleagues have developed a technique of mini-hysterotomy. The uterine opening is limited to 4 cm (compared with approx. 7 cm in the standard open procedure). Ninety-five percent of the women had intact uterine scar at delivery. Additionally, this team achieved early closure (median age 24.5 weeks) and avoided the risks of significant prematurity, median age at delivery 35.3 weeks [11]. It appears that postnatal outcomes are not only maintained using this technique but perhaps even enhanced by virtue of the earlier time of intervention [22].

Future Perspectives

Fetal repair of myelomeningocele is now established in the neurosurgical repertoire. It is now clear that myelomeningocele is not a static, exclusively congenital, malformation of the central nervous system but rather a dynamic and evolutive process involving chemical, hydrodynamic and mechanical factors that are amenable to manipulation during fetal life to the benefit of the future child. It is still unclear which surgical technique best achieves the objectives of improved CSF circulation, reversal of hindbrain herniation and neuroprotection at the repair site, whilst at the same time optimising maternal outcome.

Perhaps open and fetoscopic approaches should not be seen as mutually exclusive techniques, but both as viable and effective options depending on criteria yet to be determined.

The advent of fetal surgery for MMC has reanimated both clinical and basic science studies in neural tube defects; the topic now serves as an exemplar for translational research. The direction of travel seems to be toward earlier and less invasive techniques [53]. Developments in mechanical engineering are likely to improve endoscopic tissue handling and dissection. Tissue engineering and stem cell therapy is already being investigated with the ambition to stimulate neural regeneration [61, 62].

In any event, it will remain crucial for neurosurgeons and spina bifida clinics to engage with this rapidly developing speciality to ensure that accurate and validated clinical follow data are recorded to inform future research.

References

1. Meuli M, Meuli-Simmen C, Hutchins GM, Yingling CD, Hoffman KM, Harrison MR, Adzick NS. In utero surgery rescues neurological function at birth in sheep with spina bifida. Nat Med. 1995;1(4):342–7. http://www.nature.com/naturemedicine

2. Stiefel D, Copp AJ, Meuli M. Fetal spina bifida in a mouse model: loss of neural function in utero. J Neurosurg. 2007;106(3 Suppl):213–21. https://doi.org/10.3171/ped.2007.106.3.213.

3. Joyeux L, Engels AC, Deprez M, Khatoum A, De Bie F, Pranpanus S, Carvalho MGM, De Vleeschauwer S, Aertsen M, Patel P, Van Calenbergh F, Deprest J. Water-tightness increases reversal of hindbrain herniation and improves neuromotor function in the lamb model for spina bifida repair. Childs Nerv Syst. 2018a;34(5):2018.

4. Joyeux L, Engels AC, Van Der Merwe J, Aertsen M, Patel PA, Deprez M, Khatoun A, Pranpanus S, da Cunha MGMCM, De Vleeschauwer S, Parra J, Apelt K, Laughlin MM, Van Calenbergh F, Radaelli E, Deprest J. Validation of the fetal lamb model of spina bifida. Sci Rep. 2019;9(1):9327. https://doi.org/10.1038/s41598-019-45819-3.

5. Joyeux L, De Bie F, Danzer E, Van Mieghem T, Flake AW, Deprest J. Safety and efficacy of fetal surgery techniques to close a spina bifida defect in the fetal lamb model: a systematic review. Prenat Diagn. 2018b;38(4):231–42. https://doi.org/10.1002/pd.5222.

6. Joyeux L, Deprez M, Khatoun A, Van Kuyck K, Pelsmaekers K, Engels AC, Wang H, Da Cunha MGMCM, De Vleeschauwer S, Mc Laughlin M, Deprest J. Quantitative analysis of motor evoked potentials in the neonatal lamb. Sci Rep. 2017;7(1):16095. https://doi.org/10.1038/s41598-017-16453-8.

7. Adzick NS, Thom EA, Spong CY, Brock JW, Burrows PK, Johnson MP, Howell LJ, Farrell JA, Dabrowiak ME, Sutton LN, Gupta N, Tulipan NB, D'Alton ME, Farmer DL. A randomized trial of prenatal versus postnatal repair of myelomeningocele. N Engl J Med. 2011;364(11):993–1004. https://doi.org/10.1056/nejmoa1014379.

8. Elbabaa SK, Gildehaus AM, Pierson MJ, Albers JA, Vlastos EJ. First 60 fetal in-utero myelomeningocele repairs at Saint Louis Fetal Care Institute in the post-MOMS trial era: hydrocephalus treatment outcomes (endoscopic third ventriculostomy versus ventriculo-peritoneal shunt). Childs Nerv Syst. 2017;33(7):1157–68. https://doi.org/10.1007/s00381-017-3428-8.

9. Moron AF, Barbosa MM, Milani HJF, Sarmento SG, Santana EFM, Suriano IC, Dastoli PA, Cavalheiro S. Re: Perinatal outcomes after open fetal surgery for myelomeningocele repair: a retrospective cohort study. BJOG. 2019;126(1):131–2. https://doi.org/10.1111/1471-0528.15464.

10. Zamłyński J, Olejek A, Koszutski T, Ziomek G, Horzelska E, Gajewska-Kucharek A, Maruniak-Chudek I, Herman-Sucharska I, Kluczewska E, Horak S, Bodzek P, Zamłyński M, Kowalik J, Horzelski T, Bohosiewicz J. Comparison of prenatal and postnatal treatments of spina bifida in Poland—a non-randomized, single-center study. J Matern Fetal Neonatal Med. 2014;27(14):1409–17. https://doi.org/10.3109/14767058.2013.858689.

11. Botelho RD, Imada V, Rodrigues Da Costa KJ, Watanabe LC, Rossi Júnior R, De Salles AAF, Romano E, Peralta CFA. Fetal myelomeningocele repair through a mini-hysterotomy. Fetal Diagn Ther. 2017;42(1):28–34. https://doi.org/10.1159/000449382.

12. Belfort MA, Whitehead WE, Shamshirsaz AA, Bateni ZH, Olutoye OO, Olutoye OA, Mann DG, Espinoza J, Williams E, Lee TC, Keswani SG, Ayres N, Cassady CI, Mehollin-Ray AR, Cortes MS, Carreras E, Peiro JL, Ruano R, Cass DL. Fetoscopic open neural tube defect repair: development and refinement of a two-port, carbon dioxide insufflation technique. Obstet Gynecol. 2017;129(4):734–43. https://doi.org/10.1097/AOG.0000000000001941.

13. Graf K, Kohl T, Neubauer BA, Dey F, Faas D, Wanis FA, Reinges MHT, Uhl E, Kolodziej MA. Percutaneous minimally invasive fetoscopic surgery for spina bifida aperta. Part III: neurosurgical intervention in the first postnatal year. Ultrasound Obstet Gynecol. 2016;47(2):158–61. https://doi.org/10.1002/uog.14937.

14. Guilbaud L, Roux N, Friszer S, Dhombres F, Shah Z, Garabedian C, Jouannic JM, Vialle R, Bessières B, Di Rocco F, Zerah M. Two-port fetoscopic repair of myelomeningocele in fetal lambs. Fetal Diagn Ther. 2019;45(1):36–41. https://doi.org/10.1159/000485655.

15. Inversetti A, Van der Veeken L, Thompson D, Jansen K, Van Calenbergh F, Joyeux L, Bosteels J, Deprest J. Neurodevelopmental outcome of children with spina bifida aperta repaired prenatally vs postnatally: systematic review and meta-analysis. Ultrasound Obstet Gynecol. 2019;53(3):293–301. https://doi.org/10.1002/uog.20188.

16. Worley G, Greenberg RG, Rocque BG, Liu T, Dicianno BE, Castillo JP, Ward EA, Williams TR, Blount JP, Wiener JS, Thibadeau J, Adams JR, Hopson B. Neurosurgical procedures for children with myelomeningocele after fetal or postnatal surgery: a comparative effectiveness study. Dev Med Child Neurol. 2021;63(11):1294–301. https://doi.org/10.1111/dmcn.14792.
17. Tulipan N, Wellons JC, Thom EA, Gupta N, Sutton LN, Burrows PK, Farmer D, Walsh W, Johnson MP, Rand L, Tolivaisa S, D'Alton ME, Adzick NS, Howell L, Flak A, Hedrick H, Koh J, Rychik J, Rintoul N, Higgins R. Prenatal surgery for myelomeningocele and the need for cerebrospinal fluid shunt placement. J Neurosurg Pediatr. 2015a;16(6):613–20. https://doi.org/10.3171/2015.7.PEDS15336.
18. Elbabaa SK, Elledge R, Vlastos E. Outcome evaluation of endoscopic third ventriculostomy in infants who underwent prenatal in-utero repair of myelomeningocele: promising early results? Childs Nerv Syst. 2014;30(11):1157–68.
19. Flanders TM, Heuer GG, Madsen PJ, Buch VP, MacKell CM, Alexander EE, Moldenhauer JS, Zarnow DM, Flake AW, Adzick NS. Detailed analysis of hydrocephalus and hindbrain herniation after prenatal and postnatal myelomeningocele closure: report from a single institution. Neurosurgery. 2020;86(5):637–45. https://doi.org/10.1093/neuros/nyz302.
20. Bowman RM, Boshnjaku V, McLone DG. The changing incidence of myelomeningocele and its impact on pediatric neurosurgery: a review from the Children's Memorial Hospital. Childs Nerv Syst. 2009;25(7):801–6. https://doi.org/10.1007/s00381-009-0865-z.
21. Chakraborty A, Crimmins D, Hayward R, Thompson D. Toward reducing shunt placement rates in patients with myelomeningocele. J Neurosurg Pediatr. 2008;1(5):361–5. https://doi.org/10.3171/PED/2008/1/5/361.
22. Peralta CFA, Botelho RD, Imada V, Lamis F, Antunes DRV, Nani F, Balsalobre AGB. Fetal open spinal dysraphism repair through a mini-hysterotomy: influence of gestational age at surgery on children's ability to walk. Prenat Diagn. 2021;41(13):1634–42. https://doi.org/10.1002/pd.6051.
23. Guilbaud L, Maurice P, Lallemant P, De Saint-Denis T, Maisonneuve E, Dhombres F, Friszer S, Di Rocco F, Garel C, Moutard ML, Lachtar MA, Rigouzzo A, Forin V, Zérah M, Jouannic JM. Open fetal surgery for myelomeningocele repair in France. J Gynecol Obstet Hum Reprod. 2021;50(9):102155. https://doi.org/10.1016/j.jogoh.2021.102155.
24. Pan ET, Pallapati J, Krueger A, Yepez M, Vanloh S, Nassr AA, Espinoza J, Shamshirsaz AA, Olutoye OO, Mehollin-Ray A, De Jong H, Castillo H, Castillo J, Whitehead WE, Olutoye OA, Ayres N, Belfort MA, Sanz Cortes M. Evaluation and disposition of fetal myelomeningocele repair candidates: a large referral center experience. Fetal Diagn Ther. 2020;47(2):115–22. https://doi.org/10.1159/000500451.
25. McLone DG, Knepper PA. The cause of Chiari II malformation: a unified theory. Pediatr Neurosci. 1989;15(1):1–15. https://doi.org/10.1159/000120432.
26. Paek BW, Farmer DL, Wilkinson CC, Albanese CT, Peacock W, Harrison MR, Jennings RW. Hindbrain herniation develops in surgically created myelomeningocele but is absent after repair in fetal lambs. Am J Obstet Gynecol. 2000;183(5):1119–23. https://doi.org/10.1067/mob.2000.108867.
27. Kim I, Hopson B, Aban I, Rizk EB, Dias MS, Bowman R, Ackerman LL, Partington MD, Castillo H, Castillo J, Peterson PR, Blount JP, Rocque BG. Decompression for Chiari malformation type II in individuals with myelomeningocele in the National Spina Bifida Patient Registry. J Neurosurg Pediatr. 2018;22(6):652–8. https://thejns.org/view/journals/j--neurosurg-pediatr/22/6/article-p652.xml
28. Zarutskie A, Guimaraes C, Yepez M, Torres P, Shetty A, Sangi-Haghpeykar H, Lee W, Espinoza J, Shamshirsaz AA, Nassr A, Belfort MA, Whitehead WE, Sanz Cortes M. Prenatal brain imaging for predicting need for postnatal hydrocephalus treatment in fetuses that had neural tube defect repair in utero. Ultrasound Obstet Gynecol. 2019;53(3):324–34. https://doi.org/10.1002/uog.20212.
29. Lu VM, Snyder KA, Ibirogba ER, Ruano R, Daniels DJ, Ahn ES. Progressive hydrocephalus despite early complete reversal of hindbrain herniation after prenatal open myelomeningocele

repair. Neurosurg Focus. 2019;47(4):E13. https://thejns.org/view/journals/neurosurg-focus/47/4/article-pE13.xml

30. Appasamy M, Roberts D, Pilling D, Buxton N. Antenatal ultrasound and magnetic resonance imaging in localizing the level of lesion in spina bifida and correlation with postnatal outcome. Ultrasound Obstet Gynecol. 2006;27(5):2755. https://doi.org/10.1002/uog.2755.

31. Sherrod BA, Ho WS, Hedlund A, Kennedy A, Ostrander B, Bollo RJ. A comparison of the accuracy of fetal MRI and prenatal ultrasonography at predicting lesion level and perinatal motor outcome in patients with myelomeningocele. Neurosurg Focus. 2019;47(4):E4. https://doi.org/10.3171/2019.7.FOCUS19450.

32. Barnes KS, Singh S, Barkley A, Lepard J, Hopson B, Cawyer CR, Blount JP, Rocque BG. Determination of anatomic level of myelomeningocele by prenatal ultrasound. Childs Nerv Syst. 2022;38(5):985–90. https://doi.org/10.1007/s00381-022-05469-9.

33. Wilson RD, Johnson MP, Bebbington M, Flake AW, Hedrick HL, Sutton LN, Adzick NS. Does a myelomeningocele sac compared to no sac result in decreased postnatal leg function following maternal fetal surgery for spina bifida aperta? Fetal Diagn Ther. 2007;22(5):348–51. https://doi.org/10.1159/000103294.

34. Corroenne R, Mehollin-Ray AR, Johnson RM, Whitehead WE, Espinoza J, Castillo J, Castillo H, Orman G, Donepudi R, Huisman TAGM, Nassr AA, Belfort MA, Sanz Cortes M, Shamshirsaz AA. Impact of the volume of the myelomeningocele sac on imaging, prenatal neurosurgery and motor outcomes: a retrospective cohort study. Sci Rep. 2021;11(1):13189. https://doi.org/10.1038/s41598-021-92739-2.

35. Oliver E, Heuer G, Thom E, Burrows P, Didier R, DeBari S, Martin-Saavedra J, Moldenhauer J, Jatres J, Howell L, et al. Prenatal presence of myelomeningocele sac associated with worse neurologic sequela: evidence for prenatal stretch injury. Ultrasound Obstet Gynecol. 2019;55(6):740–6.

36. Houtrow AJ, MacPherson C, Jackson-Coty J, Rivera M, Flynn L, Burrows PK, Adzick NS, Fletcher J, Gupta N, Howell LJ, Brock JW, Lee H, Walker WO, Thom EA. Prenatal repair and physical functioning among children with myelomeningocele: a secondary analysis of a randomized clinical trial. JAMA Pediatr. 2021;175(4):e205674. https://doi.org/10.1001/jamapediatrics.2020.5674.

37. Bartonek Å, Saraste H, Samuelsson L, Skoog M. Ambulation in patients with myelomeningocele: a 12-year follow-up. J Pediatr Orthop. 1999;19(2):202–6. https://doi.org/10.1097/01241398-199903000-00013.

38. Davis WA, Zigler CK, Crytzer TM, Crytzer TM, Izzo S, Houtrow AJ, Dicianno BE, Dicianno BE. Factors associated with ambulation in myelomeningocele: a longitudinal study from the National Spina Bifida Patient Registry. Am J Phys Med Rehabil. 2020;99(7):586–94. https://doi.org/10.1097/PHM.0000000000001406.

39. Clayton DB, Tanaka ST, Trusler L, Thomas JC, Pope JC IV, Adams MC, Brock JW. Long-term urological impact of fetal myelomeningocele closure. J Urol. 2011;186(4 Suppl):1581–5. https://doi.org/10.1016/j.juro.2011.04.005.

40. Holzbeierlein J, Pope JC IV, Adams MC, Bruner J, Tulipan N, Brock JW. The urodynamic profile of myelodysplasia in childhood with spinal closure during gestation. J Urol. 2000;164(4):1336–9. https://doi.org/10.1016/S0022-5347(05)67191-1.

41. Lee NG, Gomez P, Uberoi V, Kokorowski PJ, Khoshbin S, Bauer SB, Estrada CR. In utero closure of myelomeningocele does not improve lower urinary tract function. J Urol. 2012;188(4 Suppl):1567–71. https://doi.org/10.1016/j.juro.2012.06.034.

42. Clayton DB, Thomas JC, Brock JW. Fetal repair of myelomeningocele: current status and urologic implications. J Pediatr Urol. 2020;16(1):3–9. https://doi.org/10.1016/j.jpurol.2019.11.019.

43. Brock JW, Carr NS, Adzick NS, Burrows PK, Thomas JC, Thom EA, Howell LJ, Farrell JA, Dabrowiak ME, Farmer DL, Cheng EY, Kropp BP, Caldamone AA, Bulas DI, Tolivaisa S, Baskin LS. Bladder function after fetal surgery for myelomeningocele. Pediatrics. 2015;136(4):e906–13. https://doi.org/10.1542/peds.2015-2114.

44. Brock JW, Thomas JC, Baskin LS, Zderic SA, Thom EA, Burrows PK, Lee H, Houtrow AJ, MacPherson C, Adzick NS. Effect of prenatal repair of myelomeningocele on urological outcomes at school age. J Urol. 2019;202(4):812–8. https://doi.org/10.1097/JU.0000000000000334.

45. Heye P, Moehrlen U, Mazzone L, Weil R, Altermatt S, Wille DA, Scheer I, Meuli M, Horst M. Inclusion cysts after fetal spina bifida repair: a third hit? Fetal Diagn Ther. 2019;46(1):38–44. https://doi.org/10.1159/000491877.

46. Danzer E, Thomas NH, Thomas A, Friedman KB, Gerdes M, Koh J, Scott Adzick N, Johnson MP. Long-term neurofunctional outcome, executive functioning, and behavioral adaptive skills following fetal myelomeningocele surgery. Am J Obstet Gynecol. 2016;214(2):269.e1–8. https://doi.org/10.1016/j.ajog.2015.09.094.

47. Farmer DL, Thom EA, Brock JW, Burrows PK, Johnson MP, Howell LJ, Farrell JA, Gupta N, Adzick NS. The Management of Myelomeningocele Study: full cohort 30-month pediatric outcomes. Am J Obstet Gynecol. 2018;218(2):256.e1–256.e13. https://doi.org/10.1016/j.ajog.2017.12.001.

48. Joyeux L, van der Merwe J, Aertsen M, Patel PA, Khatoun A, da Cunha MGMCM, De Vleeschauwer S, Parra J, Danzer E, Laughlin MM, Stoyanov D, Vercauteren T, Ourselin S, De Coppi P, Radaelli E, Van Calenbergh F, Deprest J. 82 Neuroprotection is improved by watertightness of spina bifida repair in the fetal lamb. Am J Obstet Gynecol. 2021;224(2):S57–8. https://doi.org/10.1016/j.ajog.2020.12.083.

49. Kabagambe SK, Jensen GW, Chen YJ, Vanover MA, Farmer DL. Fetal surgery for myelomeningocele: a systematic review and meta-analysis of outcomes in fetoscopic versus open repair. Fetal Diagn Ther. 2018;43(3):161–74. https://doi.org/10.1159/000479505.

50. Danzer E, Adzick NS, Rintoul NE, Zarnow DM, Schwartz ES, Melchionni J, Ernst LM, Flake AW, Sutton LN, Johnson MP. Intradural inclusion cysts following in utero closure of myelomeningocele: clinical implications and follow-up findings: clinical article. J Neurosurg Pediatr. 2008;2(6):406–13. https://doi.org/10.3171/PED.2008.2.12.406.

51. Hilton SA, Hodges MM, Dewberry LC, Handler M, Galan HL, Zaretsky MV, Behrendt N, Marwan AI, Liechty KW. MOMS plus: single-institution review of outcomes for extended BMI criteria for open fetal repair of myelomeningocele. Fetal Diagn Ther. 2019;46(6):411–4. https://doi.org/10.1159/000499484.

52. Etchegaray A, Cruz-Martínez R, Russo RD, Martínez-Rodríguez M, Palma F, Chavelas-Ochoa F, Beruti E, López-Briones H, Fregonese R, Villalobos-Gómez R, Gámez-Varela A, Allegrotti H, Aguilar-Vidales K. Outcomes of late open fetal surgery for intrauterine spina bifida repair after 26 weeks. Should we extend the Management of Myelomeningocele Study time window? Prenat Diagn. 2022;42(4):495–501. https://doi.org/10.1002/pd.6119.

53. Thompson D, De Coppi P. Getting earlier, smaller and regenerative: the next 10 years of in utero spina bifida repair. Prenat Diagn. 2021;41(8):907–9.

54. Heuer GG, Adzick NS, Sutton LN. Fetal myelomeningocele closure: technical considerations. Fetal Diagn Ther. 2015;37(3):166–71. https://doi.org/10.1159/000363182.

55. Pedreira DAL, Zanon N, Nishikuni K, Moreira De Sá RA, Acacio GL, Chmait RH, Kontopoulos EV, Quintero RA. Endoscopic surgery for the antenatal treatment of myelomeningocele: the CECAM trial. Am J Obstet Gynecol. 2016;214(1):111.e1–111.e11. https://doi.org/10.1016/j.ajog.2015.09.065.

56. Espinoza J, Shamshirsaz AA, Sanz Cortes M, Pammi M, Nassr AA, Donepudi R, Whitehead WE, Castillo J, Johnson R, Meshinchi N, Sun R, Krispin E, Corroenne R, Lee TC, Keswani SG, King A, Belfort MA. Two-port, exteriorized uterus, fetoscopic meningomyelocele closure has fewer adverse neonatal outcomes than open hysterotomy closure. Am J Obstet Gynecol. 2021;225(3):327.e1–9. https://doi.org/10.1016/j.ajog.2021.04.252.

57. Sanz-Cortes M, Yepez M, Torres P, Andruciolli A, Pyrali M, Espinoza J, Shamshirsaz A, Nassr AA, Whitehead W, Olutoye OO, Castillo J, Castillo H, Ostermaier KK, Belfort MA. 220: Prenatal open vs. two-port exteriorized uterus fetoscopic myelomeningocele repair.

Neurosurgical outcomes from a single center. Am J Obstet Gynecol. 2019;220(1):S160. https://doi.org/10.1016/j.ajog.2018.11.241.

58. Joyeux L, Engels AC, Russo FM, Jimenez J, Van Mieghem T, De Coppi P, Van Calenbergh F, Deprest J. Fetoscopic versus open repair for spina bifida aperta: a systematic review of outcomes. Fetal Diagn Ther. 2016;39(3):161–71. http://www.karger.com/Article/FullText/443498

59. Joyeux L, De Bie F, Danzer E, Russo FM, Javaux A, Peralta CFA, De Salles AAF, Pastuszka A, Olejek A, Van Mieghem T, De Coppi P, Moldenhauer J, Whitehead WE, Belfort MA, Lapa DA, Acacio GL, Devlieger R, Hirose S, Farmer DL, Deprest J. Learning curves of open and endoscopic fetal spina bifida closure: systematic review and meta-analysis. Ultrasound Obstet Gynecol. 2020;55(6):730–9. https://doi.org/10.1002/uog.20389.

60. Sanz Cortes M, Chmait RH, Lapa DA, Belfort MA, Carreras E, Miller JL, Samaha RBB, Gonzalez GS, Gielchinsky Y, Yamamoto M, Persico N, Santorum M, Otaño L, Nicolaou E, Yinon Y, Faig-Leite F, Brandt R, Whitehead W, Maiz N, Nicolaides KH. Experience of 300 cases of prenatal fetoscopic open spina bifida repair: report of the international fetoscopic neural tube defect repair consortium. Am J Obstet Gynecol. 2021;225(6):678.e1–678.e11. https://doi.org/10.1016/j.ajog.2021.05.044.

61. Kunpalin Y, Subramaniam S, Perin S, Gerli MFM, Bosteels J, Ourselin S, Deprest J, De Coppi P, David AL. Preclinical stem cell therapy in fetuses with myelomeningocele: a systematic review and meta-analysis. Prenat Diagn. 2021;41(3):283–300. https://doi.org/10.1002/pd.5887.

62. Watanabe M, Li H, Kim AG, Weilerstein A, Radu A, Davey M, Loukogeorgakis S, Sánchez MD, Sumita K, Morimoto N, Yamamoto M, Tabata Y, Flake AW. Complete tissue coverage achieved by scaffold-based tissue engineering in the fetal sheep model of myelomeningocele. Biomaterials. 2016;76:133–43. https://doi.org/10.1016/j.biomaterials.2015.10.051.

A New Surgical Paradigm for Postnatal Repair of Open Neural Tube Defects Using Intraoperative Neurophysiology Monitoring

Sebastian Eibach and Dachling Pang

Abbreviations

BCR   Bulbocavernosus reflex
EMG   Electromyography
IONM   Intraoperative neurophysiological monitoring
mA   Milliampere
MRI   Magnetic resonance imaging
ONTD   Open neural tube defect
SSEP   Somatosensory evoked potential
TcMEP   Transcortical motor evoked potentials

An open neural tube defect (ONTD) features an exposed, unclosed neural plate in the form of an expanded and frequently hefty neural placode. Traditional philosophy of ONTD repair aims at preserving the placode at any cost, which often means stuffing the entire thick and unwieldy but non-functional tissue into a tight dural sac, increasing the likelihood of future tethering of the spinal cord. The same philosophy of attempting to save the whole perimetry of the placode also sometimes leads to

S. Eibach (✉)
Department of Clinical Medicine, Faculty of Medicine, Health and Human Sciences, Macquarie University, Sydney, Australia

Paediatric Neurosurgery, Sydney Children's Hospital Randwick, Sydney, Australia

D. Pang
Great Ormond Street Hospital for Children, NHS Trust, London, UK

University of California, Davis, Davis, CA, USA

D. Pang, K.-C. Wang (eds.), *Spinal Dysraphic Malformations*, Advances and Technical Standards in Neurosurgery 47,
https://doi.org/10.1007/978-3-031-34981-2_3

inadvertent inclusion of parts of the squamous epithelial membrane surrounding the placode into the reconstructed product, only to form inclusion dermoid cyst causing further injury to the neural tissues. Lastly, unsuccessful neurulation of the caudal primary neural tube almost always adversely affects junctional and secondary neurulation resulting in a defective conus, often with a locally active sacral micturition centre that is isolated from and therefore lacking suprasegmental inhibitory moderation. This frequently leads to the development of a spastic, hyperactive, low-compliance and high-pressure bladder predisposing to upstream kidney damage, without benefits of normal bladder function. We are introducing a new surgical technique designed to minimise or eliminate these three undesirable complications of conventional ONTD closure.

Primary Neurulation Defect

Spinal dysraphic malformations are caused by defects of primary, junctional, or secondary neurulation—chronologically sequential and fundamentally different embryological processes involved in the formation of the central neuraxis. Primary neurulation, which is responsible for forming the brain and most of the spinal cord down to approximately the junction of the S_1 and S_2 spinal cord segments, involves the dorsal folding and midline fusion of the neural plate to form the primary neural tube. The rolling up of this neural plate, which is derived from embryonic ectoderm, encloses a central lumen. Because the two edges of the primitive neural plate are continuous with the embryonic cutaneous ectoderm on their corresponding sides, successful dorsal closure of the primary neural tube also ensures seamless fusion of the midline skin and mesodermal tissues [1]. Complete failure of primary neural tube closure must therefore result in an overt open skin defect and an exposed, unfused neural plate, constituting an open neural tube defect (ONTD).

Complete non-closure of the caudal primary neural tube, as in most ONTDs, usually leads to severe disturbance in the contiguous domains of junctional and secondary neurulation, resulting in a severely malformed and non-functional or at best poorly functional conus and sacral nerve roots, clinically presenting with neurogenic bladder and bowel dysfunction as well as varying degrees of lower limb weakness [2].

Disadvantages of Traditional Repair of Open Neural Tube Defects

Repair of ONTD traditionally aims to preserve all nervous tissue for fear of losing already paltry function, even though the exposed placode is mostly defunct and functionally disconnected from voluntary control. The philosophy of traditional closure leads to three potential ill effects that contribute to the overall late morbidity of ONTD treatment. Meticulous preservation of all neural tissue often means forcibly stuffing a disproportionately large and bulky malformed neural placode into a tight dural enclosure recreated from scant meningeal remnants. The resulting crammed spinal cord-thecal sac relationship, as seen in many postoperative magnetic resonant images (MRI), intuitively contributes to the known rate of secondary symptomatic tethering of the spinal cord in up to one third of patients (10–30%) after standard ONTD repair [3, 4].

Secondly, the obsessive fear of shaving away functional neural tissue during the detachment of the placode edges from the surrounding squamous epithelium cum arachnoid membrane sometimes inadvertently includes squamous patches that are thus rolled inside the reconstructed neural tube with the pia-to-pia neurulation step [5, 6]. Later growth of these retained squamous cells explains the occurrence of inclusion dermoid cysts [7] in up to 15% of postnatal ONTD repair [8], and in 26% following fetal myelomeningocele closure [9], causing delayed myelopathy requiring further surgery (Fig. 1).

Lastly, disturbed secondary and junctional neurulation can sometimes generate an active local sensory (from bladder wall stretch organs) and motor (bladder detrusor) circuit within the sacral cord segments that is lacking normal corticospinal inhibitory moderation and control, resulting in a spastic, hyperactive and

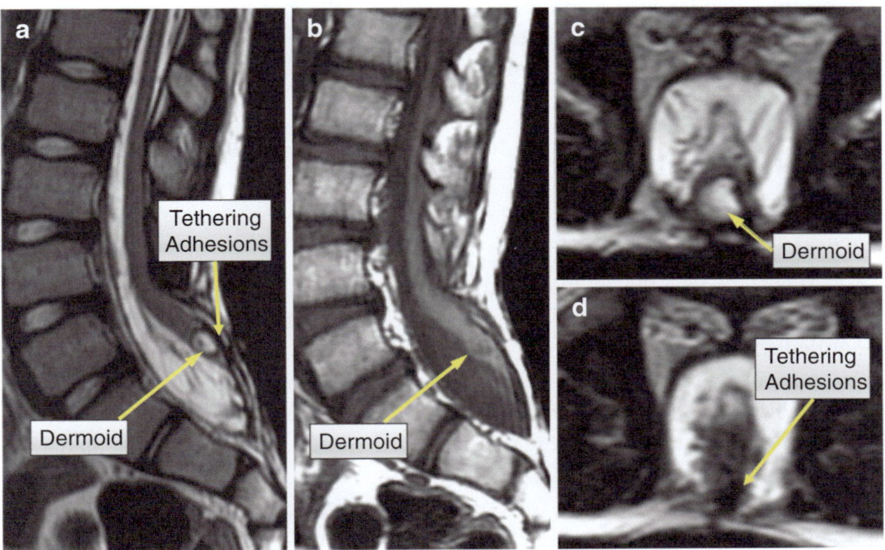

Fig. 1 MRI of a lumbrosacral ONTD 3 years after surgical closure using the traditional technique of complete placode preservation. (**a**) Sagittal T2-weighted image showing a hyperintense lesion within the dorsally imbricated neural placode which turned out to be an inclusion dermoid cyst. (**b**) Sagittal T1-weighted image shows the same lesion and a plump neural placode plastered against the dorsal dura over a wide surface. Axial T2-weighted images show the intramedullary dermoid (**c**), as well as dorsal fibrous adhesions tethering the spinal cord (**d**)

low-compliance bladder with detrusor-sphincter dyssynergia. These abnormal bladder dynamics are highly conducive to sustained massively elevated intravesicular pressures and high-grade vesicourethral reflux, and ultimately lead to repetitive pyelonephritis and chronic renal failure [10]. This type of high-pressure bladder is prognostically more hostile than a low-pressure flaccid bladder, which can be easily managed with clean intermittent catheterization [11].

Advantages of the New Paradigm for Repair of Open Neural Tube Defects

Contrary to traditional teaching, we propose a new paradigm of ONTD repair in which all non-functional malformed neural tissues unconnected to upper cerebrospinal tracts, which usually constitutes all or most of the unclosed neural placode, can be resected using careful intraoperative neurophysiological monitoring (IONM) without loss of voluntary function. This will drastically reduce the size of the preserved neural stump and create a loose cord-sac relationship, and hopefully also the likelihood of post-repair tethering. Resecting the placode *en masse* with its surrounding membranes also negates the occurrence of inclusion dermoid cysts. Eliminating the unbridled local sacral bladder circuit converts a potentially hostile hyperactive bladder into a low-pressured one easily manageable with a sensible intermittent catheterization programme. This chapter presents the surgical and IONM techniques of this new paradigm performed on a short list of patients, and their early postoperative results.

Patient Series

This series describes the postnatal surgical treatment of eight newborn infants with ONTD, in whom we resected the non-functional portion of the neural placode identified as such by direct spinal cord/placode and nerve roots stimulation, as well as by transcortical evoked motor responses to check for suprasegmental corticospinal connectivity. Any part of the placode without local function or upstream connections was resected, and the small caudal spinal cord stump artificially neurulated with pia-to-pia microsutures.

The patients were followed for pre- and postoperative neuro-urological status, and underwent assessment routinely at 3 weeks after surgery, and every 3 months thereafter. Serial magnetic resonance imaging (MRI) at 3 weeks, 6 months, and 2 years post-repair were performed. Follow-up period ranged from birth up to 3 years (mean of 24 months). Surgical closure of all ONTDs was performed within the first 48 h after birth; seven patients had surgery within the first 24 h after birth. Patient demographic and other relevant data are summarized in Table 1.

Table 1 Patient series

Case	Sex	Age	Type	Preop function	IONM findings	Operation	Immediate postop function	Shunt dependency	Syrinx	Follow-up	Late follow-up status
1	Female	2 days	Terminal	Intact S2, flaccid anal sphincter	Intact S1 and S2 (left > right), b/l anal contractions, no response at distal placode, no TcMEP to sphincter ani	Distal placode resected	Stable, CIC	VP shunt day 12	Decreasing, lower spinal cord syrinx	13 months	Stable, S2 intact, CIC
2	Female	1 day	Terminal	Intact L4, bilateral club feet, flaccid anal sphincter	b/l rectus femoris, no L5, no response over placode and distal nerve roots, TcMEP to L4	Complete placode and distal fibrotic nerve roots resected	Stable, CIC	Nil	Increasing dilated central canal of 2.8 mm	21 months	Stable, L4 intact, CIC
3	Female	1 day	Terminal	Intact S2 (right > left), brisk anal sphincter contraction to perianal stimulation	No response of most distal set of nervc roots, all responses proximal, TcMEP to sphincter ani	No resection, just neurulation	Stable, CIC	Nil	Decreasing conus syrinx	17 months	Stable, S2 intact, CIC
4	Male	1 day	Terminal	Intact L5, flaccid anal sphincter	b/l L5, S1/S2/ anal roots from proximal placode, no responses at distal placode, TcMEP to S1	Distal placode resected	Improved with new left S1, CIC	VP shunt day 13	Nil	26 months	Stable, b/l L5, left S1 only, CIC

(continued)

Table 1 (continued)

Case	Sex	Age	Type	Preop function	IONM findings	Operation	Immediate postop function	Shunt dependency	Syrinx	Follow-up	Late follow-up status
5	Male	1 day	Terminal	Intact S1, flaccid anal sphincter	No response over placode, TcMEP to S2	Complete placode resected	Improved with b/l S2, CIC	Nil	Nil	3 years	Improved, S2 intact, normal urodynamics
6	Male	1 day	Terminal	Intact L5, flaccid anal sphincter	No response over distal placode, TcMEP to L5	Distal placode resected	Stable, CIC	VP shunt day 10	Stable cervical and lower thoracic syrinx	3 years	Stable, L5 intact, CIC
7	Male	0 days	Terminal	Intact L4 (right > left), flaccid anal sphincter	Intact L5 b/l over proximal placode, right > left responses, TcMEP to L5	Distal placode resected (80%)	Improved with new b/l L5, CIC	VP shunt day 7	Nil	3 years	Stable, L5 intact, CIC
8	Female	1 day	Segmental	Intact L5, flaccid anal sphincter	Activation of all nerve roots through placode and distally, TcMEP to sphincter ani	No resection, just neurulation	Improved with new S2 function, CIC	VP shunt day 15	Increasing thoracic syrinx at 6 months	7 months	Stable, S2 intact, CIC

b/l bilateral, *CIC* clean intermittent catheterization, *IONM* intraoperative neurophysiological monitoring, *VP* ventriculo-peritoneal

Intraoperative Neurophysiological Monitoring (IONM)

Elaborate electromyography (EMG) preparations are made to capture triggered motor responses from the muscles supplied by the relevant lumbosacral nerve roots. Standard EMG needles are inserted into the rectus femoris (L_3/L_4), anterior tibialis (L_4/L_5), gastrocnemius (S_1), and abductor hallucis (S_2). Smaller-gauge (No. 27) EMG needles are inserted obliquely into the external anal sphincter through the anal verge on each side, which is insulated from the other side with a plug of dry muslin gauze so that sphincter contractions from each side can be individually evaluated [12]. All stimulations and recordings are done with the Cadwell Cascade Intraoperative Monitoring System (Cadwell Laboratories, Inc., Kennewick, WA, USA) using the Cascade Software Version 2.5.

Pad or subcutaneous needle-stimulating electrodes are placed along the shaft of the penis in males and between the periclitoral skin and the labia minora in females. Stimulation of the sensory domain (S_3–S_5) of the pudendal nerve via these electrodes generates contractions of the external anal sphincter, which is the "electric" version of the bulbocavernosus reflex (BCR), in essence, a form of H reflex within the conus useful for assessing the integrity of the central sensory-motor arc of the sacral internuncial neuronal pool apart from motor root mapping [12, 13].

Standard stimulating electrodes are placed near the posterior tibial nerve behind the medial malleolus and near the common peroneal nerve at the fibular neck to enable somatosensory evoked potentials (SSEPs) for monitoring the dorsal sensory tracts of the spinal cord segments above S_2 [12].

All motor root and direct spinal cord stimulations are done with the concentric coaxial bipolar microprobe electrode with an end-plate diameter of 1.75 mm (Medtronic Xomed, Inc., Jacksonville, FL, USA). The concentric configuration and small size of the anode–cathode complex allow extremely focused current delivery to a very small target volume, thus making the electrode ideal for fine discrimination of small and crowded electroresponsive units [14]. Stimulating currents from 0.3 to 6.0 milliamperes (mA) are used depending on target impedance. Most functional motor roots will respond to currents of 0.3–1.5 mA, though occasionally needing 2.0 mA if the roots are partially fibrotic. Direct spinal cord stimulation will require a current of 3.0 mA or higher, but seldom more than 6 mA; both sides will be recruited if the probe is placed at the midline. The stimulation frequency is usually set at 10 per second. This permits spontaneous random firing due to nerve irritation from surgical manipulation to be distinguishable from the rhythmic evoked contractions.

To elicit transcortical motor evoked potentials (TcMEP) from the external anal sphincter, the stimulation parameters are the same as for the lower limbs: a train of eight, each with a duration of 75 µs and intensity of 100–350 V. The inhalation anaesthetic concentration, for example, of sevoflurane, is usually adjusted to no higher than 0.5 minimum alveolar concentration to ensure maximum yield. Given that the BCR in infants can be variable or even unobtainable, and is also exquisitely sensitive to inhalation anaesthesia, the TcMEP of the external anal sphincter is an important adjunct for monitoring the corticospinal input to the sacral motor centre.

Surgical Technique

Using intraoperative direct spinal cord and nerve roots stimulation, we mapped the junction between functional and non-functional neural tissue on the placode, as well as that between intact and defunct nerve roots. Transcortical motor evoked potentials were then used to confirm whether the lowest functional level identified by direct cord or nerve roots stimulations was connected to the corticospinal tracts. If so, the portion of the placode with its associated roots below the functional/non-functional junction was sharply resected, and the remaining (functional) placode or stump was neurulated using pia-to-pia 8–0 nylon sutures with buried knots. If the lowest functional level of the placode by direct cord and nerve roots stimulation is below S2 but TcMEP and direct cord stimulation above S1 demonstrated no connection with the corticospinal tracts, that portion of the placode below S2 was resected, so that most or all *isolated* anal sphincter responses were eliminated. In one such case, the BCR was actually elicitable, but the anal sphincter was not activated by TcMEP, attesting that some isolated local sacral anal sphincter circuits could exist from partial but defective secondary neurulation without junctional connection to the primary neural tube above.

With drastic reduction of the placode bulk, it was always possible to perform primary dural closure and achieve a loose content-container cord-sac relationship, followed by layered soft tissues closure in the usual fashion.

Intraoperative Surgical and IONM Findings

There were seven cases of terminal ONTD (Cases 1–7) and one case of a segmental neural tube defect (Case 8) in whom the entire segmental neural placode was preserved. Amongst the seven patients with terminal ONTD, one placode was preserved in toto because of elicitable local and corticospinal responses throughout confirmed by direct stimulation and TcMEP. Two patients had placodes that had no elicitable function shown by intraoperative electrophysiology, which were thus resected completely. Four others had partially defunct placodes whose proximal functional portions only were preserved. In one of these cases, the distal placode showed isolated function of the lower sacral cord segments with locally activated anal sphincter roots but no measurable connection with the upper corticospinal tracts verified by TcMEP and direct stimulation of the normal cord just proximal to the placode. The distal placode was therefore resected.

Details of the intraoperative IONM findings and the extent of placode resection of the entire series are summarized in Table 1. Two illustrative cases from this series exemplify their functional features and different treatment strategies depending on the intraoperative IONM findings.

First Illustrative Case: Terminal Lumbar Non-functional Placode (Case #2 in Table 1)

This 1-day-old infant was born with a large, saccular open neural tube defect in the lumbosacral region. The child's preoperative examination showed moderately strong bilateral knee extension ($L_{3,4}$), but no ankle movement (L_5, S_1) or toe flaring (S_2). The weak knee flexion was made by the gracilis muscle (L_2). Both feet were fixed in talipes equinovarus deformity. The anus was patulous.

Intraoperative stimulation of individual ventral rootlets above the placode using 0.5 mA current (Fig. 2a) activated the rectus femoris muscle bilaterally but not the anterior tibialis or gastrocnemius muscle. Individual stimulation of very fibrotic and thickened nerve rootlets at the level of the placode and below elicited no response. Direct stimulation of the reddish, abnormal looking placode itself with currents as high as 6 mA elicited no muscle response anywhere. Anal contractions were never

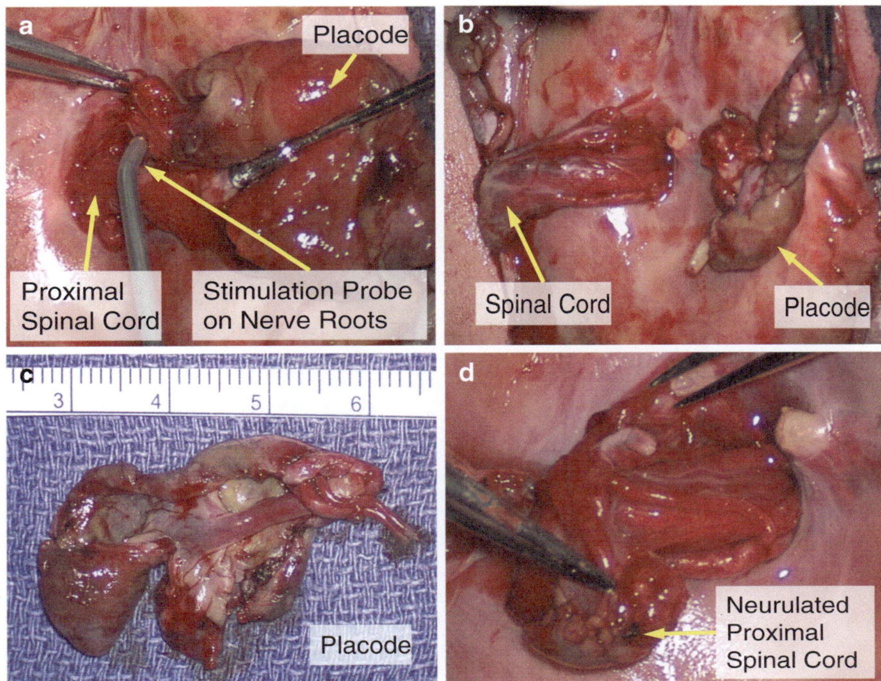

Fig. 2 Intraoperative steps of placode resection in the first illustrative case (Case 2 in Table 1). (**a**) Functional nerve roots exiting just rostral to the placode are being stimulated by a bipolar stimulation probe with a current of 0.5 mA. (**b**) The non-functional placode has been resected. (**c**) Ex vivo view of the resected placode. (**d**) Tension-free pia-to-pia neurulation of the remaining proximal spinal cord stump

obtained by placode or nerve roots stimulation (Fig. 3a). Transcortical stimulation elicited motor responses down to but not distal to the rectus femoris muscles (Fig. 3b).

The non-functional placode was resected just distal to the functional junction, which included almost its entirety, and neurulation of the trimmed-down proximal spinal cord stump was achieved in a tension-free manner (Fig. 2b–d). Primary dural closure without excessive crowding was easily accomplished. Postoperatively, the patient had neurological function unchanged from her preoperative level.

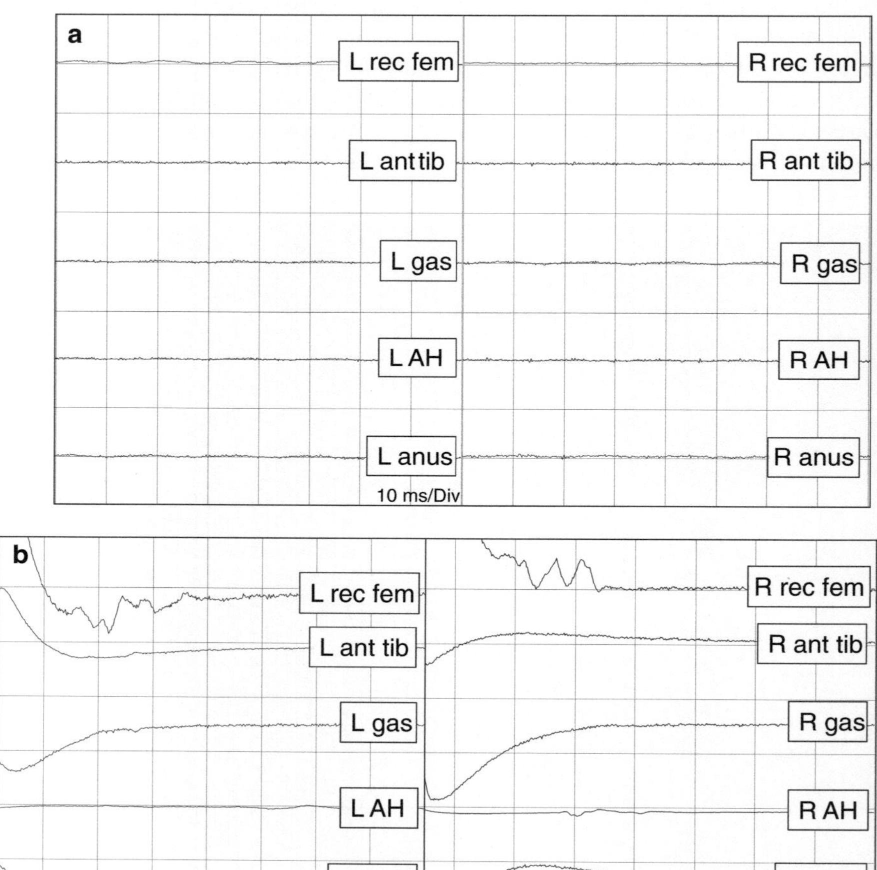

Fig. 3 Intraoperative electrophysiology of the first illustrative case (Case 2 in Table 1). (**a**) Direct stimulation of the neural placode with 6 mA elicits no EMG response in any of the lower limb muscles or anal sphincter. (**b**) TcMEP shows functional corticospinal connection to the rectus femoris muscle, but none to the tibialis anterior, gastrocnemius, abductor hallucis or external anal sphincter muscles. *AH* abductor hallucis, *ant tib* anterior tibialis, *anus* external anal sphincter, *EMG* electromyography, *gas* gastrocnemius, *L* left, *rec fem* rectus femoris, *R* right, *TcMEP* transcortical motor evoked potentials

Second Illustrative Case: Preservation of Segmental Lumbar Placode with L_5 Functional Level (Case #8 in Table 1)

This 1-day-old female infant was born with a saccular lumbar open neural tube defect measuring 2.5 × 2.5 cm (Fig. 4a). Neurological examination showed active motor functions inclusive of bilateral ankle dorsiflexion but nothing below. At surgery, ventral nerve roots were seen emanating from the underside of the exposed placode. At this point, we found that the placode tapered along its caudal extent and then continued as a fully neurulated spinal cord distally within the caudal spinal canal, indicating that this was, in fact, a segmental and not a terminal placode; that is, the lesion was a rare segmental ONTD (Fig. 4b). Direct stimulation of the placode, its associated roots, and the neurulated cord just distal to the placode using 6 mA current elicited strong contractions of the anterior tibialis, gastrocnemius and

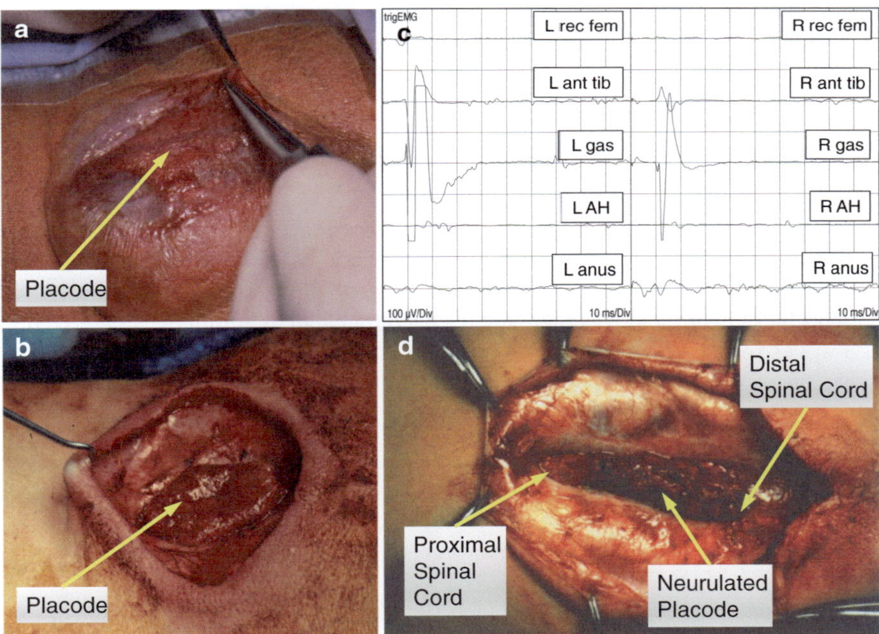

Fig. 4 Surgical steps and intraoperative electrophysiology of the segmental ONTD of the second illustrative case (Case 8 in Table 1). (**a**) Dissection of exposed neural placode from the surrounding combined membrane of arachnoid and squamous epithelium. (**b**) The placode tapers in its caudal extent and then continues as a well-formed neural tube within the distal canal, indicating its segmental nature. (**c**) Systematically mapping the spinal cord with currents up to 2 mA, from points rostral to the placode, on the placode, and just caudal to the placode, showing, successively, corresponding bilateral contractions of the tibialis anterior, gastrocnemius, abductor hallucis, and external anal sphincter muscles. (**d**) Pia-to-pia neurulation of the placode. *AH* abductor hallucis, *ant tib* anterior tibialis, *anus* external anal sphincter, *gas* gastrocnemius, *L* left, *rec fem* rectus femoris, *R* right

abductor hallucis, as well as weak twitches of the external anal sphincter on both sides (Fig. 4c). Thus, stimulating the exposed placode verified presence of motor function down to at least the S_2 cord segment or beyond. Also, TcMEP elicited responses in all muscle groups including the external anal sphincter, confirming functional corticospinal connections. We therefore preserved the entire placode and neurulated it into a slender tube (Fig. 4d). Following this, we repeated our stimulation of the placode and reaffirmed that function down to or even below S_2 was preserved. Postoperatively, the patient's neurological level improved to include S_2 function.

Histopathology of the Resected Placode

Histopathologic examination of the resected neural placodes all showed mainly fibrous stroma and blood vessels with small, scattered islands of disorganized glio-neuronal and ependymal cells. Sporadic clusters of dorsal root ganglion cells were also found in haphazard locations without appositional logic (Fig. 5).

Neurological, Urological and Imaging Follow-Up

With the new surgical paradigm, no patient experienced neurological worsening postoperatively. In fact, four out of eight patients showed improvement in neurological function, with a mean improvement of 1.25 functional levels. All patients had a neurogenic bladder with the need for clean intermittent catheterization at 3 weeks follow-up.

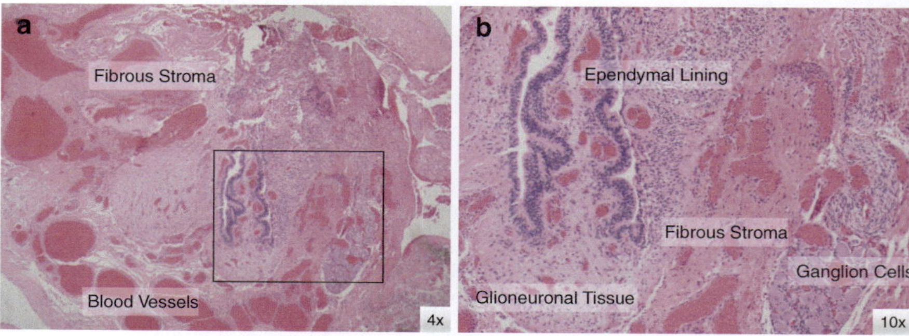

Fig. 5 Histopathology with hematoxylin/eosin-stained sections of the resected neural placode from the first illustrative case. (**a**) Low power (4 × magnification) overview shows mainly fibrous stroma and blood vessels. (**b**) High power (10 ×) magnification of squared area of (**a**) shows scattered islands of glioneuronal tissue and ependyma-lined spaces, and a misplaced dorsal root ganglion

Three patients did not need CSF diversion; of these, two had complete placode resection. Five patients had shunt-dependent hydrocephalus, for whom ventriculo-peritoneal shunts were placed between postnatal day 7 and 15.

All patients maintained their immediate postoperative neurological function throughout their follow-up. One patient (Case 5 in Table 1), who gained one neurological level from S1 to S2 immediately after surgery, improved further and had normalised urodynamic studies at 3 years follow-up, at which point CIC was deemed unnecessary. This patient had a complete placode resection, no syrinx formation and no shunt-dependent hydrocephalus. Urodynamics studies in the other seven patients did not show high-pressure bladder or detrusor sphincter dyssynergia.

In all eight patients, both the 3 weeks and 6 months MRIs showed capacious cord-dural sac relationship, all with a cord-sac ratio below 40%. The degree of capaciousness for each attenuated placode was roughly commensurate with the amount of placode reduction (Fig. 6).

Four patients (50%) had no syrinx formation, though one had a slightly dilated central canal measuring 2.8 mm. Four patients (50%) were shown to have a syrinx proximal to the repair site on MRI at 3 weeks after surgery. The diameter of the syrinx cavity decreased in two patients, remained stable in one, and increased slightly in another patient on the 6 months postoperative MRI. The one with the enlarging syrinx was the patient with segmental ONTD in whom no placode resection was done. In all four patients with syrinx, changes in syrinx size did not correlate with a change in neurological function.

No inclusion dermoid cyst was detected in any of the eight patients.

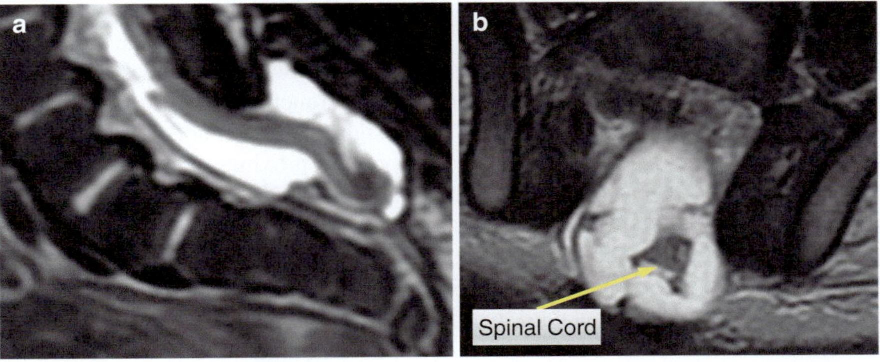

Fig. 6 Postoperative sagittal (**a**) and axial (**b**) T2-weighted MRI of the first illustrative case after resection of the non-functional placode and rendering of a slender diminutive spinal cord stump, resulting in a capacious cord-to-dural sac ratio

Discussion

Neurological deficits in ONTD depend on the level of the primary neurulation defect on the central neuraxis. In lumbar ONTD, the most common variety, the adjacent secondary neural tube is most often also severely affected or not formed at all, which explains the almost universal presence of neurogenic bladder and anal sphincter dysfunction. Experiments with *Prickle-1* knockdown chick embryo produced caudal primary neural tube defects with absent junctional and secondary neurulation. These findings strongly resemble the most common form of lumbosacral ONTDs in human, in which the caudal primary neural plate is unclosed and the adjoining secondary neural tube is at best severely malformed and non-functional, and at worst, entirely missing [15, 16].

By performing intraoperative electrophysiological mapping of the neural placodes of newborns with lumbosacral ONTDs, we strengthened the argument that the terminal neural tubes in these patients are always severely defective. These irregularly shaped, "un-conus" like tissue aggregates, with rare exception, generated no contractions in the external anal sphincter or distal leg muscles on supramaximal stimulation of their projecting nerve roots or directly on their surfaces using currents as high as 10 mA (Fig. 3a). Even in placodes that showed some response to stimulation, TcMEP usually confirmed a complete absence of meaningful suprasegmental connection with the corticospinal tracts. The utter lack of function in these defective caudal neural tubes is reflected by their chaotic histological architecture, revealed when the resected non-functional portions of these terminal placodes were examined. The scant glioneuronal content is randomly truncated by a fibrous stroma studded with large blood vessels, deranged nerve twigs, and misplaced dorsal root ganglia (Fig. 5).

Retention of this defunct but sometimes large and unwieldy placode, as taught in traditional ONTD closure, thus adds nothing to the functional status of the patient. Conversely, resection of this redundant tissue significantly reduces the bulk of the functional remainder portion of the placode or the proximal spinal cord stump, depending on the extent of resection, and therefore greatly facilitates the crucial manoeuvre of side-to-side neurulation to render a slim reconstituted pia-covered tube. More importantly, the cord-to-sac ratio also becomes more favourable (Fig. 6). Thus, future re-tethering will be less likely, an insight gained from the experience of total resection of large spinal cord lipomas [17].

In cases of segmental ONTD, as in our second illustrative case, intraoperative electrophysiology unequivocally identifies functional neural tissue caudal to and within the placode, which led to our saving the entire neural assemblage. Likewise, if the proximal portion of a terminal placode shows target response on direct placode or nerve root stimulation and possesses suprasegmental connectivity verified by TcMEP, it should be and had been saved by us while the distal non-functional portion was resected. This new approach, designed to maximize neurological function while aggressively discarding burdensome waste, therefore heavily depends on sophisticated intraoperative electrophysiology.

The non-disjunction of neural and cutaneous ectoderm in ONTD predisposes dermoid elements to be inadvertently included into the fibroneural matrix of the neurulated placode (Fig. 1). These dermoid remnants, containing viable squamous epithelial cells, may later grow and cause delayed neurological deterioration [5, 6]. This risk of inclusion dermoid should therefore be eliminated or at least drastically reduced by total or near total resection of the placode.

With the profound disturbance of secondary neurulation in lumbosacral ONTD, the sacral micturition center within the would-be conus may either be completely absent or worse, exist as an uncoordinated and hugely overactive local circuit, being disconnected from suprasegmental inhibitory moderation. The latter situation is far more detrimental because urodynamics studies regularly show sustained high intravesicular pressures, bladder wall trabeculation with loss of compliance, and severe vesicoureteral reflux, all high-risk factors predisposing to recurrent pyelonephritis and ultimately chronic renal failure [10]. Overall, an atonic low-pressure bladder is much less hostile than a high-pressure one and can be managed easily by clean intermittent catheterization. In such rare cases, removing this autonomous hyperactive sacral circuits with placode resection actually confers much more favourable long-term benefits.

Conclusion

This chapter describes a new paradigm for the postnatal repair of open neural tube defects centred on the aggressive but safe resection of the defunct portion of the unneurulated neural placode without loss of function, guided by rigorous intraoperative electrophysiology. Advantages include a more capacious cord-to-dural sac relationship and consequently a lessened risk of late spinal cord tethering, a lower incidence of inclusion dermoid cyst, and the rendering of a low-pressure bladder much less conducive to ureteral reflux and renal injury.

References

1. Schoenwolf GC, Smith JL. Mechanisms of neurulation. Methods Mol Biol. 2000;136:125–34. https://doi.org/10.1385/1-59259-065-9:125.
2. Torre M, Guida E, Bisio G, Scarsi P, Piatelli G, Cama A, Buffa P. Risk factors for renal function impairment in a series of 502 patients born with spinal dysraphisms. J Pediatr Urol. 2011;7:39–43. https://doi.org/10.1016/j.jpurol.2010.02.210.
3. Bowman RM, Mohan A, Iro J, Seibly JM, McLone DG. Tethered cord release: a long-term study in 114 patients clinical article. J Neurosurg Pediatr. 2009;3:181–7. https://doi.org/10.3171/2008.12.Peds0874.
4. Caldarelli M, Boscarelli A, Massimi L. Recurrent tethered cord: radiological investigation and management. Child Nerv Syst. 2013;29:1601–9. https://doi.org/10.1007/s00381-013-2150-4.
5. Eibach S, Moes G, Zovickian J, Pang D. Limited dorsal myeloschisis associated with dermoid elements. Childs Nerv Syst. 2017;33:55–67. https://doi.org/10.1007/s00381-016-3207-y.

6. Suocheng G, Yazhou X. A review on five cases of intramedullary dermoid cyst. Childs Nerv Syst. 2014;30:659–64. https://doi.org/10.1007/s00381-013-2281-7.
7. Thompson DNP. Spinal inclusion cysts. Child Nerv Syst. 2013;29:1647–55. https://doi.org/10.1007/s00381-013-2147-z.
8. Scott RM, Wolpert SM, Bartoshesky LE, Zimbler S, Klauber GT. Dermoid tumors occurring at the site of previous myelomeningocele repair. J Neurosurg. 1986;65:779–83. https://doi.org/10.3171/jns.1986.65.6.0779.
9. Danzer E, Adzick NS, Rintoul NE, Zarnow DM, Schwartz ES, Melchionni J, Ernst LM, Flake AW, Sutton LN, Johnson MP. Intradural inclusion cysts following in utero closure of myelomeningocele: clinical implications and follow-up findings clinical article. J Neurosurg Pediatr. 2008;2:406–13. https://doi.org/10.3171/Ped.2008.2.12.406.
10. Timberlake MD, Jacobs MA, Kern AJ, Adams R, Walker C, Schlomer BJ. Streamlining risk stratification in infants and young children with spinal dysraphism: vesicoureteral reflux and/or bladder trabeculations outperforms other urodynamic findings for predicting adverse outcomes. J Pediatr Urol. 2018;14:319.e311–7. https://doi.org/10.1016/j.jpurol.2018.05.023.
11. Elzeneini W, Waly R, Marshall D, Bailie A. Early start of clean intermittent catheterization versus expectant management in children with spina bifida. J Pediatr Surg. 2019;54:322–5. https://doi.org/10.1016/j.jpedsurg.2018.10.096.
12. Pang D. Electrophysiological monitoring for tethered cord surgery. In: Yamada S, editor. Tethered cord syndrome. Stuttgart: Thieme Medical Publisher; 2010. p. 199–209.
13. Pang D. Intraoperative neurophysiology of the conus medullaris and cauda equina. Childs Nerv Syst. 2010;26:411–2. https://doi.org/10.1007/s00381-010-1112-3.
14. Pang D, Zovickian J, Oviedo A. Long-term outcome of total and near-total resection of spinal cord lipomas and radical reconstruction of the neural placode: part I-surgical technique. Neurosurgery. 2009;65:511–28. https://doi.org/10.1227/01.NEU.0000350879.02128.80.
15. Dady A, Havis E, Escriou V, Catala M, Duband JL. Junctional neurulation: a unique developmental program shaping a discrete region of the spinal cord highly susceptible to neural tube defects. J Neurosci. 2014;34:13208–21. https://doi.org/10.1523/JNEUROSCI.1850-14.2014.
16. Eibach S, Moes G, Hou YJ, Zovickian J, Pang D. Unjoined primary and secondary neural tubes: junctional neural tube defect, a new form of spinal dysraphism caused by disturbance of junctional neurulation. Childs Nerv Syst. 2017;33:1633–47. https://doi.org/10.1007/s00381-016-3288-7.
17. Pang D, Zovickian J, Wong ST, Hou YJ, Moes GS. Surgical treatment of complex spinal cord lipomas. Childs Nerv Syst. 2013;29:1485–513. https://doi.org/10.1007/s00381-013-2187-4.

Focal Spinal Nondisjunctional Disorders: Including a Discussion on the Embryogenesis of Cranial Focal Nondisjunctional Lesions

Sui-To Wong and Dachling Pang

Introduction

Disjunction, the separation of the neuroepithelium (NE) from the surface epithelium (SE), is one of the major processes in the embryogenesis of the primary neural tube (NT). Not surprisingly, failure of it to happen (nondisjunction) with consequential clinically identifiable anomalies is not so rare [1, 2]. Nondisjunction (ND) can occur anywhere along the dorsal midline of the primary NT, from the supraoptic recess to the S1 or S2 spinal cord [3, 4]. ND also usually occurs over a focal, or limited, segment of the primary NT and be the principal cause of an anomaly [1, 2]. In this group of anomalies, called focal nondisjunctional disorders, failed disjunction is the primary culprit in their embryogenesis, although it may also occur simultaneously with and adjacent to other embryogenetic defects such as premature disjunction lesions, one involving the timing of disjunction, the other the actual mechanism of disjunction [5, 6]. On the other hand, ND can be a component of a more severe embryogenetic defect, involving a longer segment of the primary NT, such as in myelomeningoceles or anencephaly. In these severe forms of anomalies, ND is a secondary feature, due to failure of the preceding primary neurulation events; they are not further discussed in this chapter.

Even though the spinal cord and the brain can both be afflicted by focal nondisjunctional disorders, their clinico-pathological manifestations vary, due to

S.-T. Wong
Department of Neurosurgery, Tuen Mun Hospital, Hong Kong, China

D. Pang (✉)
University of California, Davis, Davis, CA, USA

Great Ormond Street Hospital for Children, NHS Trust, London, UK

© The Author(s), under exclusive license to Springer Nature Switzerland AG 2023
D. Pang, K.-C. Wang (eds.), *Spinal Dysraphic Malformations*, Advances and Technical Standards in Neurosurgery 47,
https://doi.org/10.1007/978-3-031-34981-2_4

their different developmental characteristics—the brain predominantly has an expansile growth, but the spinal cord a longitudinal one.

Focal nondisjunction (FND) in the spinal segment of the primary NT results in a normal or near-normal spinal cord, except for the presence of a tract anchoring the dorsal surface of the spinal cord to the base of a characteristic skin lesion. The chief clinical manifestation is tethering of the spinal cord by this tract and, depending on its cellular constituents of the tract, may be accompanied by dermal sinus tissues. Herniation of neural tissue is rarely a problem.

With FND of the cranial region of the primary NT, the major divisions of the brain remain grossly well developed, but there is a midline skull defect of various sizes. Clinical manifestation depends on the size of this skull defect and the tissues traversing it, such as frank herniation of brain tissue or collection of dermal sinus tissue. Here, tethering is not a concern.

This chapter aims to give an updated summary of the conditions that have been grouped under the common embryogenetic mechanism of FND, and extend the scope of 2 previous articles on focal spinal nondisjunctional disorders to include a discussion on the embryology of cranial FND [5, 6]. Focal spinal nondisjunctional disorders (FSND) consist of congenital spinal dermal sinus tract (CSDST), limited dorsal myeloschisis (LDM), and combined lesions [1, 2, 7–12]. Focal cranial nondisjunctional disorders include congenital cranial dermal sinus tract, atretic encephalocele, and at least some of the true encephaloceles.

Embryogenetic Mechanisms of Focal Nondisjunctional Disorders

Normal Primary Neurulation

Primary neurulation, the formation of the primary NT, the primordium of the brain and the spinal cord down to the S1 or S2 level, occurs during the third and fourth post-fertilization weeks. It consists of 4 main processes occurring sequentially at each axial level of the embryo. They are the (1) formation of the neural plate, (2) shaping of the neural plate, (3) bending of the neural plate, and (4) closure of the neural groove (Fig. 1) [13]. By the Carnegie system, these processes begin at stage 7 when the neural plate can first be visualized [14]. The last process, closure of the neural groove, starts at the hindbrain/upper cervical region in humans and propagates both rostrally and caudally [13], resulting in the closure of the rostral neuropore at Carnegie stage 11, and closure of the caudal neuropore at Carnegie stage 12 (Fig. 2) [14]. During this process, fusion of the neural folds and complete separation of SE from NE take place at the dorsal midline. It consists of a complex sequence of events at the tissue level which occur in an overlapping manner that cannot be unlinked from the preceding processes, i.e. bending of the neural plate, formation of the paired neural folds, and their convergence towards the dorsal midline [13, 15–17].

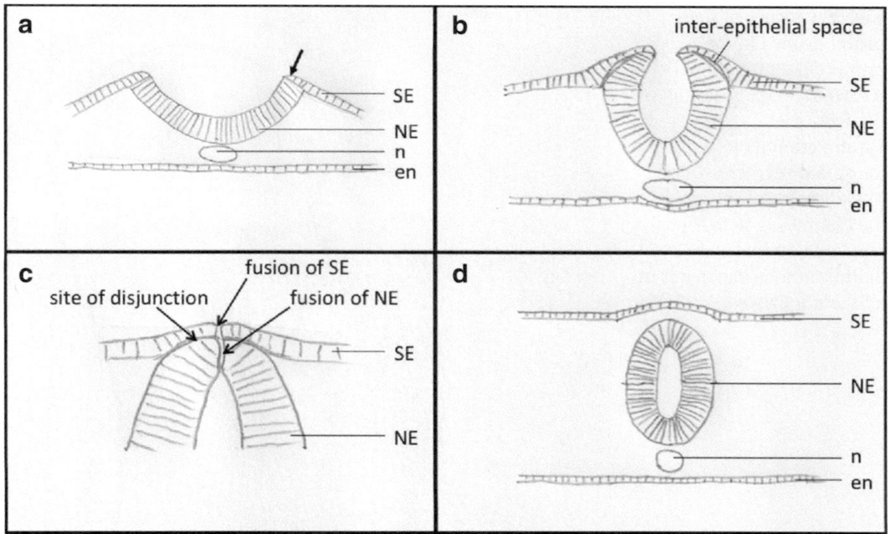

Fig. 1 Normal primary neurulation. Diagrams showing the major steps in closure of the neural groove in an axial level. (**a**) Elevation of the neural folds (arrow). (**b**) Progressive elevation of the neural folds. Delamination at the neuroepithelium—surface epithelium interface. (**c**) Components involved in the final phase in closure of the neural groove. (**d**) Closed neural tube at an axial level. *en* endoderm, *n* notochord, *NE* neuroepithelium, *SE* surface epithelium

The sequence of primary neurulation events are as follows (Fig. 1) [13, 15–17]:

1. *The formation of an overlapping SE and NE junction:* When the neural plate first develops, NE cells and SE cells lie side by side on the same plane at its border. As the paired neural folds progressively elevate and converge towards the dorsal midline, the NE cells enlarge in height and drag the flattened SE cells onto their dorsal surface. In effect, the 2 epithelia are connected over a broad, overlapping surface of several cells' thickness.

2. *Delamination:* An inter-epithelial space then gradually develops in the middle part of this broad interface of the 2 epithelia. The basal lamina of the 2 epithelia however remains continuous at the ventral point (ventro-lateral extreme of their contact). Thus, when the inter-epithelial space expands, it acquires a crescent shape. As the 2 neural folds approach each other to close the dorsal midline gap, the inter-epithelial space extends further dorsally towards the dorsal midline. The basal lamina at the lateral most contact point of the 2 epithelia also gradually breaks down, separating the 2 epithelia here, and the inter-epithelial space becomes an "open" space. A new basal lamina then forms on the original inter-epithelial surfaces of each of the 2 epithelia. As the inter-epithelial space continues to enlarge towards the dorsal-most meeting point of the 2 epithelia, the epithelia ultimately separate completely, thereby consummating the process known as disjunction.

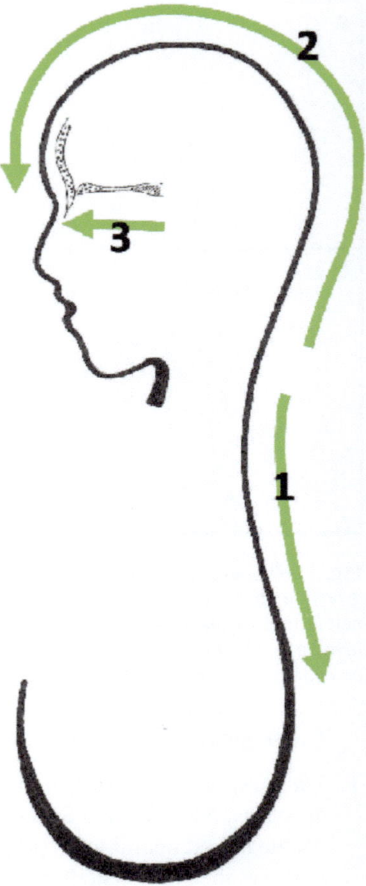

Fig. 2 Closure of the neural groove in the primary neural tube with reference to the anatomy of the foetus. 1: Unidirectional closure in the spinal segment. 2 and 3: Bidirectional closure in the cranial segment. Focal nondisjunctional malformations can occur in all these locations

3. *Fusion at the dorsal midline:* Fusion of the SE and NE layers with their respective counterpart on the opposite side of the midline takes place simultaneously with disjunction. Fusion is preceded by apposition of the two opposing sets of epithelia at the tips of the two neural folds, followed by intercellular adhesion at points of contact. The initial contact areas are often discontinuous from superficial to deep [18], and it is likely that fusion of the two epithelial layers proceeds independently of each other [17]. Using chick embryos, Schoenwolf in 1982 concluded that fusion completed first in the SE [19]. However, van Straaten in 1993, also using chick embryos, demonstrated that there was no fixed priority of completion of fusion in the two layers [17].

It is obvious that the final steps of delamination (disjunction) and fusion of the two epithelia are topographically and chronologically tightly knit, but the fine details of their inter-relationship are still not fully elucidated. What is well established is that in normal embryos, complete closure of the neural groove at any axial level is marked by the presence of a continuous basal lamina under the SE across the dorsal midline, and a continuous sheath of basal lamina around the NE (primary neural tube) at that level [20].

There are two subtle details of these intercalated processes that are important to our embryogenetic hypotheses: First, fusion of the two epithelial layers likely proceeds independently of each other [17]. Second, although the exact timing of epithelial fusion and disjunction is unknown, intuitively, fusion of the epithelia must precede disjunction of the SE and NE. The answer may have to rely on dynamic observation at the ultrastructural level, which at the present time is still unattainable [21].

On the Caudal End of the Primary Neural Tube

The notion that the caudal end of the primary NT is the S1 or S2 segment of the spinal cord is mainly based on O'Rahilly and Müller's study on the somitic level of the final caudal neuropore closure site in human embryos [4, 22–24]. In this respect, human embryos are different from other animals' [22–24]. In O'Rahilly and Müller's last publication on this issue in 2003, they settled on somite 31 as the caudal end of the primary NT in human, albeit retained the qualifier "approximately". Somite 31 corresponds to S2 spinal ganglion, thus the S2 spinal cord. In the embryonic period proper, the spinal cord has not ascended, the S2 spinal cord lies at the S2/S3 vertebral level [23]. The findings in a few clinical examples of junctional neurulation defects support O'Rahilly and Müller's "S1 or S2 level" conclusion [25, 26]. Ironically, the discovery of junctional neurulation has complicated, in a taxonomy sense, our definition of the caudal end of the primary NT [25]. The caudal neuropore has a unidirectional closure in the rostral-to-caudal direction. O'Rahilly and Müller defined the caudal end of the primary NT as the final closure site of the caudal neuropore (Fig. 2). However, since the dorsal aspect of the junctional NT closes at its dorsal midline in the same manner as the primary NT and is a direct extension from the dorsal neural groove of the primary NT, the final closure site of the caudal neuropore at least partially involves the junctional NT. Thus, FND lesions are not restricted to the primary NT but the caudalmost location of the dorsal neural groove closure and can therefore occur in the junctional NT.

Molecular mechanisms initiating the transitions between primary neurulation, junctional neurulation, and secondary neurulation and therefore the spinal cord levels of the primary, junctional, and secondary NTs are still poorly understood. In all 3 types of neurulation, the 2 key steps are the genesis of neural progenitor cells from the primordial cell pool and the morphogenesis of the induced neural progenitor cells into the NT. The types of neurulation are defined based on the pattern of their morphogenesis. Junctional neurulation, being the middle link, is important to our understanding of the transitions. During junctional neurulation, *Prickle-1* expression at the node-streak border regulates the polarized deposition of fibronectin on the surface of cells and in the basement membrane, thus bringing about the orderly morphogenesis of the junctional NT [25]. Yet, little is known about what governs the "space-time" of the transitions between primary, junctional, and secondary neurulation. Elucidating their underlying molecular mechanisms might give us some insights as to how caudal the dorsal neural groove closure process might reach in individual cases.

Relevant Features in the Rostral End of Primary Neural Tube

Unlike the caudal neuropore, the rostral neuropore has a bidirectional neural groove closure process (Fig. 2) [27]: One direction starts at the hindbrain/upper cervical junction and runs rostrally. At its rostral end, the roof of the primary NT formed from this caudal-rostral zip-like closure of the neural groove forms the dorsal lip of the rostral neuropore. The rostral neuropore also closes in a rostral-to-caudal direction, starting from the rostral tip of the neural plate, which corresponds to the preoptic recess/rostral limit of the chiasmatic plate. The roof of the primary NT thus formed is called the terminal lip of the rostral neuropore [27]. The rostral portion of this terminal lip forms the embryonic laminar terminalis. The anterior portion of the embryonic laminar terminalis gives rise to the "postnatal" laminar terminalis and the posterior portion, part of the commissural plate [3, 27]. The final closure site of the rostral neuropore, called situs neuroporicus, is where the terminal lip and the dorsal lip meet and is at the commissural plate in the middle of the embryonic laminar terminalis [28]. The commissural plate gives rise to the corpus callosum, anterior commissure, and commissura fornicis [29].

At the microscopic level, the final fusion at the dorsal midline in the cranial region follows the same schema as in the rest of the primary NT. Listed here are some local features in the cranial segment that might be relevant to the study of FND: (1) Concerning the sequence of the fusion of SE and NE, the SE seems to fuse first in the dorsal lip, while both SE and NE layers fuse simultaneously in the terminal lip. (2) There are 2 layers of cells in the SE of the terminal lip at the time of fusion, but only one layer in the rest of the primary NT [27]. (3) There might be variations in the timing of when the basement membranes of the SE and NE become widely separated in the embryonic cranial dorsal midline [30].

Regarding embryonic-postnatal anatomical correlation in the median plane, the SE and mesenchyme overlying the dorsal midline of the rostral primary NT, from its rostral pole to the rhombencephalon, correspond to the extraneural tissue of the anterior fossa (anterior to the tuberculum sellae) to the nasion (3 in Fig. 2) and then through the inion to the suboccipital raphe (2 in Fig. 2) (Fig. 2). At the skin-bone level, the situs neuroporicus likely corresponds to the fonticulus frontalis, which is the interposition between the nasal process of the frontal bone and the nasal bones. The terminal lip therefore corresponds to the midline of the anterior cranial fossa. This postulation is supported by data derived from a mouse study [31], human embryo observations [4], examinations of anencephalic foetuses [32], and clinical observations in congenital nasal masses [33]. In mouse and human embryos, the situs neuroporicus is at the level of the nasal primodium. In typical anencephalic foetuses, the skull base is present despite absence of the cranial vault likely due to the presence of closure at the terminal lip. In congenital nasal masses arising from the anterior corpus callosum, the lesions extend through the skull between the frontal and nasal bones.

In the postnatal form, the abovementioned anatomical correction is obscured by the development of the complex dural anatomy—the falx cerebri, the tentorium, and their dural sinuses.

Faults in Embryogenesis in Focal Nondisjunctional Disorders

The embryogenesis of all FND lesions are due to faults occurring at a focal point during the last phases of neural groove closure, characterized by nondisjunction and incomplete fusion of NE and/or SE at a limited segment anywhere along the dorsal midline of the future brain down to the S2 spinal cord level [34–37]. This general schema is the basis of several anatomical phenotypes of FND malformations, depending on the exact aberrant behaviours of the primordial SE and NE cells involved. In addition, the matured features of these FND phenotypes are determined by the individual or combined errors of the primordial SE and NE cells, as well as of the adjacent mesoderm and neural crest cells (Fig. 3) [16, 38, 39].

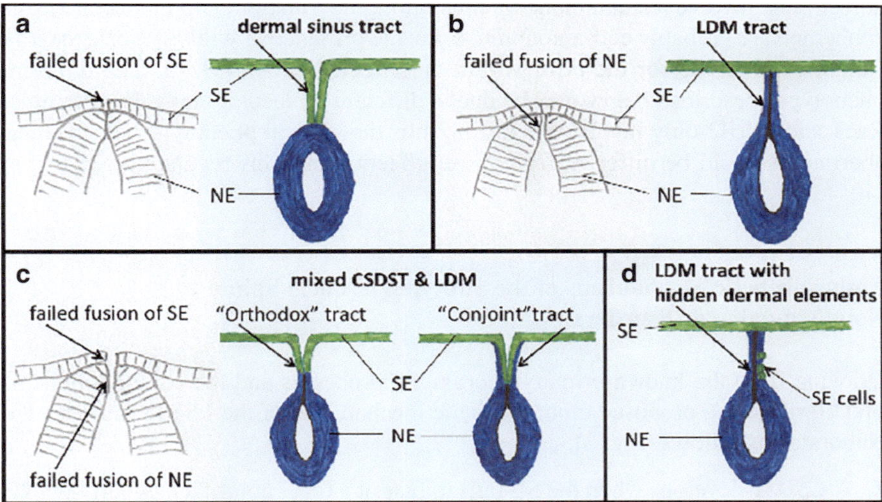

Fig. 3 Proposed embryogenetic mechanisms for different types of focal spinal non-disjunctional disorders. (**a**) Congenital spinal dermal sinus tract (CSDST). (**b**) Limited dorsal myeloschisis (LDM). (**c**) Mixed CSDST and LDM-"Orthodox" type and "Conjoint" type. (**d**) LDM with hidden dermal elements. *NE* neuroepithelium, *SE* surface epithelium

Molecular Mechanisms of Focal Nondisjunctional Malformations

At the molecular-genetic level, the mechanism of primary neurulation has only been partially elucidated. The different stages of primary neurulation have different key molecular players [40].

As proposed above, the underlying faulty molecular events in FND disorders are likely confined to those related to fusion of the epithelia and delamination/disjunction occurring at the dorsal midline. Known molecular processes involved in the fusion of the epithelia include polymerization of actin filaments in cellular protrusions and adhesive interactions between cell surface proteins.

A group of regulator proteins that may be targets in the genesis of FND disorders is the Rho GTPases, including Rac1 and Cdc42. Both Rac1 and Cdc42 are involved in the regulation of actin filaments [40, 41], while EphrinA-EphA receptor interactions have been implicated in neural fold adhesion. EphrinA proteins, which are linked to plasma membrane by a glycophosphatidylinositol anchor, and EphA receptors, which are integral membrane proteins, were found to be expressed at the apices of neural folds just prior to onset of epithelial fusion [42]. As for the molecular mechanisms of disjunction, there is even scarcer information. One possible point of aberration leading to nondisjunction may occur during the caspase-dependent apoptosis of the cells at the SE–NE border [40, 43].

There are two general points about defective molecular mechanisms in FND lesions: (1) to account for the "limited" extent of a FND lesion, a causative molecular defect must involve a small clone of cells during neurulation; and the mechanisms concerned are probably cell-autonomous, i.e. the presence of wild-type cells nearby cannot compensate for the error within the affected cells [40]. (2) The different phenotypes described below may be due to different molecular faults. For example, Rac1 and Cdc42 only involve SE fusion; thus the clinical phenotypes due to their aberrations could be different from those affecting proteins regulating NE fusion [40, 41].

Embryogenetic Mechanisms of the Subtypes of Focal Spinal Nondisjunctional Disorders

Drawing from the known primary neurulation processes and the configurations of FND lesions, the proposed embryogenetic mechanisms of the FSND subtypes are elaborated as follows (Fig. 3):

1. A *CSDST* develops when the SE fails to fuse at a focal point. The underlying NE has fused by some intercellular protrusions, but disjunction at this focal point between the two epithelia does not happen. In this scenario, closure of the primary neural tube immediately cranial and caudal to this focal nondisjunction spot is unhindered, but at this focal spot, the gaping SE is persistently linked with the NE. This link, a midline gap in the converging SE and, below it, between the dorsal scleromyotomes in opposite sides of the embryo, remains very narrow.

Further unimpeded development of the surrounding normal full-thickness dorsal myofascial tissues skirting the midline strip progressively sets the primary neural tube into its normal, primarily intraspinal location. However, a dorsomedian tract of SE tissue persists as the original link between the closed primary neural tube and the still slightly gaping epithelial surface. The tract is firmly anchored on the SE side because its component cells are still essentially part of the surface epithelium, but its deep-end attachment to the NE cells after closure of the neural groove may not be solid. The deep end of the tract could therefore be detached from the underlying neural tube by cellular migrations and tissue development during normal development of the neural crest cells, scleromesoderm, and meninges, so that the inner anchorage of the tract may end short of the spinal cord but on the meninges or even the outer musculofascial layers.

2. A *LDM* develop when the fusion of the NE fails at a focal point, but the overlying SE fusion has at least been established by some intercellular adhesions, and disjunction at this focal point also does not happen. Like the reverse of the development of a CSDST, the SE gap is closed, but because NE fusion and disjunction never occur at this focal point, the NE here remains linked to the SE. This link, now in the form of a narrow developing tract, runs from the midline gap in the converging NE through the dorsal scleromyotomes from opposite sides of the embryo. Further unimpeded development of the surrounding normal full-thickness dorsal myofascial tissues around this midline tract also progressively sets the primary neural tube into its normal, primarily intraspinal location.

   However, a dorsomedian tract of NE tissue (vs. SE tissue in CSDST) persists as the original link between the closed epithelial surface and the focally gaping primary neural tube [43]. This essentially neural tract is anchored to the undersurface of the SE, and affects the normal integration of mesodermal tissue at that focal spot to result in the characteristic cutaneous stigmata of LDM (see below).

3. A tract with *combined LDM and CSDST* develops when fusion of NE and SE both fail and disjunction never happens, often culminating in an *"orthodox"* pattern, with the outer tract consisting of SE while the inner portion of the tract containing NE tissue. The "pulling forces" along the outer and inner portions of the tract during embryogenesis will determine the relative proportion of the 2 kinds of tissues in the final malformation. However, a *"conjoint"* configuration may also form, where the entire tract is lined by both SE and NE elements. These mixed entities are rare, and may also easily elude detection [8, 10].

4. As for *LDMs with hidden dermal element*, in which the LDM stalks or tracts are studded with scattered dermal elements without a dermal sinus tract, the origin of such dermal elements could be from dislodged SE cells somehow being included during the formation of the LDM stalk, or from pluripotent cells near the dorsal midline [1, 2, 8].

5. *FSND with spinal cord lipoma*: Both LDMs and CSDSTs have been known to be associated with spinal cord lipomas, either directly adjacent to the lipoma or continuous with it. Since both transitional and dorsal lipomas probably originate

from *premature* disjunction during the same embryogenetic stage as nondisjunction, it is not surprising that nondisjunction and premature disjunction disorders may coexist [1, 2].

6. *FSND with split cord malformation*: The dermal sinus tract or fibroneural stalk found in some cases of split cord malformation may in fact be the remnant of the dorsal portion of an anomalous ecto-endodermal fistula resulting from aberrant early gastrulation [44, 45], which is the embryogenetic basis for split cord malformation. Very rarely, examples of LDM involving one hemicord of a split cord malformation have been reported [46].

Embryogenetic Mechanisms of Cranial Focal Nondisjunctional Disorders

As with FSNDs, FND can occur in the cranium along the rostral end of the embryonic dorsal midline. All the morphological subtype malformations found in FSNDs are embryogenetically feasible in the cranial segment, including the association with lipoma and "split cord" malformation (up to the midbrain/diencephalon junction) [47]. Morphologically, the major difference between cranial and spinal FND malformations is the constituents and thickness of the derivatives from the surrounding mesodermal elements in the final construct.

Pathological Anatomy and Clinical Manifestations of FSND

Variations in the exact cellular types and histological configurations of FSND lesions during development give rise to the spectrum of different focal nondisjunctional disorders. Partial atresia of a tract may lead to certain variants of the full forms [48], while perturbations in the physical milieu, such as hydrostatic pressure within the embryo, could produce the corresponding patho-anatomical FSND subtypes.

The "level" of a FSND lesion should also reflect the spinal cord level of the initial causative nondisjunctional error in the embryo, and accordingly should correspond to the level of the laminar defect through which the fibroneural stalk or sinus tract passes.

Pure CSDST

Pathological Anatomy

The essential feature of a CSDST is a dorsal midline dermal sinus tract—a narrow tubular structure lined by squamous epithelium [49, 50]. The size of the ostium of this tract on the skin is variable but usually small (Fig. 4). The depth through which

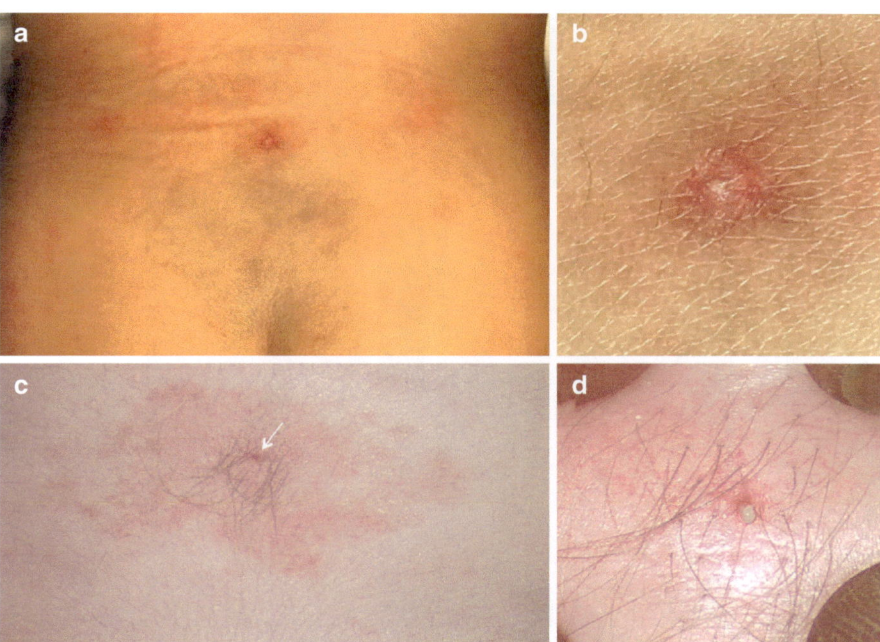

Fig. 4 (**a**) Dermal sinus ostium, appeared as a pin-point area of dry scaling with surrounding red discoloration, but without soft tissue swelling. (**b**) Magnified view of (**a**). (**c**) Dermal sinus ostium, appeared as a dot of dark discoloration with surrounding hypertrichosis and pigmentation keratin material could be seen with light compression. (**d**) Magnified view of (**c**)

the tract penetrates is also variable; over 60% end intradurally, and some are firmly attached to the spinal cord (Figs. 5, 6 and 7) [5].

Concerning the CSDSTs' location along the vertebral column, over 60% of them are in the lumbosacral spine; the rest are distributed over the thoracic and cervical regions [5]. The shape of a sinus tract on the sagittal plane varies depending on its level of origin, because the spinal cord ascends along the vertebral column for a fair distance during development due to their discrepant growth rates. A lumbosacral CSDST typically takes on a V-shape with the apex pointing at exactly the laminar level of its nondisjunctional error; its subcutaneous tract descends caudally from the skin lesion to reach the lamina, and from thence it ascends towards the thecal sac. With more rostrally situated lesions, the subcutaneous tract becomes progressively more horizontal until it points cranially towards the dura in cervico-thoracic lesions. At the skin level, other skin stigmata may sometimes accompany the sinus ostium (Fig. 4). At the laminar level, the tract may pass through the interspinous ligament, or through a bifid spinous process or lamina. The tract then penetrates the dura but can also run between the dural layers for a short length before becoming intradural. Within the thecal sac, it may be adherent to the nerve roots or filum and, until proven otherwise, one should always assume all sinus tracts reach the spinal cord.

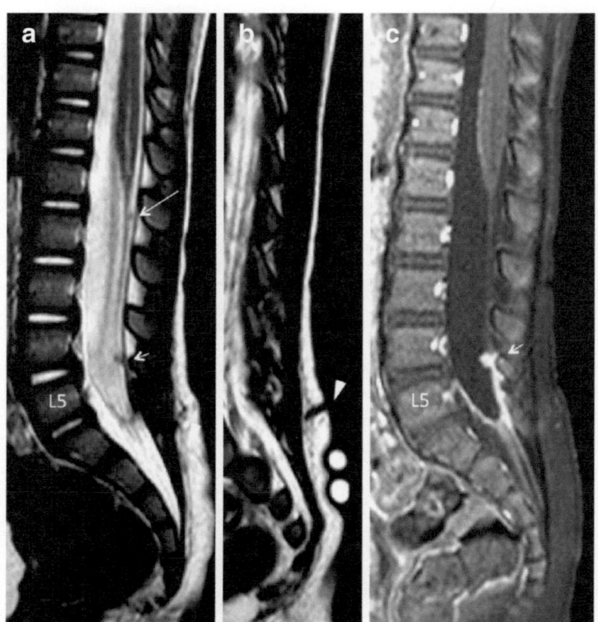

Fig. 5 MRI images of a 22-month-old with a dermal sinus tract, which as confirmed intraoperatively, has the skin ostium at L5 spinous process level (Fig. 4a, b), passes along the caudal aspect of L5 laminae, and terminates on the dorsal surface of the conus. (**a**) Mid-sagittal T2-weighted MRI image showing a tiny T2 hypointense intradural nodule at L1/L2 vertebral level (long arrow) and another slightly larger one at L4 vertebral level (short arrow). The intradural dermal sinus tract is beyond the resolution power of MRI. (**b**) Paramedian sagittal T2-weighted MRI image showing a dermal sinus tract from the skin ostium extending into the subcutaneous fat (arrow head). (**c**) T1-weighted MRI with gadolinium injection image, corresponding to (**a**), showing that only the L4 lesion (short arrow) and the end of the thecal sac become enhanced due to active inflammation

Anywhere along the sinus tract, a dermoid cyst may form from existing keratin material, and it can even be intramedullary (Fig. 8). In a report of ten intramedullary spinal dermoid cysts, nine had a traceable CSDST [51]. The rare occurrence of spinal dermoid cyst without a sinus tract is probably due to isolated sequestration of pluripotent SE cells or atresia of the outer tract [48].

Histologically, a dermal sinus tract is lined by keratinizing stratified squamous epithelium (Fig. 9a, b). Other components in variable abundance include hair follicles and shafts, mesenchymal derivatives such as blood vessels and fibrous tissue (Fig. 9a–c), and occasionally even nerve fibres. Keratin material fills the lumen of the tract and the cavity of dermoid cysts (Fig. 9d). Sometimes, the lumen of part of the tract may be obliterated (Fig. 9c). In slender tracts, a transitional zone of epithelial to non-epithelial tissues can be observed over the tract's deep end (Fig. 9e). Within the CSDST, inflamed granulation tissue containing mixed neutrophils, plasma cells, lymphocytes, and histiocytes is consistently found

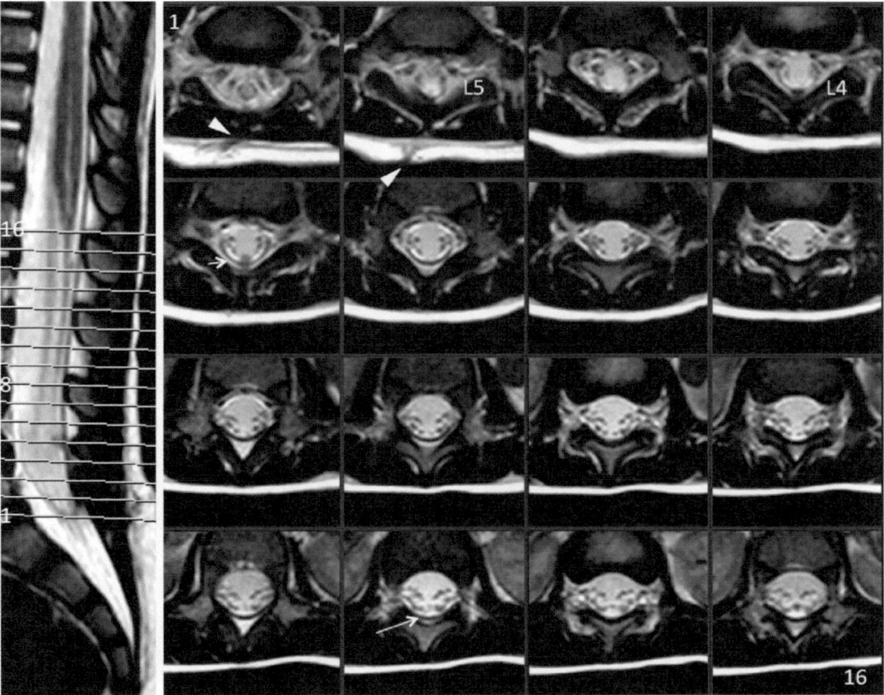

Fig. 6 Right panel: 16 serial T2-weight MRI axial cuts over the lumbosacral region of the patient shown in Fig. 4. Only the L4 nodule (short arrow), the skin ostium and subcutaneous tract (arrow heads), and vaguely the L1/L2 nodule (long arrow) are demonstrable by MRI. Left panel: T2-weighted MRI image with cut lines numbered 1–16. *L4* left lamina of L4 vertebra, *L5* left lamina of L5 vertebra

(Fig. 9a–c) [49, 52, 53]. It is due to chemically induced inflammation from keratin accumulation, and may also be secondary to bacterial infections from the sinus tract's communication with the skin surface.

Clinical Manifestations

The age of presentation has a wide range; in most series, the mean is 3 years or below, with some patients first diagnosed in their 30's or even 50's [5]. The commonest presentation is skin stigmata, usually a cutaneous pit, frequently associated with pigmentation, haemangioma, skin tag, subcutaneous lipomas, or hypertrichosis (Fig. 4). A prominent subcutaneous lipoma should arouse the suspicion for an associated spinal cord lipoma, and hypertrichosis for split cord malformation. In many published series, over 40% of patients had neurological deficits involving limbs and/or bowel and bladder. In infected cases and in patients

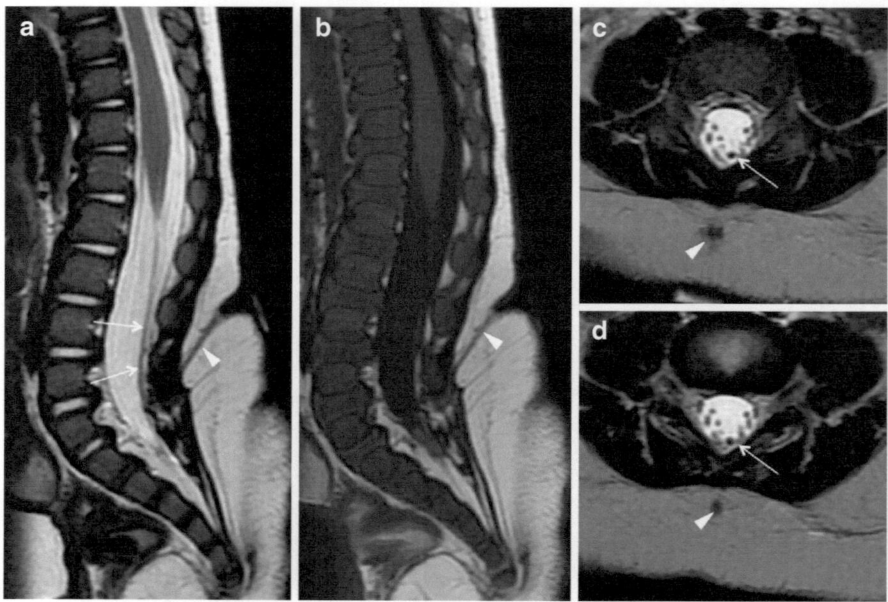

Fig. 7 MRI images of a 20-month-old with a dermal sinus tract. (**a, c, d**) T2-weighted MRI images. (**b**) T1-weighted MRI image. Although there is marked abnormal signal at the skin level, the skin ostium is tiny (Fig. 4c, d). There is a 2 vertebral levels difference between the skin ostium and where the tract located at the laminar level. The intradural tract (long arrows) appears as a structure that is slightly thicker and more T2 hypointense than normal nerve roots. Arrow heads = the subcutaneous portion of the dermal sinus tract

harbouring large intradural epidermoid/dermoid cysts, neurological deficits may erupt catastrophically [5].

In clinical practice, actual discharge from a sinus ostium is uncommon, seen only in 25% of cases. Even rarer is the presence of inflamed skin surrounding an obviously infected ostium or a deep-seated abscess, which occurs in less than 15%. Paradoxically, in some series, a history of recurrent meningitis or active meningitis is found in up to 40% of cases [5].

Pure LDM

Pathological Anatomy

The two constant clinic-radiological features of all LDMs are (1) a cutaneous stigma and (2) an underlying fibroneural stalk anchoring the spinal cord to the skin lesion (Fig. 10). The cutaneous marker, a pearly crater of abnormal covering composed mainly of squamous epithelium, commonly called a "cigarette-burn mark", is due to hindrance on normal skin development by the stalk's attachment to the undersurface

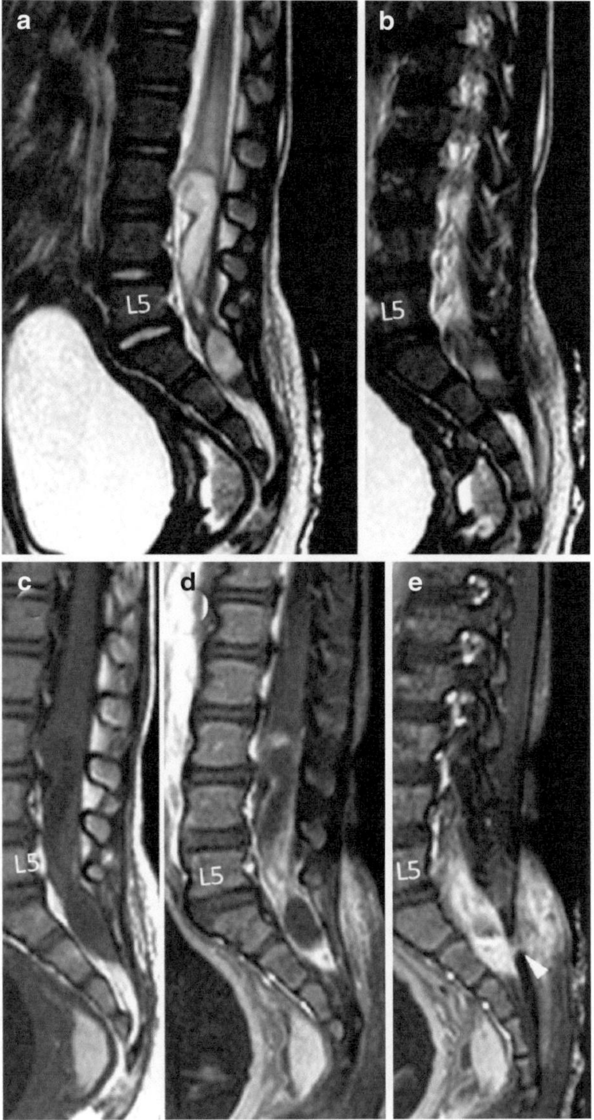

Fig. 8 MRI images of a 25-month-old with a large intradural dermoid cyst. (**a, b**) T2-weighted images. (**c**) T1-weighted image. (**d, e**) T1-weighted with gadolinium injection. The dermoid cyst, spanning 5 vertebral levels, extends from L3 to S2. It is heterogeneous in signal intensity, but the main bulk of it is T2-hyperintense, mildly T1-hypointense, and demonstrates periphery gadolinium enhancement. There is also marked gadolinium enhancement in the subcutaneous tissue signifying active inflammation. The intradural dermoid cyst communicates with an outside dermal sinus tract at the caudal aspect of the S1 laminae (white arrow head in **e**)

of the SE (Fig. 3). In all instances, the fibroneural stalk, extending from the deeper side of the abnormal skin, ultimately merges with the spinal cord. Only rarely have examples of a discontinuous stalk been observed [48]. In all LDMs, the spinal cord is therefore tethered to the surface myofascial tissue by the fibroneural stalk [54–56] and by the meningeal and other mesenchymal investments condensed around the stalk. The merge point of the stalk with the spinal cord is always above the conus, indicative of this being due to faulty primary neurulation [1, 2]. Lesions arising

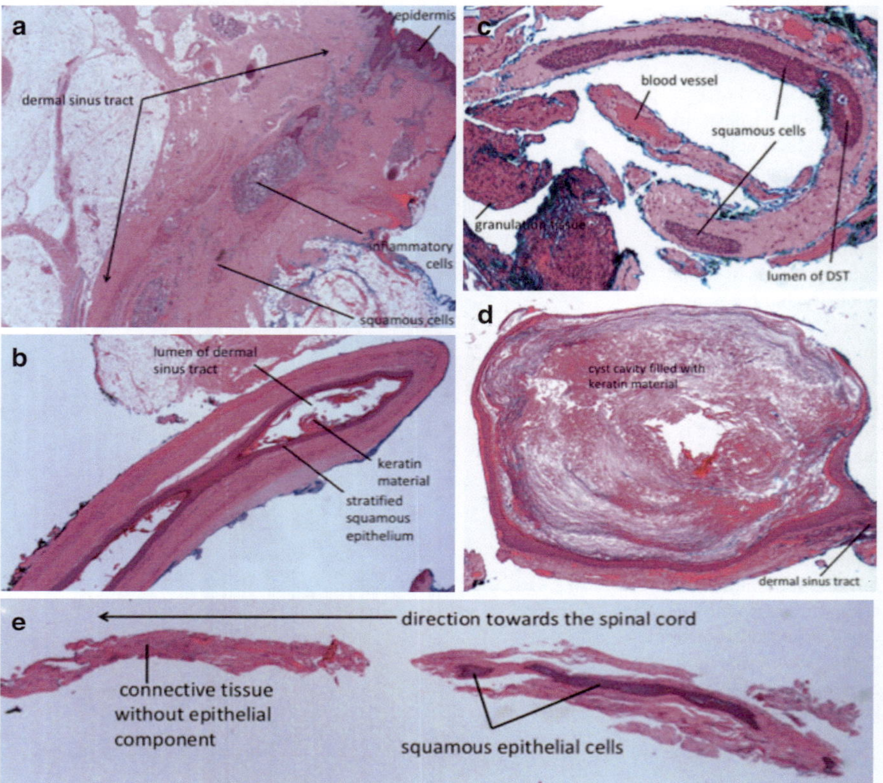

Fig. 9 Histological slides. (**a**) Section through the most superficial portion of a dermal sinus tract. (**b**) The portion of the dermal sinus tract in the intraoperatively identified subcutaneous tissue. (**c**) The intradural portion of a dermal sinus tract (DST). (**a**) The intradural portion of a DST. (**d**) A dermoid cyst formed along a slender dermal sinus tract (the L1/L2 lesion in Fig. 5). (**e**) The deepest end of a dermal sinus tract where a transition from epithelialized tissue to connective tissue totally devoid of it can be seen. (Haematoxylin and eosin stain)

from secondary neurulation defects, but mimicking the morphology of a LDM should therefore not be classified as a true LDM [34, 37].

LDMs can be categorized by the external appearance of their skin lesion into flat (non-saccular) or saccular (Fig. 10). *The flat LDM* is recognisable either by a simple pin-point *pit* or a wider *crater* with "non-skin" squamous epithelium. Internally, the fibroneural stalk passes through the deep fascia, a bifid lamina or the interspinous ligament, and the dura (Fig. 11a–e). The intradural stalk of a lumbosacral lesion is seen, on magnetic resonance imaging (MRI), as a separate longitudinal structure dorsal to the filum and, more rostrally, attached to the dorsal surface of the conus (Fig. 11a). At the stalk-cord union site (merge point), the cord takes on a trapezoid shape on axial MRI (Fig. 11b). The fibroneural stalk is V-shaped on the sagittal plane when it is in the lumbosacral region, similar to the CSDST (Fig. 12), but it

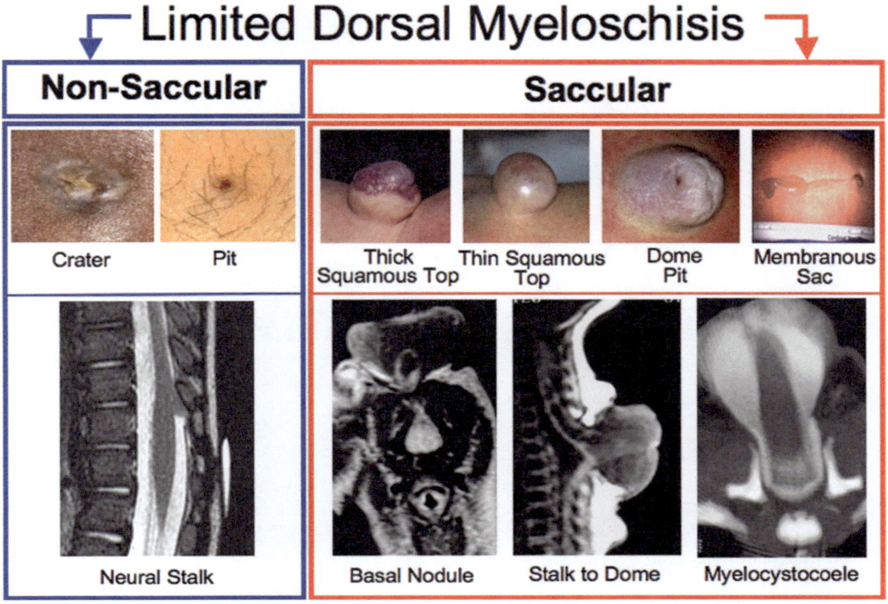

Fig. 10 Classification of LDM into non-saccular and saccular types, according to the 2 universal features of LDMs, one external, one internal. The top images depict the various skin signatures of either crater, pit, or the subtypes of sacs. The bottom images feature the internal fibroneural connections between the skin lesion and the spinal cord

becomes progressively horizontal and then slants upwards when located more cranially (Fig. 13). The tethering effect to the cord can be very obvious when the fibroneural stalks are stout (Fig. 14), or when the cord is tented dorsally at the stalk-cord merge point (Fig. 15). In rare cases, the stalk appears to pull the cord archly towards the skin lesion to the extent that the cord seems to have displaced the overlying bone and myofascial layers (Fig. 16). In all these examples, the apparent dynamism of the tethering is obvious.

The saccular LDM begins life with the same basic embryogenetic architecture as the flat LDM, but the increasing hydrodynamic pressure of cerebrospinal fluid (CSF) soon changes its anatomical configuration drastically. CSF may be forced up along the slender dural sleeve surrounding the stalk, or through the potential space within the bi-leaf core of the fibroneural stalk to reach and distend the overlying skin into a fluctuant sac. Internally, the "sac" of saccular LDMs can have 3 types of content. First, the entire sacis part of a *segmental myelocystocele*: When the portion of the cord bearing the dorsal myeloschisis has an associated hydromyelia, the central lumen of the fibroneural stalk may be distended by CSF into a large myelocystocele housed in an epithelium-covered sac (Fig. 17). This type is most commonly found in the cervical region (Figs. 18, 19 and 20) [55–58]. Second, the sac contains *basal neural nodules*: When there is no hydromyelia, the fibroneural stalk and its central lumen remain compressed and narrow in its deeper course, but

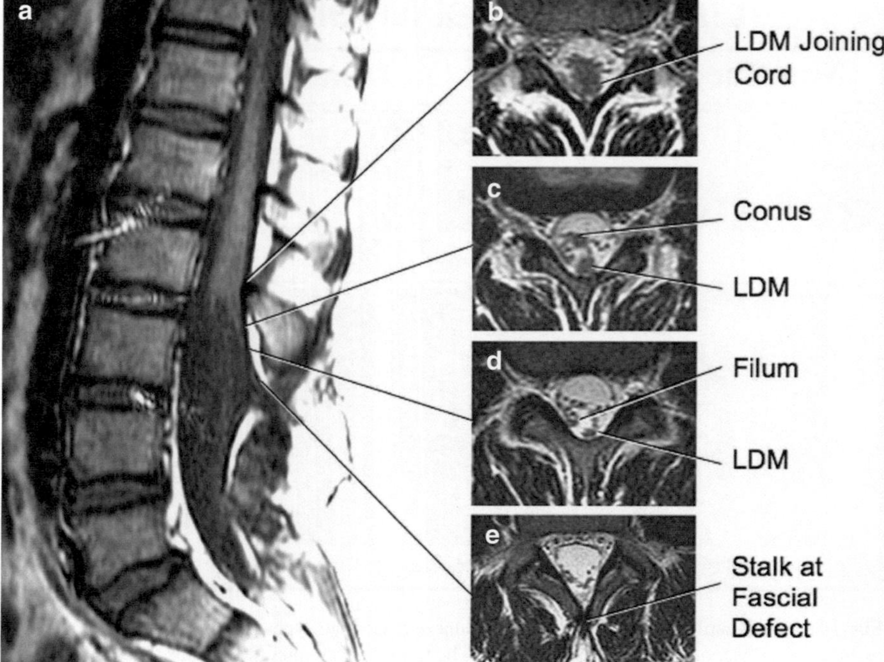

Fig. 11 Lumbar non-saccular (flat) LDM: (**a**) Sagittal MR showing subcutaneous fibroneural stalk going through laminar defect opposite $L_{3/4}$, entering dura opposite L_3, and joining spinal cord at L_2. (**b**) Axial image where LDM stalk joins spinal cord. Note trapezoid shape of the cord-stalk junction. (**c**) Intradural LDM stalk dorsal to the conus (low-lying). (**d**) Intradural LDM stalk dorsal to thickened filum. (**e**) Extradural LDM stalk at laminar defect

the superficial portion of the stalk swells into a fluid sac with two basal neural nodules at its base, while retaining the original nondisjunctional attachment to the cutaneous epithelium (Figs. 21 and 22) [44, 54, 55, 59]. Third, the sac contains a slender fibroneural stalk traversing the CSF sac to reach its dome (*stalk-to-dome* subtype). In all saccular LDMs, the normal meninges around the neural tube extends dorsally to ensheath the fibroneural stalk be it slender or part of a myelocystocele and projects to reach the SE. CSF squeezes into this dural fistula and ultimately distends the thinner, less well-supported squamous epithelial membrane on the surface into a CSF-filled, skin-based but epithelium-capped sac. Strands of the fibroneural stalk always traverse the fluid cavity of the sac to reach the part of the dome bearing the edge of the crater, conveniently identifying the original nondisjunction site (Fig. 23).

Depending on the fluid pressure and the thickness of the apical epithelium and adjacent skin, the sac wall varies from the coarse, purplish, corrugated cap in the not-so-turgid tubular structures in many cervical saccular lesions, to the translucent membrane topping a tense sac in the lumbar region, and finally to the giant,

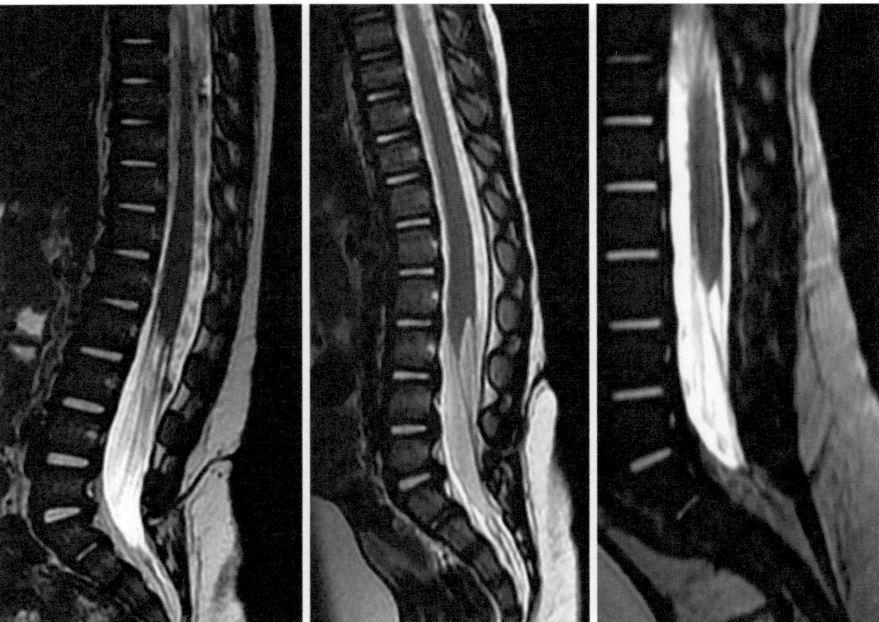

Fig. 12 Three cases of lumbar flat LDMs with V-shaped course of the LDM stalks: Left: Crater is at $L_{4/5}$, stalk enters thecal sac at S_1, and joins spinal cord at upper margin of L_2. Middle: Crater at $L_{3/4}$, stalk enters dura probably at L_5/S_1 and joins spinal cord at L_2. Right: Crater at $L_{4/5}$, stalk enters dura around L_5/S_1 and joins spinal cord at L_3

diaphanous bubble. A transitional form between saccular and flat LDMs can be seen in some flat LDMs with an intermittently ballooning central crater, due to transient rises in CSF pressure during straining (Fig. 24).

As with CSDST, registration of the spinal level of LDMs can be difficult. The challenge is due to the great differences in the level of the skin lesion, the level where the fibroneural stalk passes through the lamina or penetrates the dura, and where it merges with the spinal cord. In the largest LDM series published [1, 2], the vertebral level where the stalk merges with the spinal cord was chosen as the level of the LDM because it is usually the most unequivocal feature on MRI. The locations of the LDMs in that series are shown in Fig. 25, while the distribution of the types of LDMs is depicted in Fig. 26. Over two-thirds of the LDMs in that series are located in the lower half of the spinal cord [1, 2].

Histologically, the central feature of all LDM stalks is neuroglial tissue, a hallmark of the stalk's origin from the NE. It is either in large elongated swaths containing scattered neurons within a glial core (Fig. 27a), or in nests embedded in dense fibrous tissue (Fig. 27b). Also found in every stalk is a profuse network of peripheral nerves randomly admixed with the glial nests, but in some cases, nerves are seen emanating from a central core of neuron-containing glia likened to an abortive spinal cord (Fig. 27c). Large nodules of dorsal root ganglion cells are seen

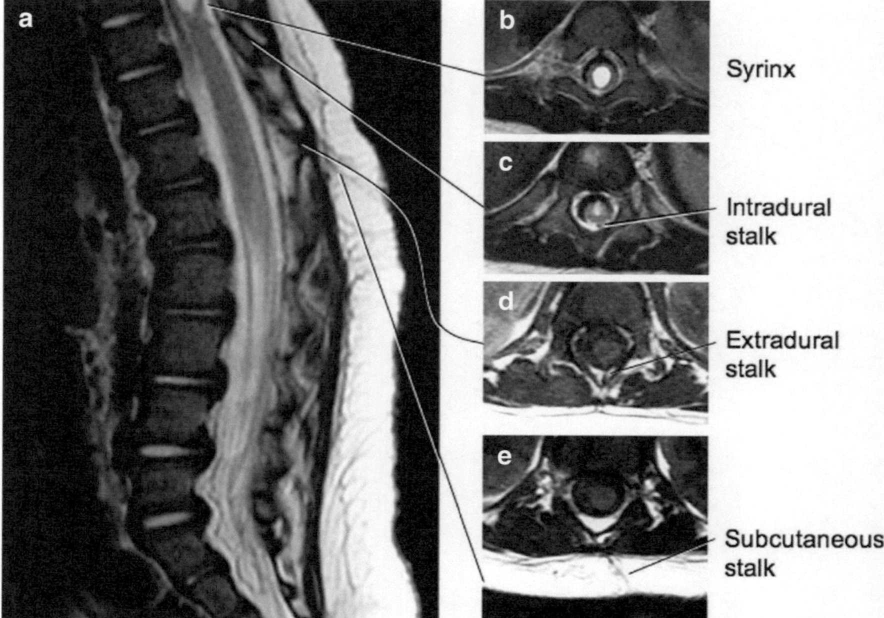

Fig. 13 Upward coursing LDM stalk in a thoracic flat LDM. (**a**) Sagittal image shows skin crater at L_1, extradural stalk at T_{12}, dural entrance of the stalk above T_{12}, and joining of stalk to spinal cord at T_{10}. (**b–e**) Show axial image of the LDM stalk at corresponding points shown in (**a**)

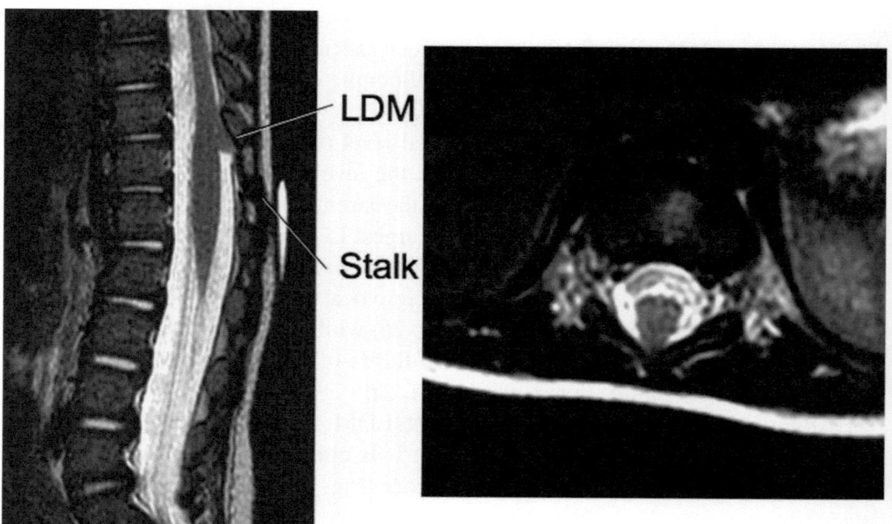

Fig. 14 Thick upward slanting fibroneural stalk in a thoracolumbar (T_{11}/T_{12}) LDM

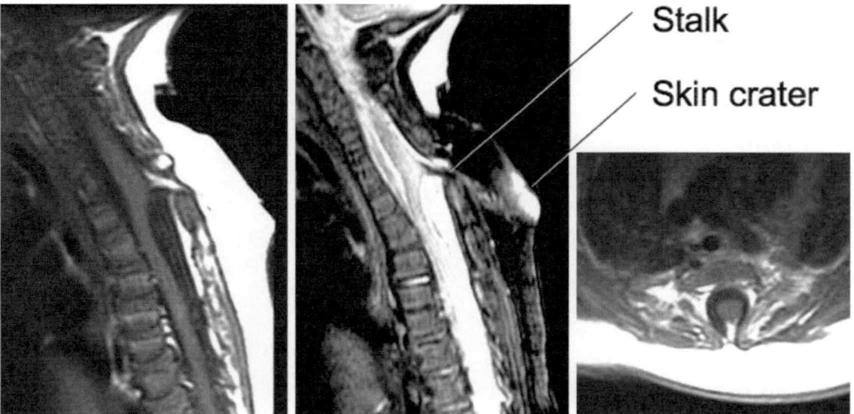

Fig. 15 Upper thoracic crater type LDM showing dorsal tenting of both the dural sac and spinal cord at the site of the stalk-cord junction, giving the appearance of taut tethering of the cord. Left: T_1 sagittal MR; Middle: T_2 sagittal MR; Right: axial MR. Note skin crater, subcutaneous tract and intradural course of the stalk are well shown on the T_2 sagittal image. Also, fat is seen within the stalk

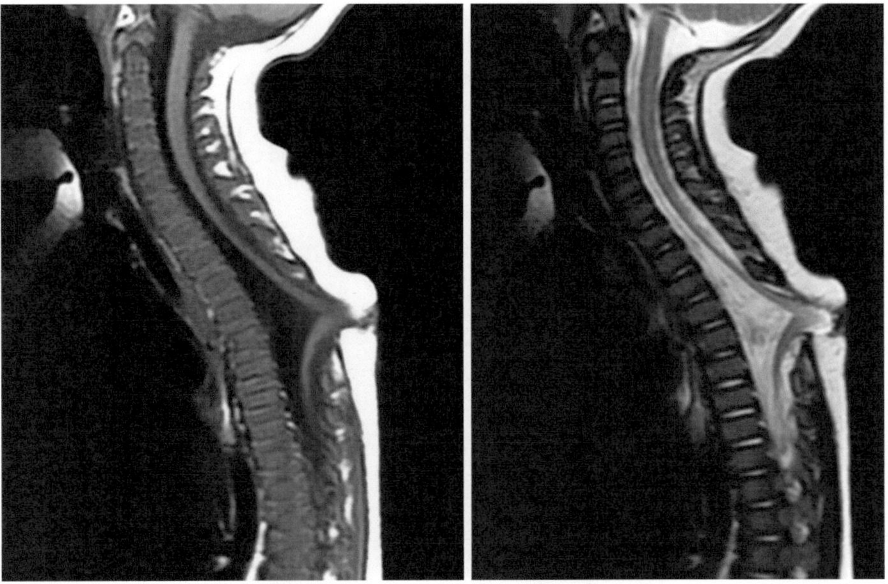

Fig. 16 T_5 LDM with non-saccular skin crater showing extreme dural displacement and kinking of the thoracic cord presumably due to "pull" by a short, stout fibroneural stalk. Left: T_1 sagittal MRI. Right: T_2 sagittal MRI. This child had early neurological deficits

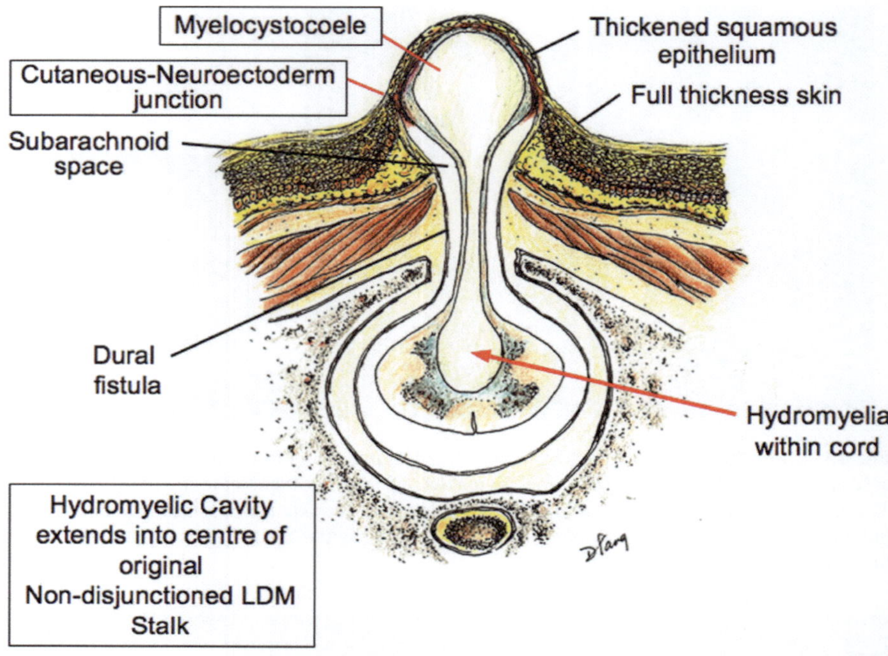

Fig. 17 Formation of saccular LDM with segmental myelocystocele. Fluid from hydromyelic cavity in the underlying spinal cord dissects through the potential tubular space within the original cutaneo-neuroectodermal tract and subsequently balloons out into an ependyma-lined myelocystocele, a sac within an outer sac of distended subarachnoid CSF. The sac is covered by a full-thickness skin base and a thickened, distinctly different squamous epithelial dome

Fig. 18 CT myelogram of a cervical saccular LDM with segmental myelocystocele. The myelocystocele sac does not contain contrast material, which remains in the subarachnoid space

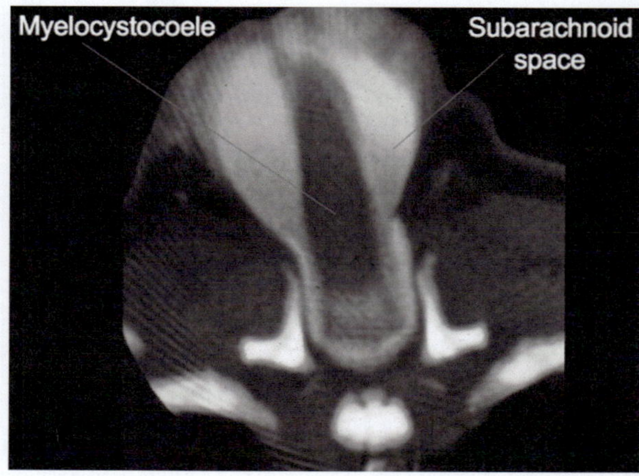

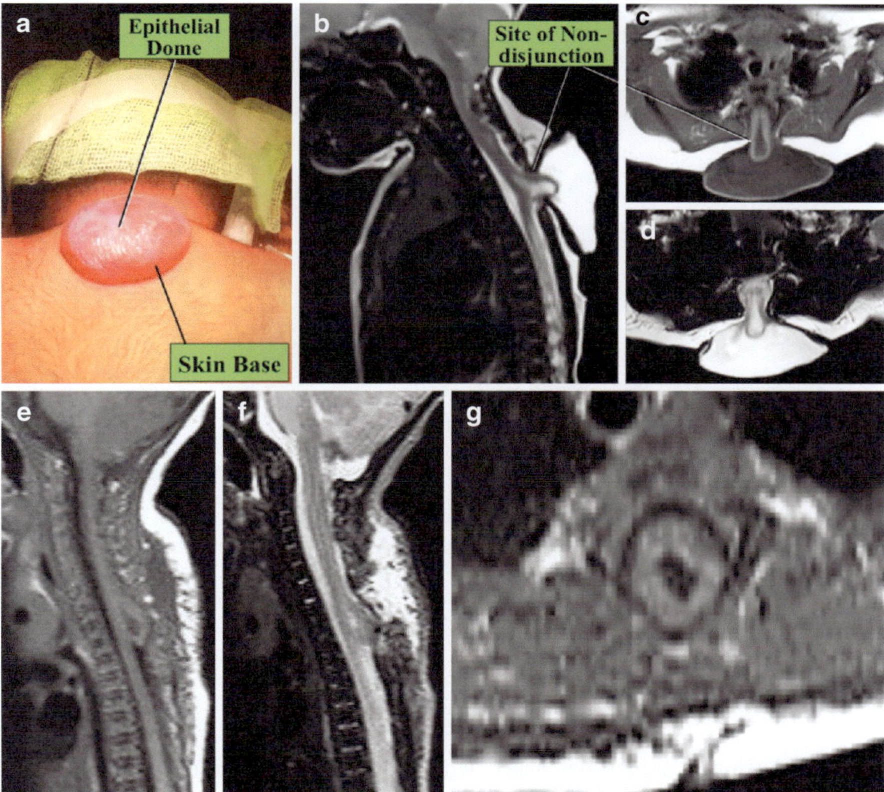

Fig. 19 High thoracic saccular LDM with segmental myelocystocele. (**a–d**) Pre-operative. (**a**) Photo showing the sac with the epithelial dome. (**b**) Sagittal T2-weighted MRI. (**c**) Axial T1-weighted MRI. (**d**) Axial T2-weighted MRI. (**e–g**) Postoperative MRI images. (**e**) Sagittal T1-weighted MRI. (**f**) Sagittal T2-weighted MRI. (**g**) Axial T1-weighted MRI

in some cases, attesting to the occasional entrapped neural crest stem cells during formation of the neural stalk (Fig. 27d). Pacinian corpuscles (Fig. 27e) seen amongst some of these nerves suggest they are indeed sensory axons. Evidence of mesenchymal condensation around the lengthening neural stalk is shown by the almost universal inclusion of numerous fibrous bands, skeletal muscle, fat (Fig. 28a), and prominent vascular channels sometimes in the form of a vascular glomus (Fig. 28b). Glioependymal tissue lines the sac cavities in cases of segmental myelocystoceles (Fig. 28c). The cutaneous "cigarette-burn mark" has the histological appearance of a thick pseudostratified squamous epithelial layer with engorged vascularity, abundant nerve fibres, and an abnormal collagen fibre matrix. The unevenness of its surface is due to the wrinkling effect of the surrounding rugged epidermis and dermis (Fig. 29) [60, 61].

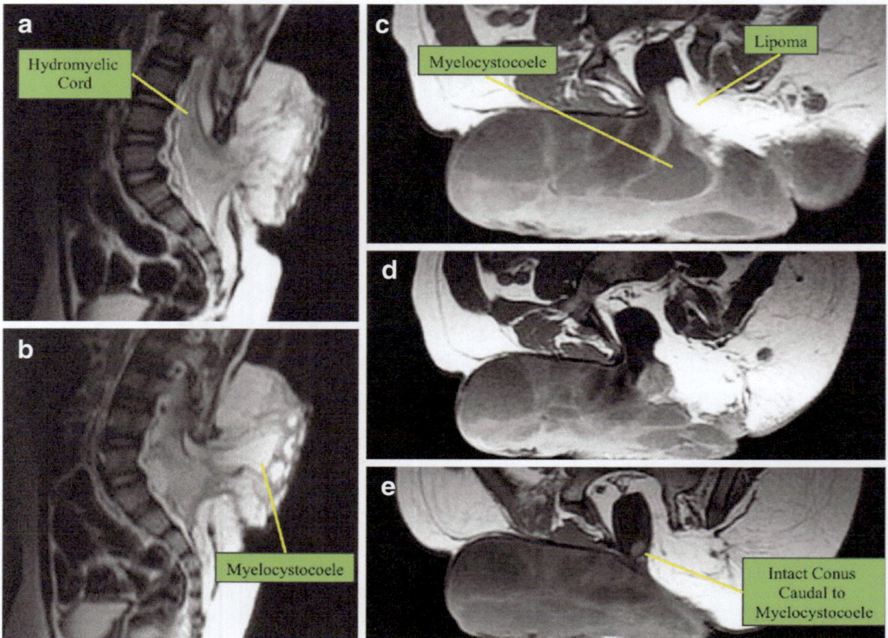

Fig. 20 Lumbar saccular LDM with segmental myelocystocele and lipoma in a 2.5-year-old boy. (**a**, **b**) Sagittal T2-weighted MRI. (**c–e**) Axial T1-weighted MRI

The question is sometimes asked what constitute the minimum criteria for a diagnosis of LDM. It has been shown that there are patients with clinical and radiological features of LDM (Figs. 30 and 31) and most of its histological features including periphery nerve fibres, but no glial tissue within the stalk (Fig. 32) [60–62]. In many of these patients, melanocytes are also a prominent feature. Since periphery nerves and melanocytes are neural crest derivatives, and neural crest cells are located in the primary neural folds close to the SE/NE junction, a nondisjunctional stalk might easily drag with it neural crest progenitor cells without neuroglial progenitor cells [13, 16, 38, 59]. Thus the diagnosis of LDM can probably be applied in these patients with periphery nerve fibres but no glioneuronal tissue within the stalk.

Clinical Manifestations

Most LDM patients also present at a young age. In a series with a total of 63 patients [1], the mean age at presentation of 56 children was 5.9 years; and that of 7 adults was 28.2 years.

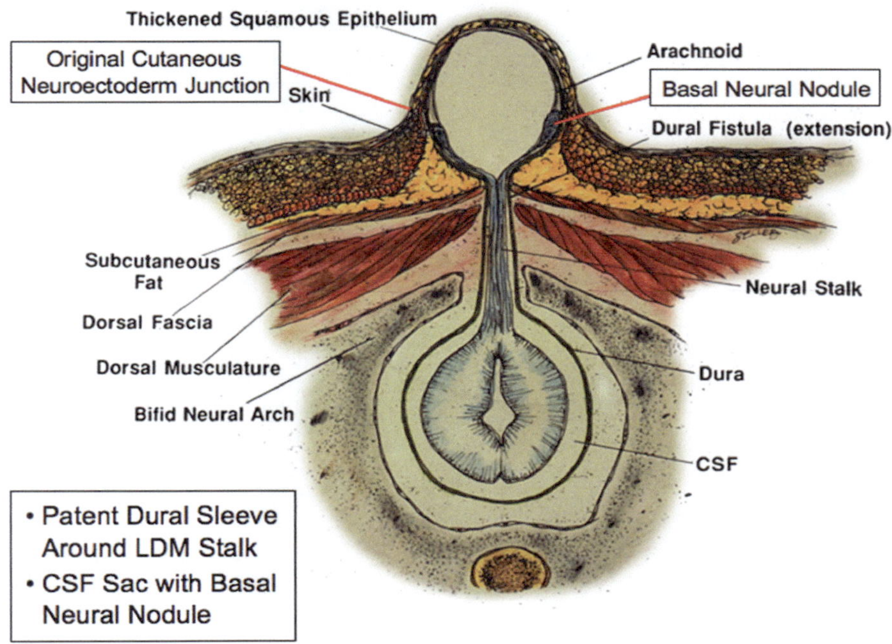

Fig. 21 Formation of a saccular LDM with basal neural nodule. In these cases, CSF dissects along the dural fistula ensheathing the fibroneural stalk and balloons out the less well-supported midline epithelial layer to give a CSF-filled sac, whose base is skin-covered. The neuroectoderm at the original site of non-disjunction swells to become the basal neural nodule

Fig. 22 Cervical saccular LDM with basal neural nodule within the base of the CSF sac at the original non-disjunction site between cutaneous and neural ectoderms

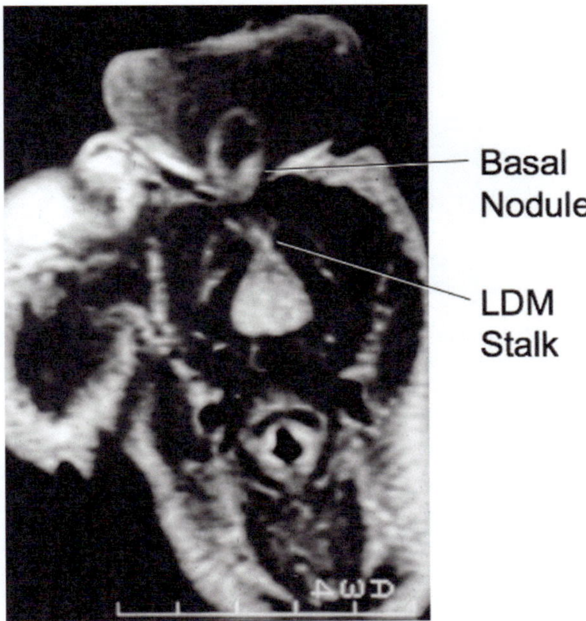

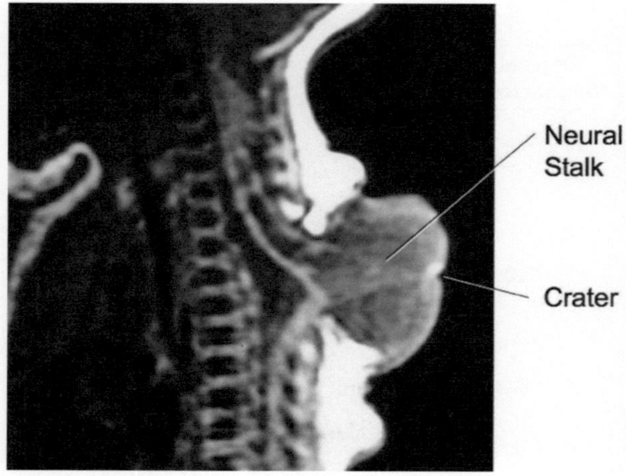

Fig. 23 Thoracic saccular LDM with neural stalk that traverses the CSF sac and reaches the small skin crater at the top of the cystic dome, presumably the original site of disjunction failure

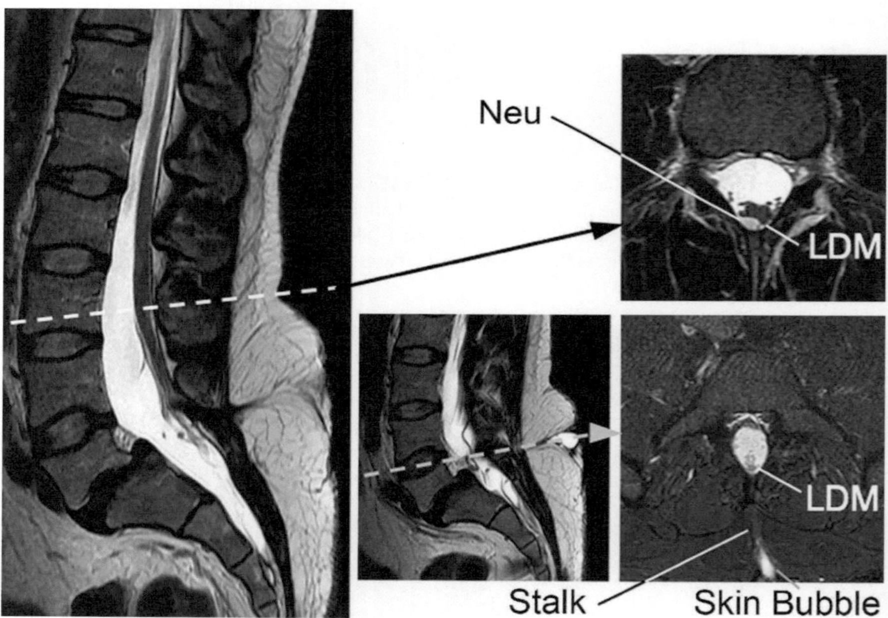

Fig. 24 Lumbar LDM showing a CSF-filled "bubble" topped by squamous epithelium that distends only on straining. Note site of cord-stalk union is with slight dorsal "hump" on the cord outline, and a neurenteric cyst (Neu) right at this site

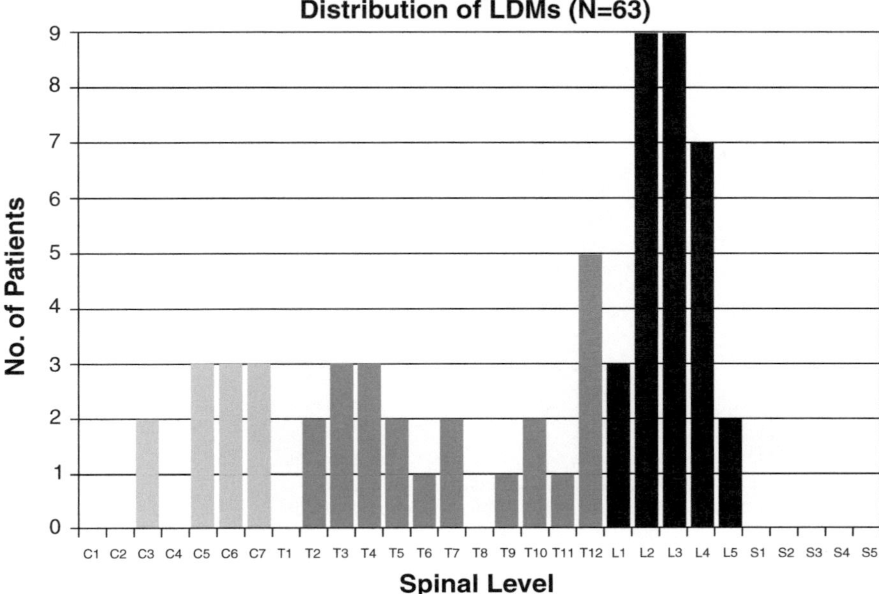

Fig. 25 Distribution of LDMs along the spinal axis. Designation of location is determined by the vertebral level where the fibroneural stalk attaches to the spinal cord. Note the two peaks at L_2–L_4 and C_5–C_7 and the absence of sacral lesion

Cutaneous Markers

About half of LDM patients are neurologically intact at presentation, which underscores the importance of the cutaneous marker as an initial diagnostic clue [1, 2]. The "pathognomic" cutaneous marker in both flat and saccular LDMs is a confined area of abnormal epithelium over the dorsal midline. In flat LDMs, the cutaneous lesion can be a conspicuous crater or a tiny pit. (*1*) *Crater*: The commonest skin abnormality in flat LDMs is a sunken crater on the flat skin surface covered by pinkish squamous epithelium (Fig. 33a, b), often with elevated skin margin (Fig. 33c) and sometimes surrounded by a capillary haemangioma with irregular corrugated borders (Fig. 33d) or by hyperpigmented skin (Fig. 33e). There are occasionally long hair emanating from the crater (Fig. 33f), and some craters are edged by hooded overhanging skin (Fig. 33g). In several examples, the crater is adjacent to an area of wrinkly, over-stretched skin that periodically distends with CSF on dependent posturing or straining (Fig. 34a). Very rarely, the centre of the crater is adorned with a CSF-filled blister (Fig. 34b), which is a transitional form between flat and saccular

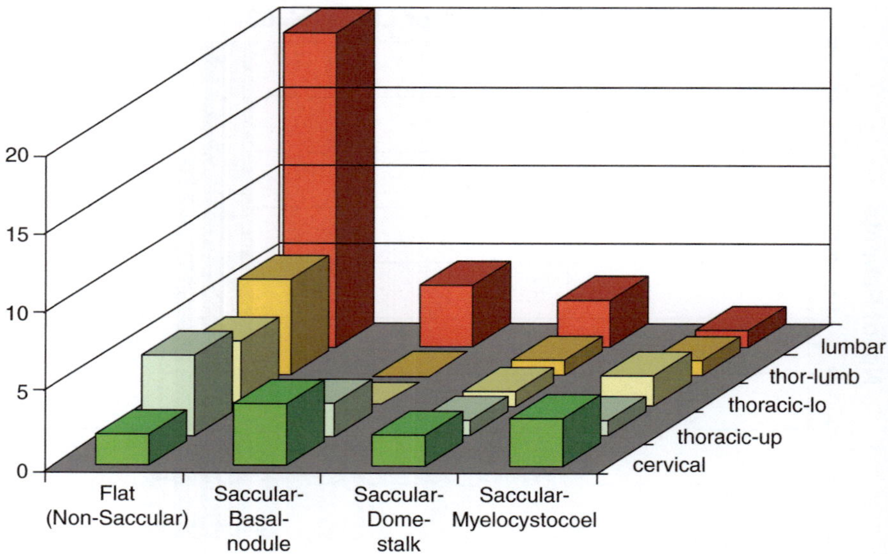

Fig. 26 Distribution of the 4 types of LDM classified according to external and internal features and assorted by regions of the spinal axis. The 4 types are flat (non-saccular), saccular with basal neural nodule, saccular with neural stalk reaching the cyst dome, and saccular with segmental myelocystocele. Note preponderance of the flat LDM in the lumbar and lower thoracic regions. Saccular types are seen in both cervical and lumbar segments. The regions of the vertebral column are coded as: cervical (C1–C7); thoracic-up (T1–T5); thoracic-lo (T5–T11); thor-lumb (T12–L1); lumbar (L1–L5)

lesions. (2) *Pit*: The most subtle skin abnormality in a flat LDM is a small midline pit with no other unusual features (Fig. 35), easily missed on cursory examination, and might be confused with a CSDST ostium. Sometimes the pit situates within a capillary haemangioma. Pit lesions are usually found in low thoracic and lumbar cases.

Externally, saccular LDMs usually appear as a skin-based sac, but rarely as a translucent membranous sac. (1) *Skin-based sac*: The sac wall is thick, skin-based with a dome that is distinctly abnormal skin. The appearance of the dome cover can be roughly subdivided into three subtypes. One subtype has a wide top of purplish, raw-looking, thick-stratified squamous epithelium (Fig. 36a). A second subtype has a much smaller, pale, discrete, puckered crater of squamous epithelium on the dome (Fig. 36b). A third subtype has a small, almost imperceptible patch of ultra-thin epithelium on the apex of the relatively delicate skin-based dome (Fig. 36c). (2) *Membranous sac*: This type should be managed urgently as an "open" spinal dysraphic lesion, but the fibroneural stalk should not be missed. An example is a tubular, CSF-filled sac made of a diaphanous membrane resembling thickened arachnoid,

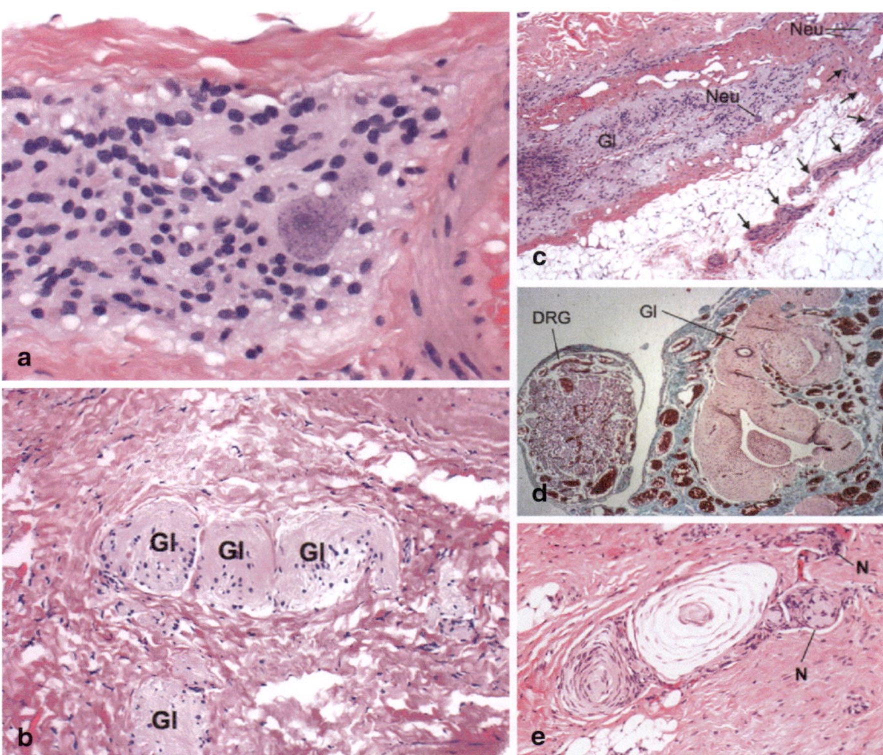

Fig. 27 Histopathology of LDM stalk. (**a**) Core of glial tissue with a large neuron, framed by fibrous tissue. (**b**) Nests of glial tissue (Gl) embedded in a dense fibrous matrix. (**c**) LDM stalk showing a longitudinal glial core (Gl) containing neurons (Neu). A peripheral nerve (arrows) issues forth at right angle to the glial core as from a "real" spinal cord. (**d**) LDM stalk containing glial tissue (Gl) and a large dorsal root ganglion (DRG). (**e**) Peripheral nerves (N) with Pacinian corpuscle within LDM stalk. Pacinian corpuscle in the stalk indicates the nerves involved in LDM formation are indeed sensory nerves likely from the adjacent neural crest

protruding through a 4-mm skin-lined dorsal defect (Fig. 37). The base of this sac has a shallow collar of skin similar to the skin-based sacs. The locations and types of the cutaneous lesions are summarized in Table 1.

It is noteworthy that other cutaneous markers of dysraphism such as hypertrichosis, capillary haemangioma, or misaligned gluteal crease are never seen alone in LDM without the quintessential epithelial crater or pit. The pearly midline crater in a non-saccular LDM thus remains the single most important diagnostic clue for LDM, especially before the development of neurological symptoms.

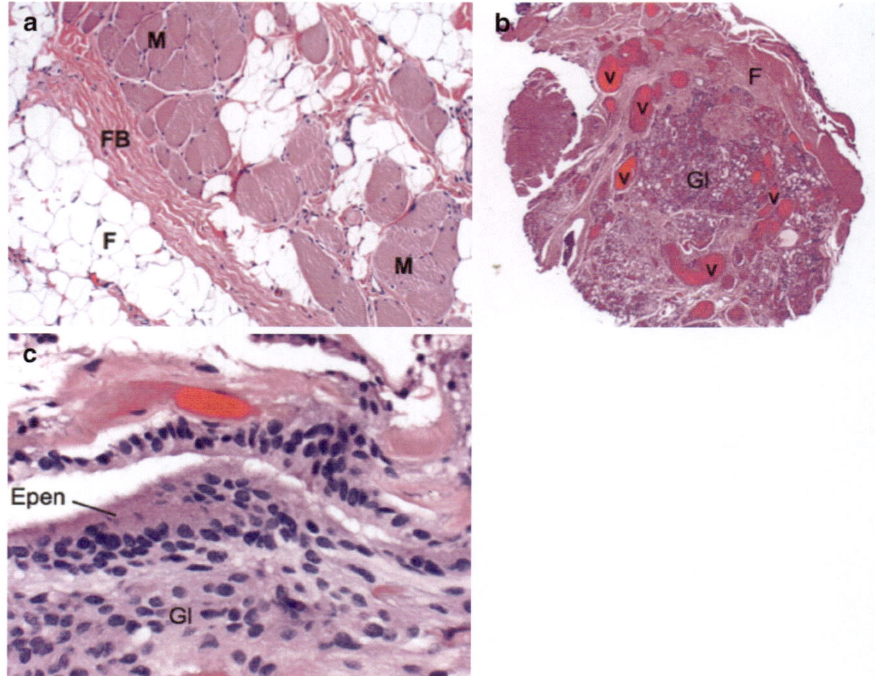

Fig. 28 Histopathology of LDM stalk. (**a**) LDM stalk containing skeletal muscle (M), fat (F), and fibrous band (FB). (**b**) LDM stalk containing prominent blood vessels (V) within a core of glial tissue (Gl), and fibrous bands (F), in the form of a vascular glomus. (**c**) Glioependymal lining of a segmental myelocystocele in a lumbar saccular LDM. *Epen* ependyma; *Gl* glial tissue

Fig. 29 Histological slide of a skin "cigarette burn mark" showing increase vascularity, plenty of nerve fibres (yellow arrows), and a different collagen pattern, comparing to the adjacent normal dermis. Yellow dashed line marks the border between normal and abnormal dermis. Gross appearance of the skin lesion is shown in Fig. 30a. (Haematoxylin and eosin stain)

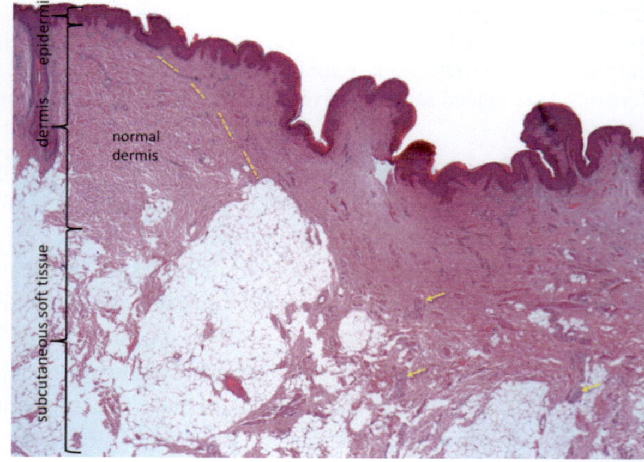

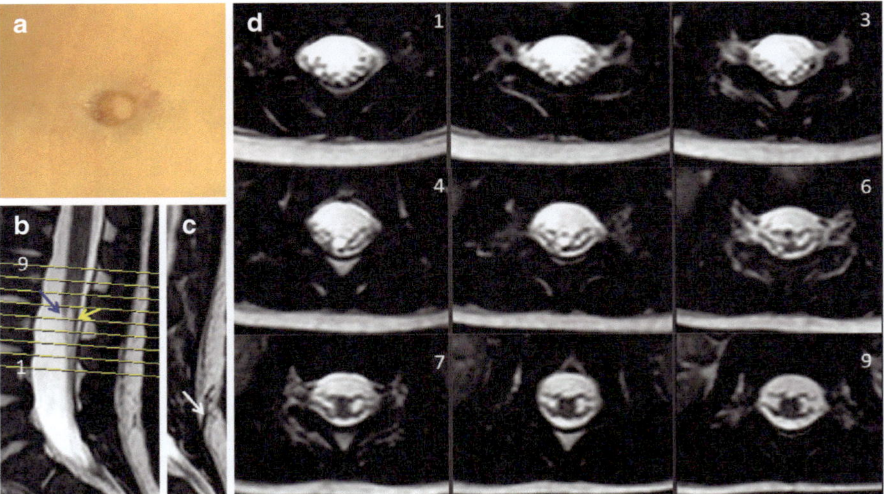

Fig. 30 A case of "clinical and radiological" LDM. (**a**) Cigarette burn mark. (**b**) Mid-sagittal T2 weighted MRI image showing the intradural portion of the LDM stalk (yellow arrow). Blue arrow = the conus. (**c**) Sagittal MRI just next to (**b**) showing the subcutaneous portion of the stalk (white arrow). (**d**) Axial T2-weighted MRI images corresponding to the cut lines in (**b**)

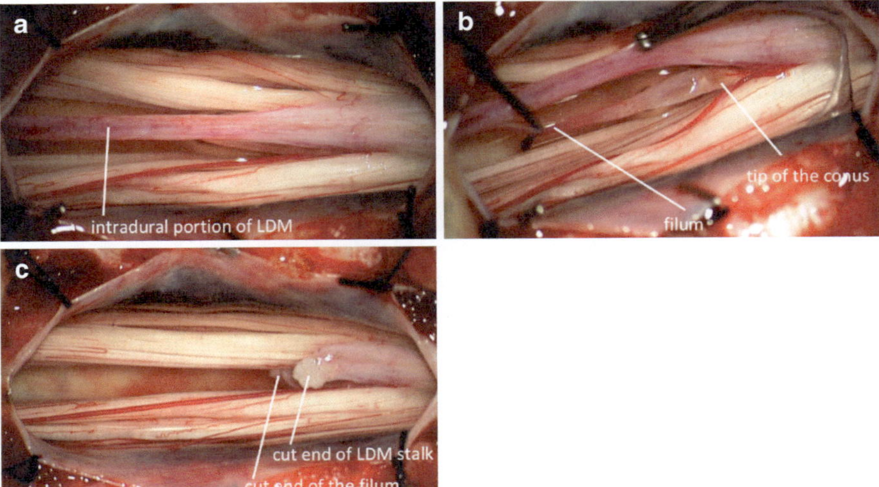

Fig. 31 Intra-operative photographs showing excision of a LDM with a L2L3 laminoplasties. Pre-operative MRI images and the skin lesion are shown in Fig. 30. The skin lesion was traced to the supraspinous ligament of S1 only; the S1 laminae were untouched. This kind of limited exposure thus left a small segment of the LDM stalk in situ

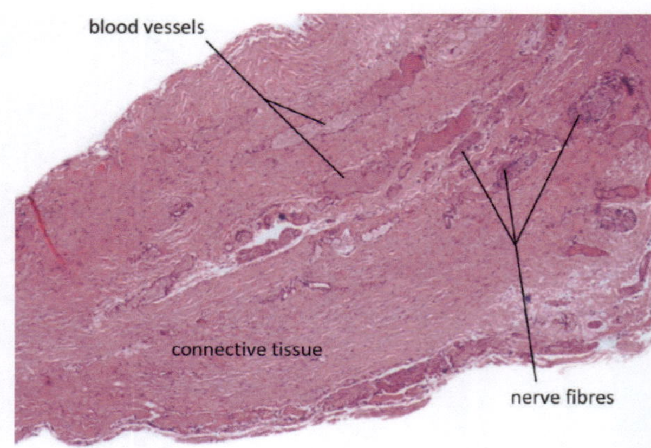

Fig. 32 Histological slide of the intradural portion of a LDM stalk showing the presence of nerve fibres and blood vessels. Intraoperative photograph is shown in Fig. 31. (Haematoxylin and eosin stain)

Neurourological Findings

LDMs cause neurological deficits solely by their tethering effect, which vary in kind and severity determined by the spinal level of the LDM. In general, LDM patients tend to have milder disability than patients with other forms of dysraphic malformations such as split cord malformations and spinal cord lipomas. In Pang et al.'s series [2], half of the LDM patients had neurological deficits at presentation. About 10% of patients had significant weakness and neuropathic bladder, and the rest of the patients had mild or tolerable neurological or urological deficits, with relatively little hindrance to their lifestyle. The correlations between the types of deficits and locations of the LDMs are summarized in Table 2. The proximity of tension to the relevant cord segments does seem to correspond with the kind of deficits. For example, only cervical lesions produce hand and arm weakness; leg weakness is seen in only 9% of cervical lesions, but 22% in upper thoracic lesions, 38% in thoracolumbar lesions, and 50% in lumbar lesions; and bladder dysfunction is seen in approximately 15% of lower thoracic and lumbar lesions but not in cervical or upper thoracic lesions. Lumbar LDMs close to the conus are perhaps more treacherous because they more often implicate the bladder yet are more likely to be occult.

Similar to other cord tethering entities, the probability of neurological injury increases with longitudinal growth of the spine and with age. Pang et al. [1, 2] demonstrated that older patients with LDMs had a tendency to present with more severe neurological and urological disabilities and that infants and young children were more likely to be neurologically normal (Figs. 38 and 39). Regression analysis of neurological severity against age shows without doubt that LDM is a progressive disease (Fig. 38). Neurological deterioration was observed in all 4 adolescents who had had longitudinal follow-up and delay of surgery of 1–9 years.

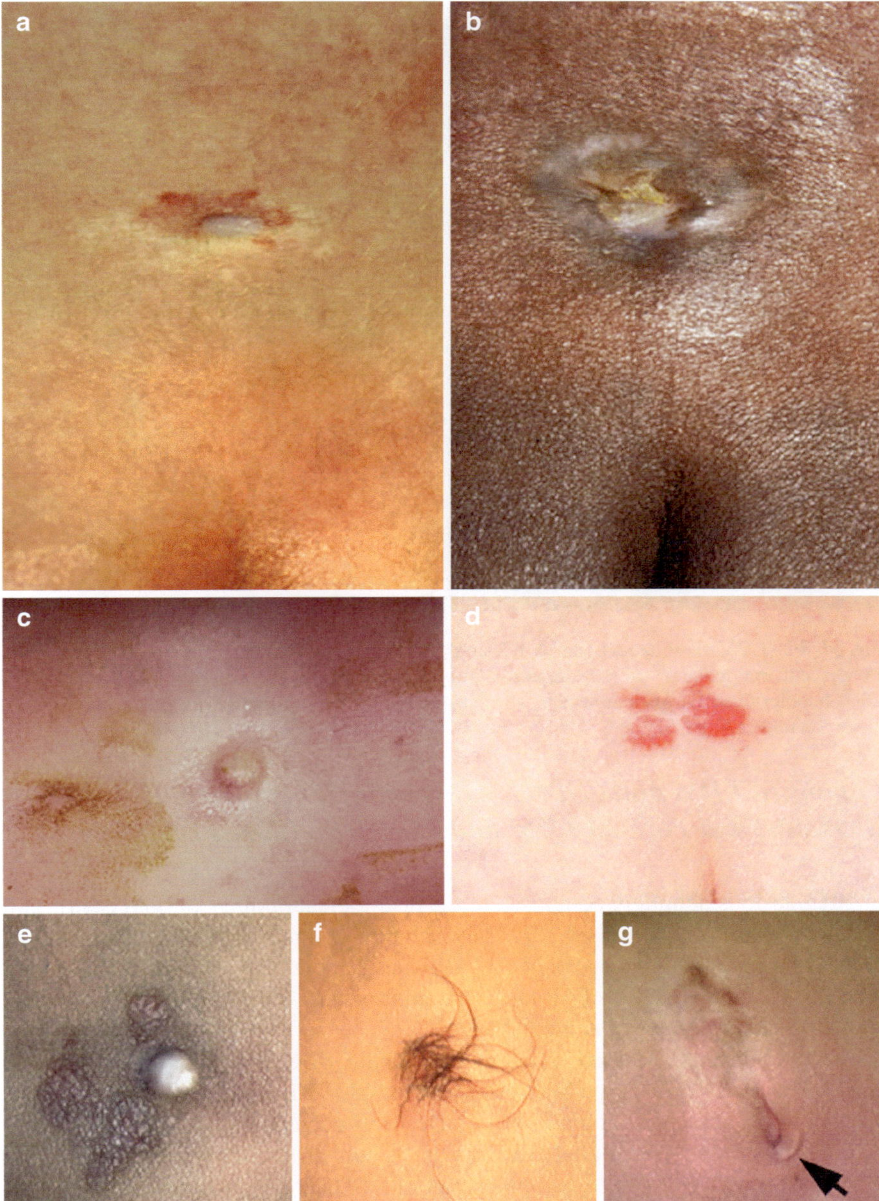

Fig. 33 Flat type skin lesions in LDM: (**a**) Sunken crater of pale squamous epithelium. (**b**) Sunken crater of pale epithelium. (**c**) Squamous epithelial crater with rim of elevated skin borders. (**d**) Crater surrounded by prominent capillary haemangioma with irregular corrugated borders. (**e**) White non-melanotic, epithelial crater with surrounding hyperpigmented skin. (**f**) Crater covered with long hair arising from the rim of surrounding full-thickness skin. (**g**) Crater with surrounding skin overhang (arrow)

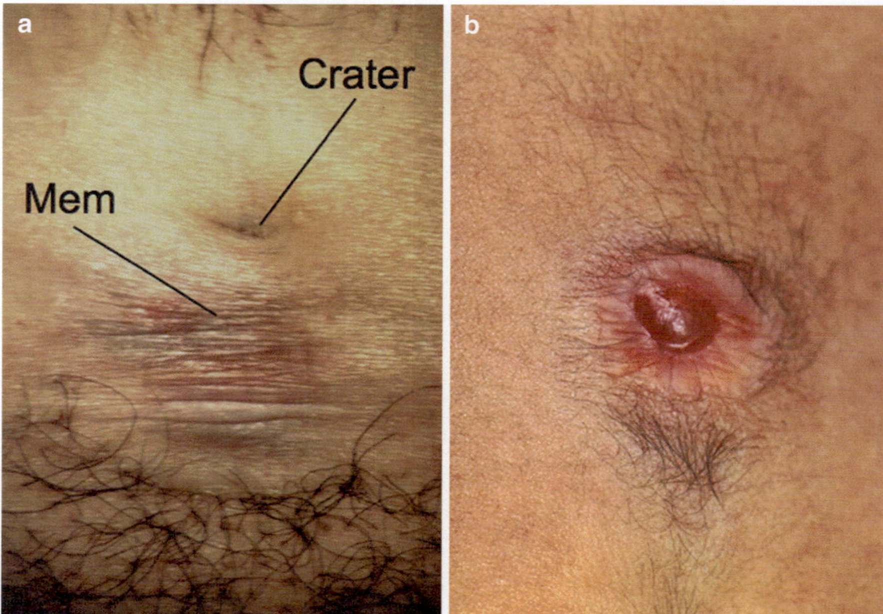

Fig. 34 Flat LDMs with transitional skin lesions: (**a**) Lumbar LDM with a flat epithelial crater and an adjacent area made of stretchable, non-skin epithelium (Mem) that distends into a small CSF-filled bubble when the patient strains. (**b**) Pink epithelial crater slightly distended into a small blister by underlying CSF

Combined LDM and CSDST, LDM with Hidden Dermal Elements, and Parallel LDM and CSDST in Close Proximity

In 2013, lesions definitely composed of the histological findings of both LDMs and CSDSTs were first described [2]. They are rare compared to the pure forms of LDMs and CSDSTs. In a series of 75 LDM cases, there were 5 cases of this mixed type [8]. In another series of 51 cases that consisted of 40 LDMs and 11 CSDSTs, another 5 cases were documented [10].

Macroscopically, a mixed lesion of LDM and CSDST can mimic either of the pure forms. Even cystic type has been observed [10]. Thus, their recognition relies on histology. Three histological types have been documented. In the "orthodox" type, the dermal and neuroglial elements are in tandem in their respective embryologically orthodox order, i.e. an outer tract of CSDST and an inner tract of LDM elements (Fig. 40) [10]. In the "conjoint" type, the entire FSND tract is lined by both SE and NE elements (Figs. 41, 42 and 43). The most treacherous mixed lesions, "LDM with hidden dermal elements", have been observed in which the dermal

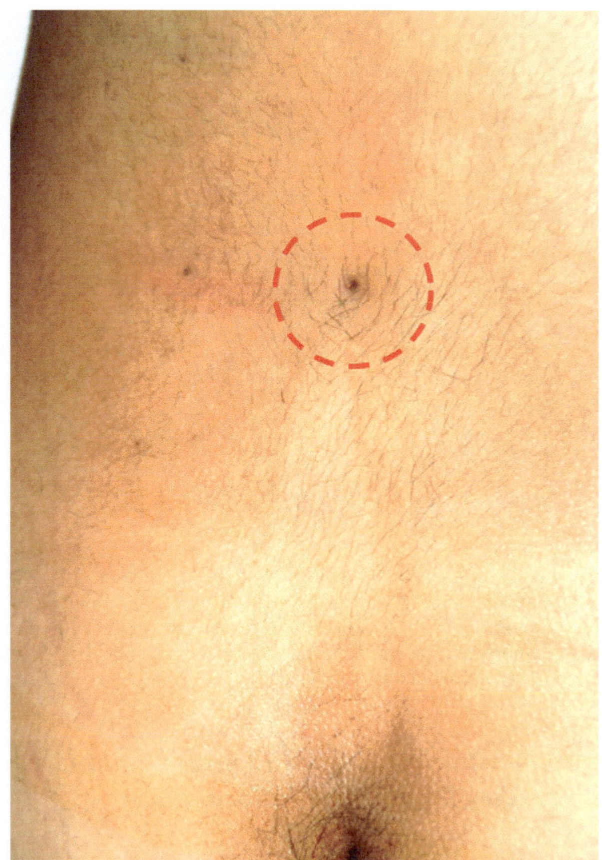

Fig. 35 Subtle pit (within circle) in a flat lumbar LDM with no surrounding exuberance

elements form microscopic squamous epithelial islands within the neuroglial tissue of an otherwise proper LDM tract (Fig. 44) [8, 53]. Rarely, parallel LDM and CSDST tracts can co-exist in close proximity from skin to spinal cord (Fig. 45).

The most salient implication in clinical practice with the discovery of these combined types, especially the subtle ones, is that such mixed lesions cannot be reliably exonerated at the time of surgery without benefit of histology. Retained dermoid elements within part of the LDM stalks that were left behind at surgery have been known to enlarge into he and compressive dermoid cysts years after the initial operation of partial LDM stalk resection [8]. Thus, it seems prudent that in all cases of suspected LDM, the entire tract is removed from skin to spinal cord. In addition, all FSND patients should have a delayed post-operative MRI to rule out a recurrent dermoid cyst.

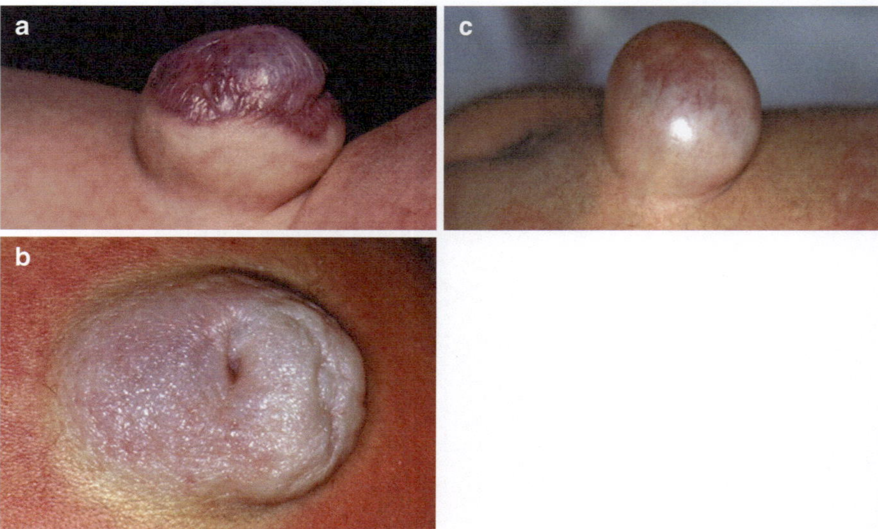

Fig. 36 Saccular skin lesions in LDM: (**a**) a cervical saccular LDM with full-thickness skin at the base and coarse, thick, corrugated purplish squamous epithelial top. Cervical saccular lesions are usually not turgid. (**b**) An upper thoracic saccular LDM with mostly skin except for a dome crater of squamous epithelium. (**c**) A turgid lumbar saccular LDM with a skin base and a translucent "non-skin" epithelial top

FSND with Spinal Cord Lipomas, Split Cord Malformations, and Other Dysraphic Malformations

FSNDs have been observed to occur with other dysraphic or paradysraphic malformations such as spinal cord lipomas, myelomeningoceles, neurenteric cysts, split cord malformations, and even a lesion with the LDM stalk involving only one hemicord of a split cord malformation [46] (Table 3) (Fig. 46). In such cases, the complex anatomy of the other malformations usually dominates the pathological anatomy of the composite malformation, for a pure FSND lesion is structurally more subtle unless it is an CSDST with a large intradural dermoid/epidermoid cyst.

The clinical manifestations of these composite malformations also follow the usual course of the associated anomalies, especially when there are only LDM elements without dermoid cyst. However, if present, the dermal elements can have significant late adverse impact due to their inherent risks of inflammation, infection, proliferation producing mass effect, and recurrence if not totally excised. One should therefore always be vigilant for hidden dermal elements when dealing with any spinal dysraphic malformations.

Fig. 37 Lumbar LDM with membranous sac: (**a**) Large ruptured sac made of diaphanous membrane. (**b**) Close-up of the base showing a small skin defect through which protrudes a tubular basal neural nodule. (**c**) The entire LDM is exposed at surgery to show basal neural nodules (BN), subcutaneous tract, and intradural stalk (S) attached to the spinal cord

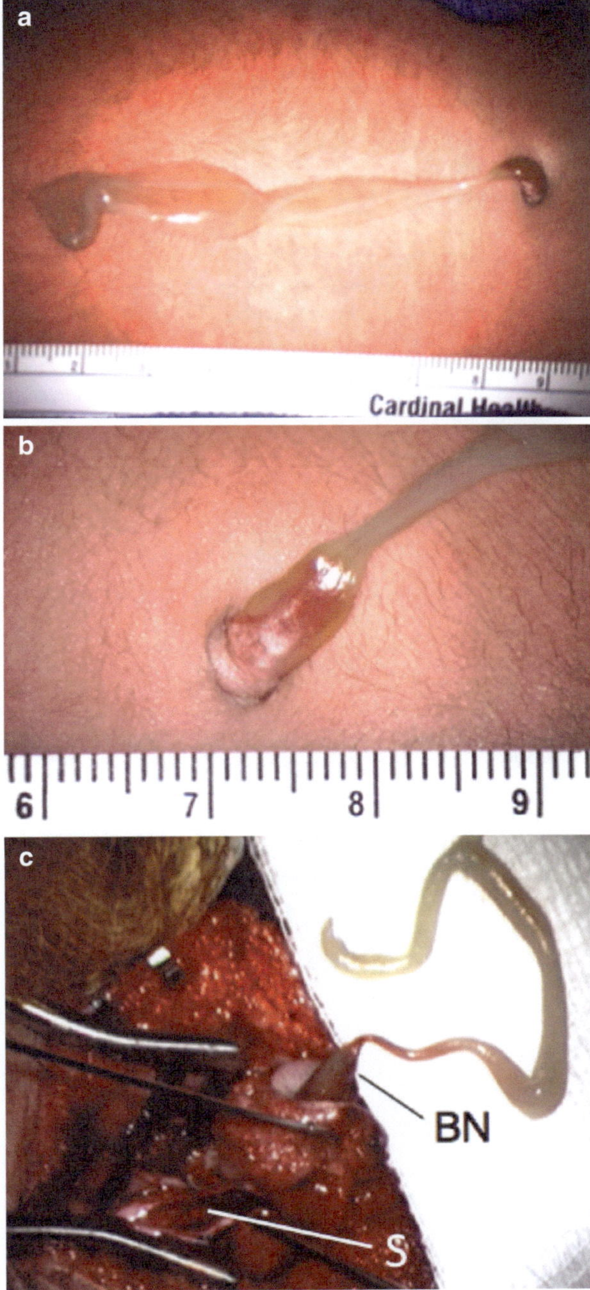

Table 1 Skin lesions in LDM in different LDM locations ($n = 63$)

LDM location[a]	Skin lesions in LDM			
	Crater	Pit	Saccular	Membranous sac
Cervical	2	0	9	0
Thoracic-upper	3	2	4	0
Thoracic-lower	4	0	3	0
Thoracolumbar	4	2	2	0
Lumbar	16	4	6	2

(From Pang et al. 2013, [2])

[a]The regions of the vertebral column are coded as: cervical (C1–C7); thoracic-upper (T1–T5); thoracic-lower (T5–T11); thoracolumbar (T12–L1); lumbar (L1–L5)

Table 2 Types of neurological deficits in different LDM locations ($n = 63$)

Neurological status	Number of patients assorted by LDM location				
	Cervical (11)	Thoracic upper (9)	Thoracic lower (7)	Thoracolumbar (8)	Lumbar (28)
Normal	4 (36%)	2 (22%)	4 (57%)	4 (50%)	14 (50%)
UE weakness/ sensory loss	7 (64%)	2 (22%)			
LE weakness	1 (9%)	2 (22%)	3 (43%)	3 (38%)	14 (50%)
LE sensory loss		1 (11%)	2 (31%)	1 (13%)	8 (29%)
Spastic legs	4 (36%)	4 (44%)	2 (31%)		
Back pain			1 (25%)		3 (13.6%)
Foot deformity					2 (9.1%)
Scoliosis			2 (31%)	1 (16.6%)	1 (4.5%)
Neurogenic bladder			1 (25%)	1 (16.6%)	4 (18%)
Abnormal URD			1 (25%)	1 (16.6%)	2 (9.1%)

(From Pang et al. 2013, [2])

LE lower extremity, *UE* upper extremity, *URD* urodynamics

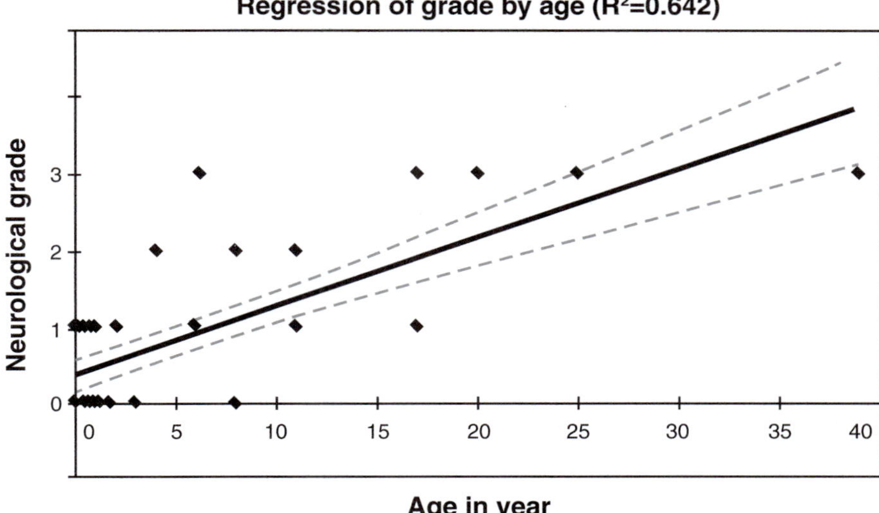

Fig. 38 Linear regression analysis between neurological grade * and patient age shows a logistical tendency for older patients with LDM to present with higher grades of neurological deficits. (Correlative coefficient $R^2 = 0.642$). *Neurological grading system in LDM: Grade 0: No deficits or symptoms. Grade 1: Mild upper or lower extremity weakness, or pure sensory deficits +/− pain. Grade 2: Moderate to severe upper or lower extremity weakness ± sensory deficits, or neurogenic bladder without weakness. Grade 3: Upper or lower extremity weakness + neurogenic bladder. (From Pang et al. 2013, [25])

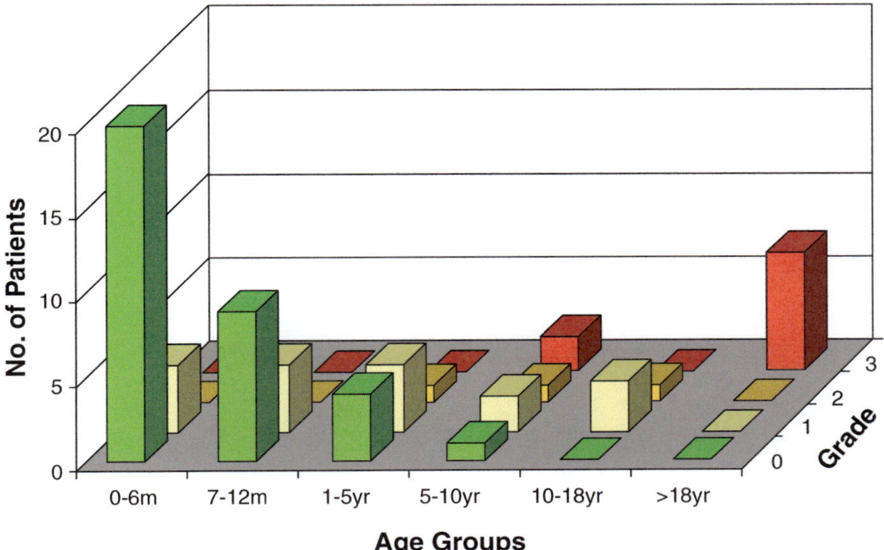

Fig. 39 Clustered bar graphs showing neurological grade assorted by patients' age-groups (birth to 6 months; 6–12 months; 1–5 years; 6–10 years; 11–18 years; and over 18 years) within each neurological grade of 0–3. There is a preponderance of younger children with the better neurological grades and preponderance of older patients with the worse grades

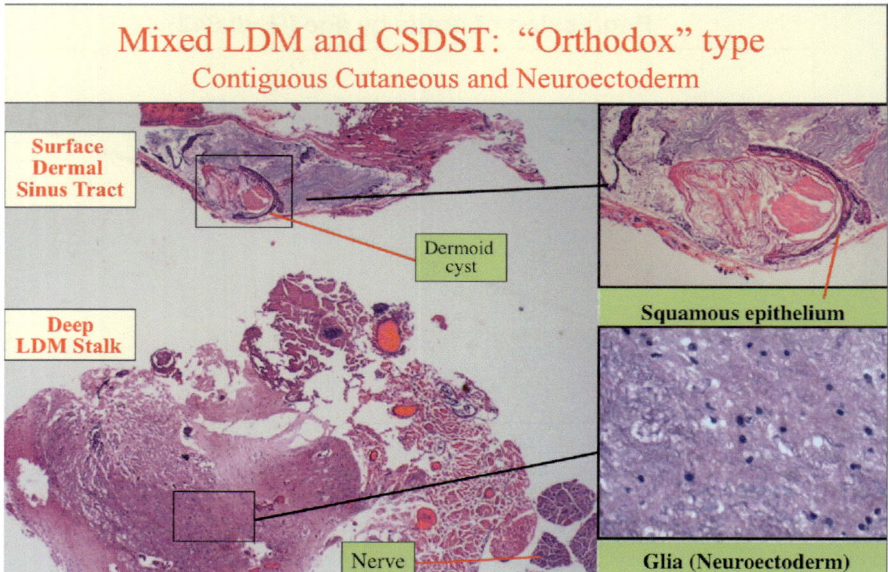

Fig. 40 Histological constituents of a mixed LDM-CSDST stalk of the "orthodox" type. Its superficial portion is of typical dermal tissue lying in tandem with its deeper portion containing mainly glioneuronal tissue. Insets showing both tissues in high power. (Haematoxylin and eosin stain)

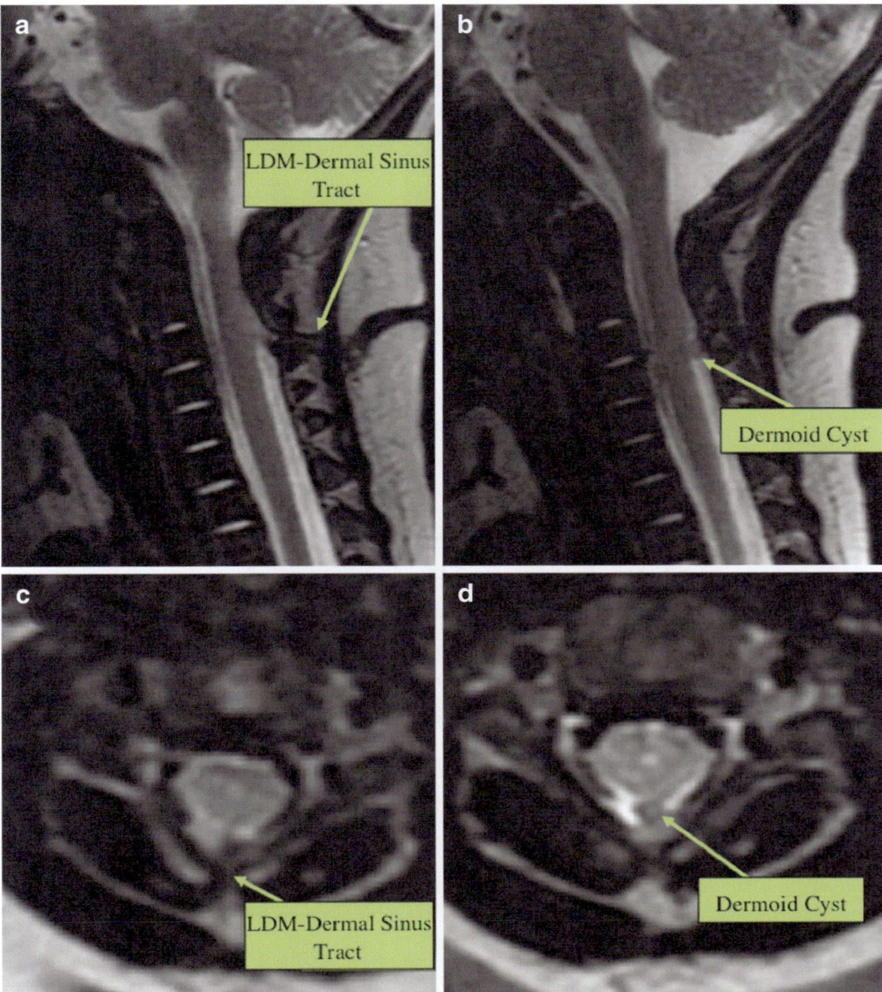

Fig. 41 MRI images of a 3-month-old girl with a mixed LDM and CSDST-"Conjoint" type. The diagnosis was made based on intraoperative and histological findings (Figs. 42 and 43). MRI images can only show a tract extending from the skin to the spinal cord but cannot confirm the components of the tract. (**a**, **b**) Sagittal T2-weighted MRI images. (**c**, **d**) Axial T2-weighted MRI images

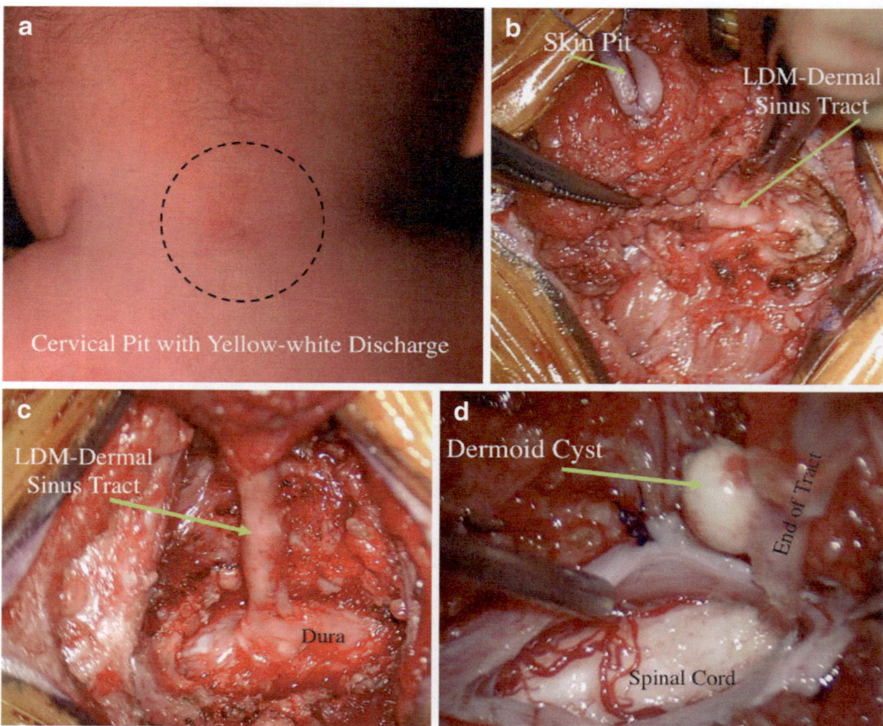

Fig. 42 Intraoperative photos of a patient (Fig. 41) with a mixed LDM and CSDST-"Conjoint" type. (**a**) Skin pit, (**b**, **c**) dissection of the extra-dural portion of the tract. (**d**) Photo taken at the moment before complete detachment of the tract from the spinal cord

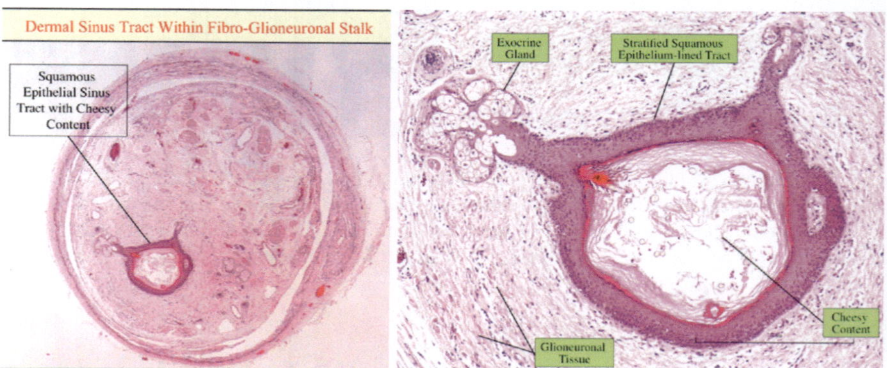

Fig. 43 Histological slides of a patient (Fig. 41) with a mixed LDM and CSDST-"Conjoint" type showing the presence of a dermal sinus tract within a fibro-glioneuronal stalk. (Haematoxylin and eosin stain)

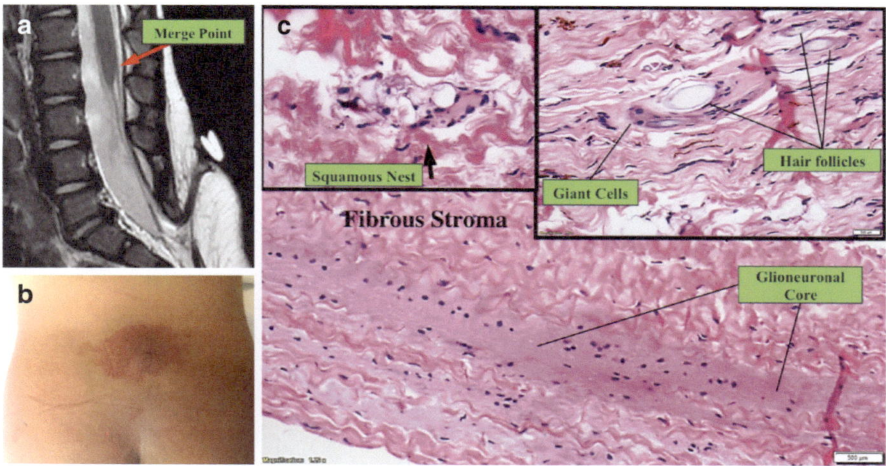

Fig. 44 A 15-month-old with a LDM with hidden dermal elements. (**a**) Sagittal T2-weighted MRI showing the appearance of a classic lumbar LDM. (**b**) Photo showing a crater and surrounding haemangioma. (**c**) Histological slide showing a stalk with glioneuronal core and derivatives of squamous epithelium. (Haematoxylin and eosin stain)

Fig. 45 Intraoperative photos showing the presence of a LDM and a CSDST in parallel

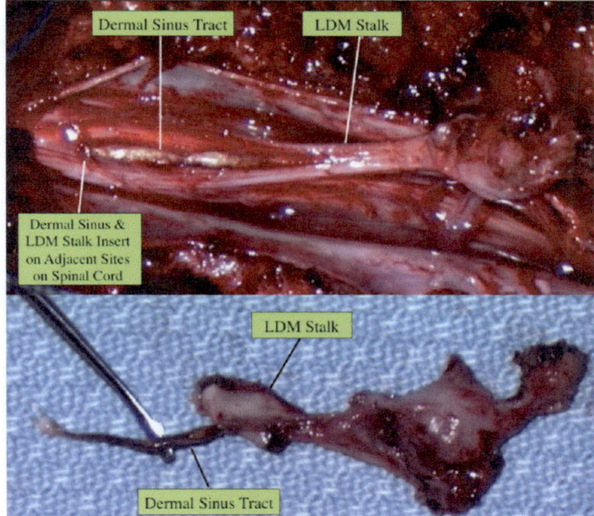

Table 3 Associated anomalies in LDM ($n = 63$)

| | LDM location | | | | |
Anomalies	Cervical (11)	Thoracic upper (9)	Thoracic lower (7)	Thoracolumbar (8)	Lumbar (28)
SCM	4	1			1
Terminal lipoma		1			1
Dorsal lipoma		1		2	3
Thickened filum	2	1		3	21
Neurenteric cyst					1
Syringomyelia		1		1	
Chiari II	3	2			
Hydrocephalus	6				
Dermal sinus			1	1	1
Velum interpositum cyst		1			
Vertebral/rib fusion		2	1		

(From Pang et al. 2013, [2])

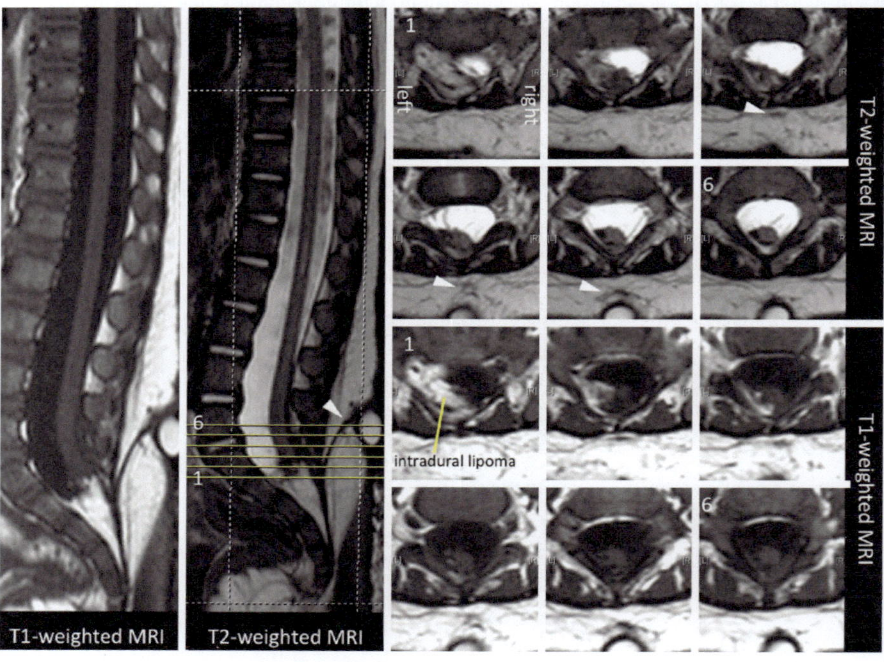

Fig. 46 MRI images showing a LDM associated with a transitional spinal cord lipoma in a 11-month-old. The axial cuts are numbered according to the cut-lines on the T2-weighted mid-sagittal MRI image. Arrow head = the subcutaneous portion of the LDM stalk. The stalk was confirmed intraoperatively to pass through bifid S1 and S2 laminae

Evaluation of FSND

As in all patients with suspected dysraphic lesions, a thorough clinical history and physical examination are paramount to elicit the symptoms and signs of neurological deficits related to the types and spinal level of the lesions, past or active infection, and clues to the existence of associated anomalies. Urological assessment is also essential and should include urinalysis, ultrasonography of the urinary system, voiding cystourethrogram, and urodynamic studies.

MRI is the imaging technique of choice to delineate the details of the pathological anatomy of the various malformations. 3T MRI may especially be informative for composite lesions [63]. MRI findings suggestive of FSND are as follows: (1) A tract linking the skin and the spinal cord even it does not appear continuous (Figs. 5, 6, 7 and 11); (2) posteriorly tacked-up spinal cord (Figs. 11, 12, 14, 15 and 16); and (3) a cystic lesion over the dorsal midline (Figs. 8, 13, 18, 22, 23 and 24). When FSND is suspected on the MRI, the entire path of the tract must be traced from the skin through subcutaneous tissue, lamina, dura, and to the spinal cord. The constituents of the tract are interpreted as much as possible (Fig. 46). Any cyst along its course or in the vicinity is particularly noted (Figs. 8, 13, 18, 22, 23 and 24), as is the presence of any associated anomalies especially spinal cord lipoma and split cord malformation. Lastly, the whole spinal axis should be surveyed for the rare coexistence of multiple FSNDs in the same spine (Fig. 47).

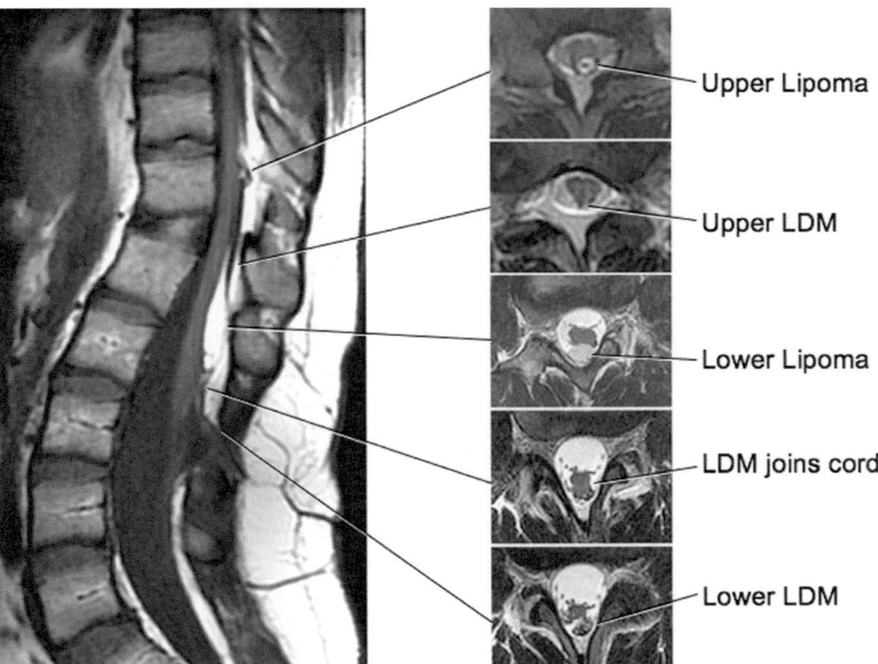

Fig. 47 Double LDMs, both crater type, with accompanying dorsal lipomas. The lower LDM is at $L_{2/3}$, and upper LDM is at T_{12}. Both accompanying lipomas are just rostral to the LDM stalk

However, in spite of it being the mainstay of investigation, the reliability of MRI in delineating FSNDs is far from absolute. For example, a small tract can be below its resolution (Fig. 6) [53, 64], and it cannot always differentiate a CSDST from a LDM, except when the CSDST becomes inflamed and exhibit abnormal enhancement of the tract, the wall of a constituent cyst, or the adjacent meninges (Fig. 5) [52]. All are essential information for surgical planning.

Management of FSND

All FSNDs can cause functional impairment by tethering of the spinal cord, while CSDST or any of its mixed forms pose the additional risks of inflammation, infection, mass effect, and even secondary hydrocephalus if left untreated. Early surgery should be performed in all patients with CSDST and in symptomatic patients with LDM. In asymptomatic children with pure LDM, we also strongly recommend surgery to obviate the dreadful consequences of late and unrecognized neurological deterioration especially involving bladder function. Observation by serial MRI is probably only suitable for patients with equivocal MRI findings or perhaps in asymptomatic adults.

For CSDST patients with active infection and neurological deficits, urgent surgery covered with appropriate antibiotics should be done. However, if infection is not accompanied by neurological deficits, surgery should be deferred until the infection has been treated with antibiotics and local therapy.

Surgery

The main aims of surgery in all FSNDs are to completely untether the spinal cord and to remove all epithelial elements if present. For pure forms, a narrow laminectomy for exposure is usually adequate. Laminoplasty is an option, and dural grafting is rarely necessary. In cases with a large intradural dermoid cyst, however, wider bony exposure is usually needed. The extent of longitudinal exposure must include the span between the skin lesion and where the tract joins the spinal cord, which is usually apparent on MRI where the cord outline suddenly becomes trapezoid instead of the normal ovoid. In uncertain cases, the skin should be widely draped to accommodate for extension of the incision. If the lesion is in the lumbosacral region, the filum terminale may be thickened and should be cut during treatment of the FSND, so that appropriate provision must be made for more caudal exposure.

Surgical Technique for CSDST

The patient is put in a prone position, the sinus ostium identified, and the laminae of the planned laminectomy confirmed with fluoroscopy (Fig. 48). A standard midline longitudinal skin incision with a small elliptical island around the ostium is made.

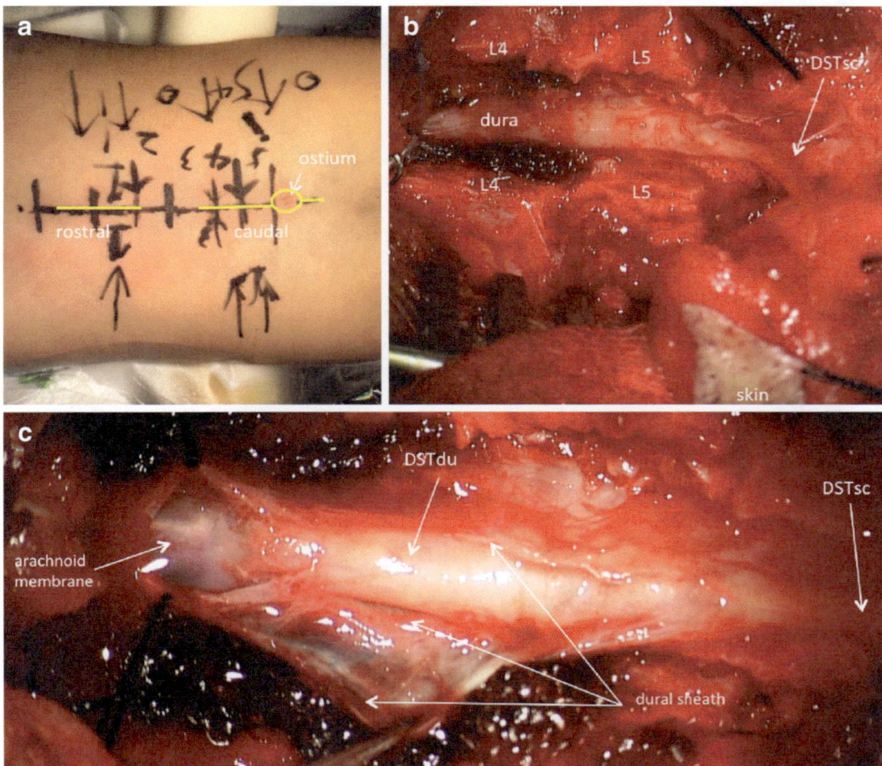

Fig. 48 Intra-operative photographs showing excision of a dermal sinus tract (DST) with skip laminectomy technique (MRI images of this patient are shown in Figs. 4 and 5). (**b–g**) Caudal. (**h–k**) Rostral wound. (**a**) Skin preparation. Yellow lines = skin incisions. Numbers in black on skin = levels of lumbar spinous processes. (**b**) L4L5 laminectomy has been done. The subcutaneous portion of the DST (DSTsc) merging with the dura has been fully exposed. (**c**) Photography taken after opening the dural sheath enveloping a portion of DST that is lying in the dura mater (DSTdu). (**d**) Photography showing the arachnoid membrane entry site of the DST. (**e**) After opening the arachnoid membrane, the intradural portion of the DST (DSTintradural) and keratin material are seen. (**f**) The DSTdu has been removed. The DSTintradural is seen adhering to the filum. (**g**) The caudal portion of the DST has been completely removed via the L4L5 laminectomy. (**h, i**) Operative exposure via a T12L1 laminectomy. (**h**) is the T12 side of the exposure; (**i**) the L1 side. A dermoid cyst along a slender DST (DSTrostral) is shown in (**i**). The DSTrotral was then cut at the yellow cross, and the cyst with the portion of DST under the intact L2 and L3 laminae delivered from this exposure. The sub-millimetre thickness of the DST testifies to the difficulty in detecting them with MRI. (**j, k**) Complete removal of the deep end of the DST from the dorsal midline of the spinal cord

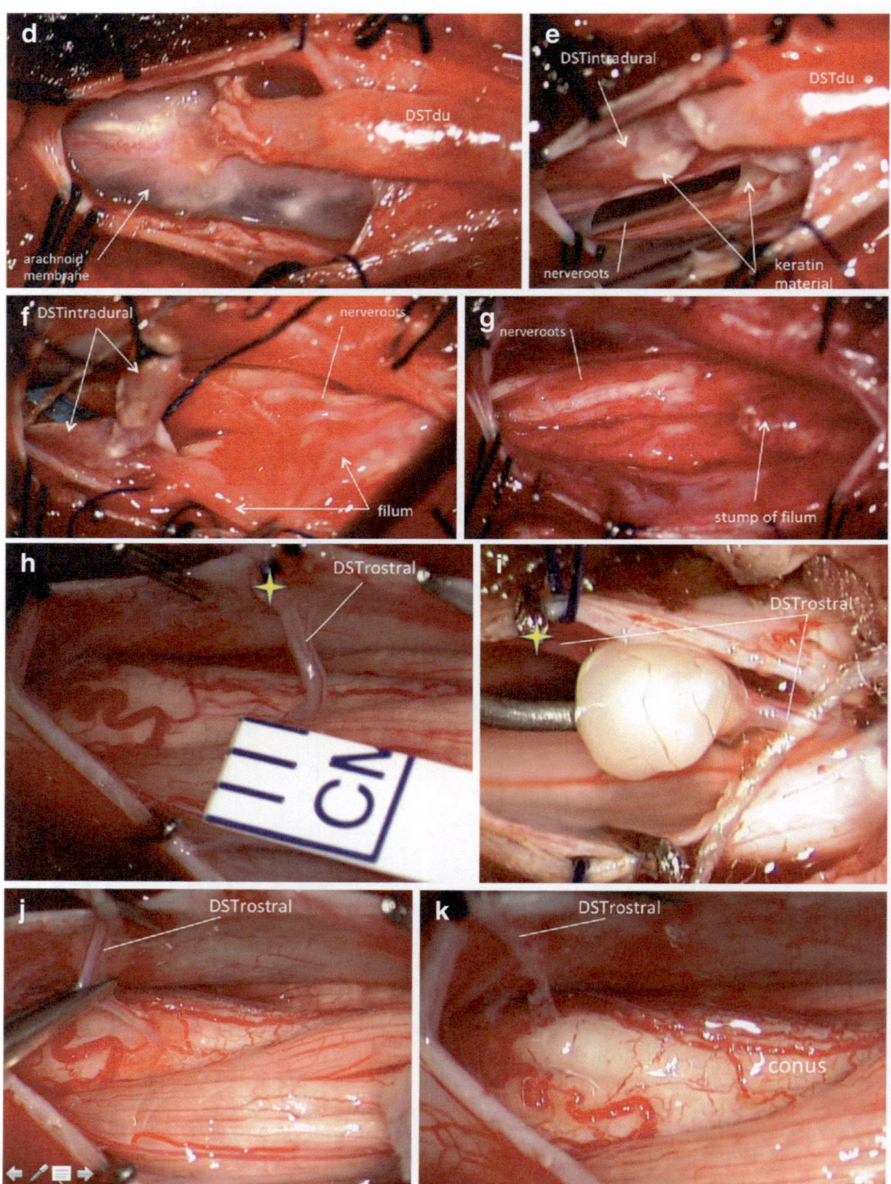

Fig. 48 (continued)

The tract is then traced from superficial to deep through the subcutaneous layers and deep fascia, to reach the bifid spinous process or through the interspinous ligament. The laminectomy is then carried out carefully around the tract. Dissection of the tract should be done under magnification to minimize the possibility of leaving behind residuum [52]. The dura should always be opened unless the surgeon is absolutely certain that the tract ends outside the dura. When the tract goes intradural, a cuff of dura needs to be excised with the tract, and the tract should be traced to its terminal end on the spinal cord. Often the tract becomes attenuated and loosely perches on the surface of the cord. Adequate bony exposure must be done without compromise to display the full extent of the tract. If a long tract truly spans many laminar levels, skip laminectomy technique should be considered in which some laminae between the tract's dural entry point and its spinal cord attachment site are strategically kept intact. The whole CSDST tract can be carefully delivered through the laminectomy gaps after its deep intradural attachments are completely freed (Fig. 49). In most cases, primary closure of the dura usually suffices.

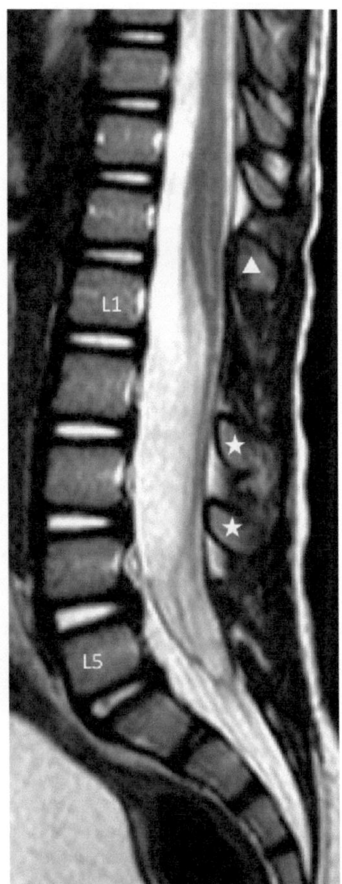

Fig. 49 Mid-sagittal MRI image showing the post-operative appearance of a skip laminectomy technique in which T12 laminoplasty, L1 laminectomy, and L4L5 laminectomy were done. White triangle = laminoplasty level. White star = intact laminae level

The sinus tract may expand along its course or terminate in an epidermoid or dermoid cyst. Cysts located extradurally are readily excised. For large intradural cysts, refined microsurgical techniques are required for their complete removal since the cyst wall is notoriously adherent to nerve roots and the pia (Figs. 50 and 51). Microbial cultures from adjacent areas should be obtained, and post-operative antibiotics should be given until negative growth is confirmed.

Surgical Technique for Flat LDM

The surgical strategy for flat LDMs is akin to that for CSDST. Following a standard midline skin incision, the pit or skin crater is excised and the stalk at the base of the skin lesion is carefully dissected out and traced through the defects in the myofascial layers, laminae or interspinous ligament (Fig. 52a). To provide good exposure of the stalk-spinal cord junction for a safe excision, at least one level of laminectomy both rostral and caudal to the stalk-spinal cord merge point should be planned (Fig. 52b). Again, if the stalk spans multiple levels, the skip laminectomy technique is desirable.

A midline durotomy is made, centred upon the dural entry of the fibroneural stalk, and extended according to the track of the stalk as shown on the MRI. The

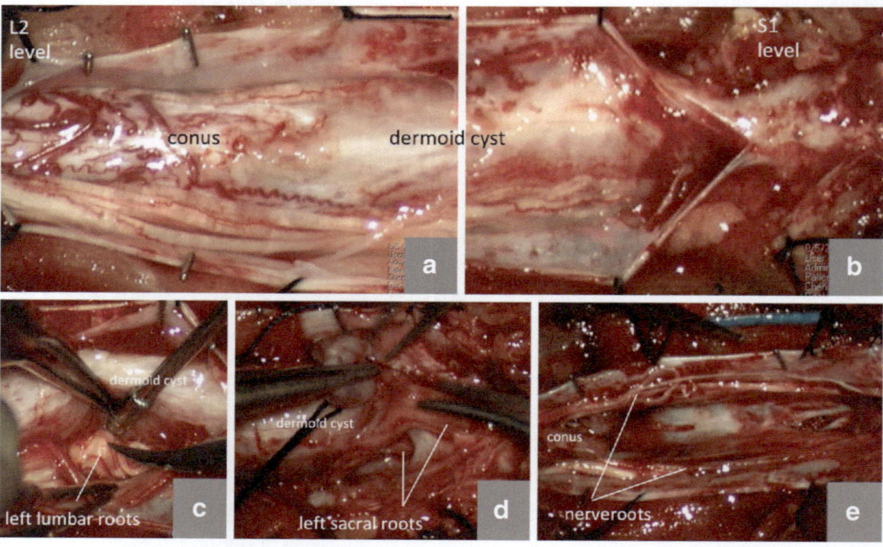

Fig. 50 Intra-operative photographs showing complete excision of an intradural dermoid cyst via L2–L5 laminoplasties and S1 laminectomy (MRI images are shown in Fig. 8). (**a, b**) Surgical view after opening of dura. The dermoid cyst appears to merge with the conus and nerve roots. The dermoid cyst communicates with the skin ostium via a dermal sinus tract at the S1 laminar level. (**c, d**) Dissection to free the nerve roots from the wall of the dermoid cyst. (**e**) Excision cavity after complete excision of the dermoid cyst

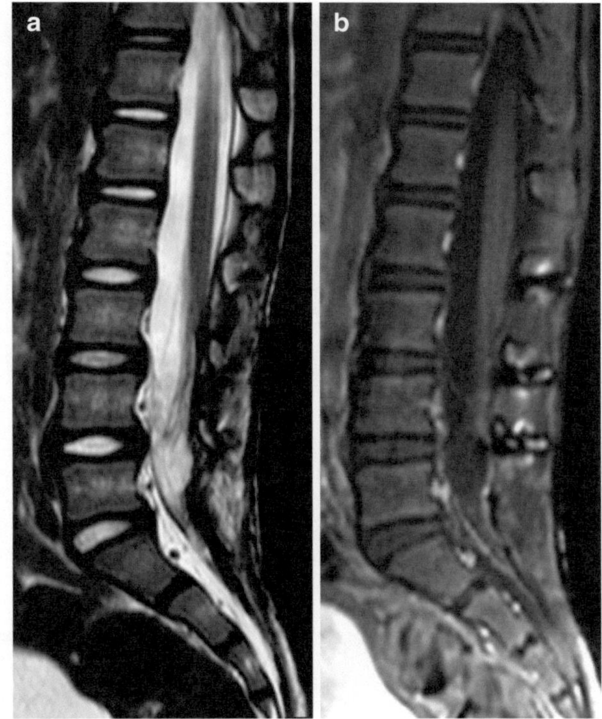

Fig. 51 6-year post-operative MRI images (of the patient shown in Figs. 8 and 50) showing no recurrence of the dermoid cyst and post-laminoplasty changes. (**a**) T2-weighted MRI. (**b**) T1-weighted MRI with gadolinium injection

usually slender stalk is most often attached to a discrete linear spot or cleft on the dorsal midline of the cord at the merge point (Fig. 52c). It is simply cut flush with the cord surface (Fig. 52d, e). Any peripheral nerve twigs, blood vessels, and fibrous bands encircling the neural stalk are similarly cut. Once the intradural stalk had been disconnected from the cord, the entire stalk with its skin appendage is resected en bloc (Fig. 52f).

The LDM stalk may be exceedingly slender and attaches to the cord in a small confined midline scar (Fig. 53), or the stalk flares out into a wider hold on the cord so that the cut edge on the cord resembles a gaping fish mouth (Fig. 54). The stalk may also contain a glomus of vascular channels (Fig. 55), or its deep end expands into tentacles of blood vessels that sprawl on the cord surface (Fig. 56a, b). Rarely, the stalk attachment is stout and deceptively complex, and the dorsal roots surround it like a cuff (Fig. 57a, b). These attachments are cut flush as above, but sparing the surrounding nerve root, to reveal a large base of raw spinal cord (Fig. 57b). Rarely, it is necessary to approximate the pial edges of the large raw bed of a pure LDM to eliminate a potentially adherent surface susceptible to re-tethering (Fig. 58). The dura can usually be closed primarily.

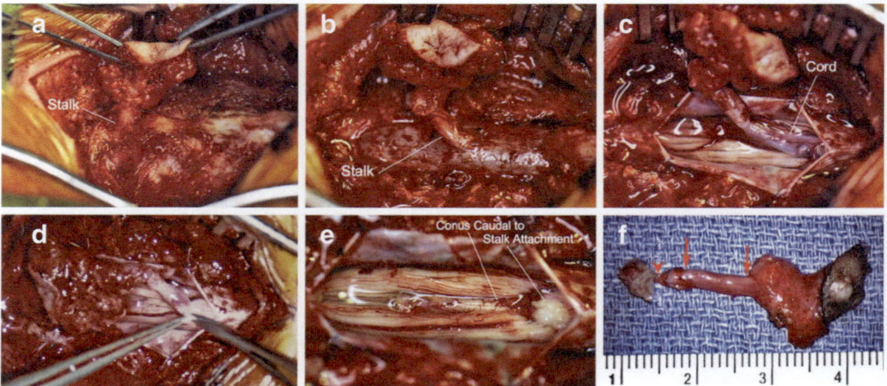

Fig. 52 Surgical resection of a lumbar crater-type flat (non-saccular) LDM. (**a**) Ellipse of resected skin crater and subcutaneous tract going through defect in lumbodorsal fascia. (**b**) Extradural stalk and dural fistula. (**c**) Intradural exposure showing stalk-cord union. (**d**) Resection of stalk flush with cord surface. (**e**) Normal conus caudal to stalk attachment site. (**f**) En bloc specimen showing, from right to left, skin ellipse bearing pale epithelial crater, the subcutaneous portion bearing fat, the extradural portion of the stalk (between arrows), intradural stalk (between arrow and arrow head), and an exuberant cuff of tissue on the cord

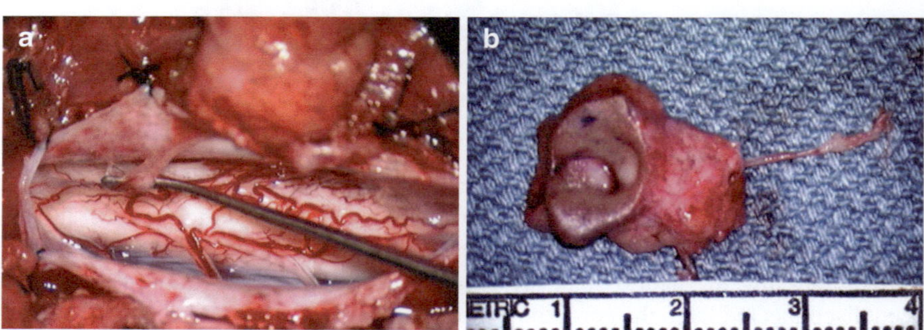

Fig. 53 Exceedingly slender LDM stalk: (**a**) Stalk attaches to discrete spot on dorsal cord surface. (**b**) En bloc specimen shows large complicated skin crater and the very slender LDM stalk

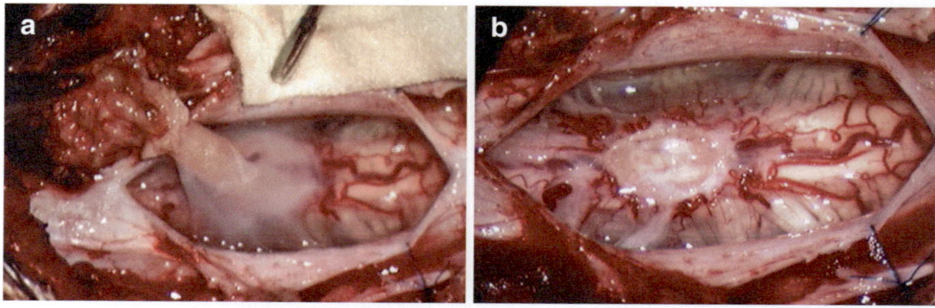

Fig. 54 Moderate-sized LDM stalk: (**a**) stalk has a flared-out cord attachment. (**b**) Stalk resection leaves a fish-mouth shaped scar

Fig. 55 Long LDM stalk with vascular glomus (at tip of forceps)

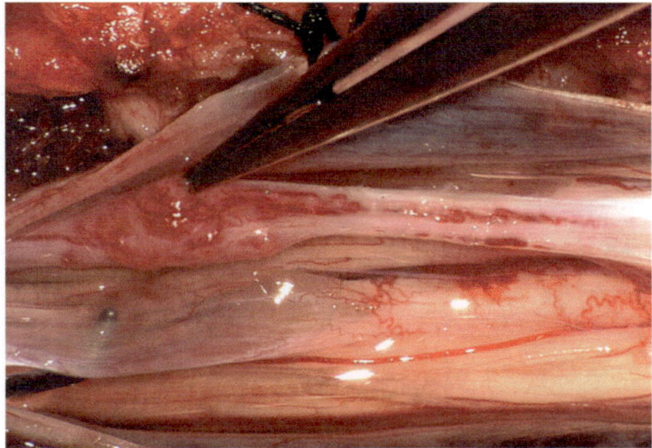

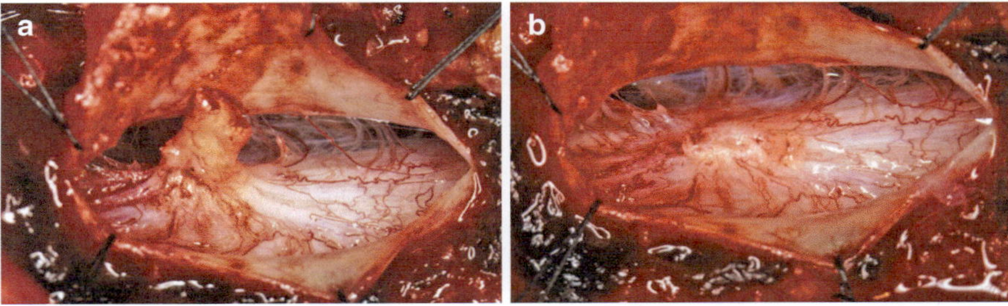

Fig. 56 Moderately thick LDM stalk with exuberant tentacles of blood vessels that seem to crawl on to the dorsal surface of the spinal cord. (**a**) Before LDM resection. (**b**) After LDM stalk resection showing centripetal distribution of the blood vessels

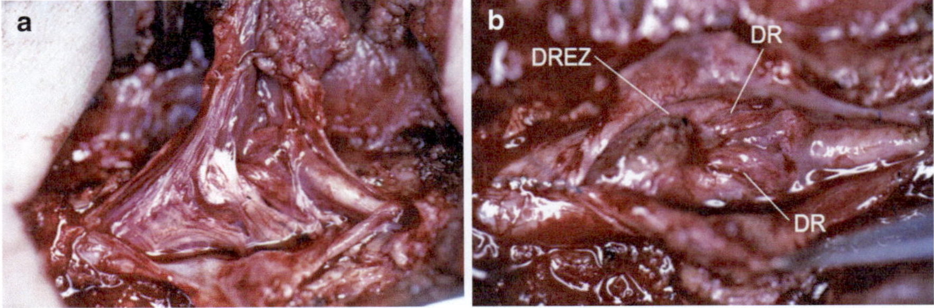

Fig. 57 Thick, complex-looking fibroneural stalk in a lumbar non-saccular LDM: (**a**) Lesion contains dysplastic spinal cord tissue, large blood vessels, ample skein of non-functioning nerves, and thickened folded membranes. Spinal cord is lifted dorsally by the tethering effect. (**b**) Bizarre arrangement of dorsal roots (DR) and dorsal root entry zone (DREZ) surround a large flat myeloschistic scar after stalk resection

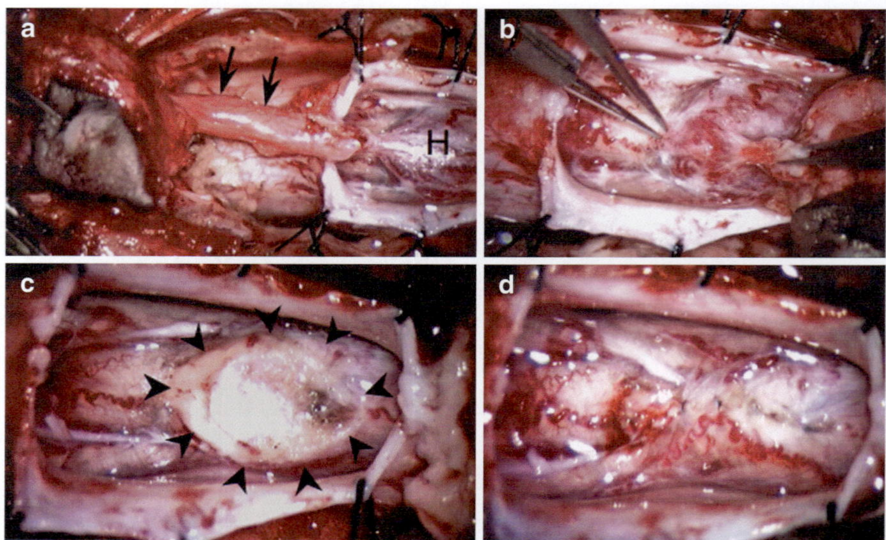

Fig. 58 Crater type lumbar LDM: (**a**) lumbar LDM stalk (arrows) with a very prominent hump (H) of abnormal tissues on the cord. (**b**) Resection at the base of this hump. (**c**) Resection produced a very large scar (outlined by arrowheads). (**d**) Dorsal pia-to-pia approximation of scar with 8-O nylon sutures

Surgical Technique for Saccular LDMs

The operative technique for tackling the internal structures of LDMs is basically the same whether the LDM is saccular or flat. The minor differences between handling the two types lay in the initial superficial soft tissue dissection. For the saccular LDMs, a large skin ellipse is made at the sessile base of the sac to expose the dural funnel where the narrow dural fistula fans out to form the sac at the skin level (Fig. 59a). The dural fistula is then traced to the laminar level as with the flat LDM (Fig. 59b).

For the basal nodule type of saccular LDM, the sac is entered near the base to locate the basal neural nodule (Fig. 59c) and the subjacent fibroneural stalk within the dural fistula, where it is traced to its attachment to the cord and removed (Fig. 59d, e). Saccular LDMs with very thick stalks that traverse the sac to reach the dome are exposed from the spinal cord side up towards the top (Fig. 60). The base of the stalk is then disconnected from the cord surface. In large saccular lesions with slender stalks that may be hard to find, the sac is opened at the dome and the fibroneural stalk is located at the base of the abnormal skin crater and then traced back to the spinal cord surface where it is transected (Fig. 61). In saccular LDM with segmental myelocystoceles, the stalk may be longer than expected and its cut end

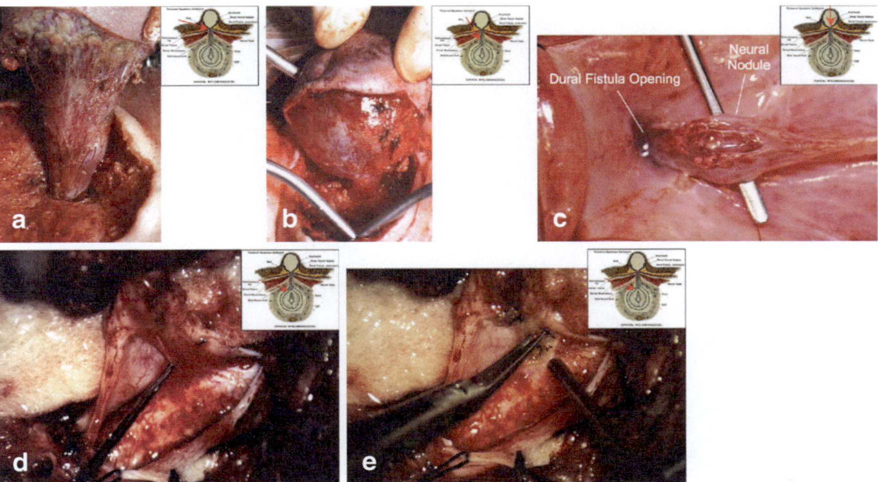

Fig. 59 Large cervical saccular LDM. (**a**) Exposure of the dorsal fistula at the level of the nuchal fascial defect. (**b**) The neck of the sac passing through large laminar defect. (**c**) The sac is opened from the top; basal neural nodule and the dural fistula opening (into the cyst) are seen through the cavity. (**d**) Dural fistula opened into the main thecal sac, showing the thin fibroneural stalk inserting on to the dorsal spinal cord. (**e**) Stalk being resected. All insets show exact level of the exposure

Fig. 60 Thoracic saccular LDM with the fibroneural stalk (displayed by instrument) traversing the sac cavity and reaching the dome of the sac

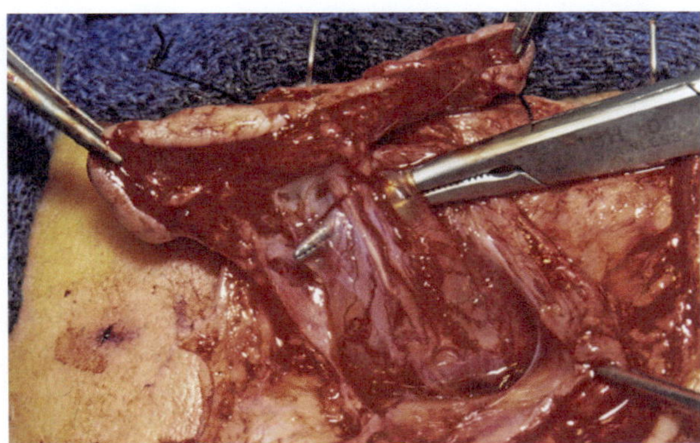

can often be traced directly into the hydromyelic cavity of the cord (Figs. 62 and 63). The defunct portion of the extruded neural "trumpet" near its origination point on the "parent" cord, after verification of no-function with intraoperative electrophysiology, can then be resected sharply from the cord surface, whose gaping cut edges are then neurulated with 8–0 nylon microsutures.

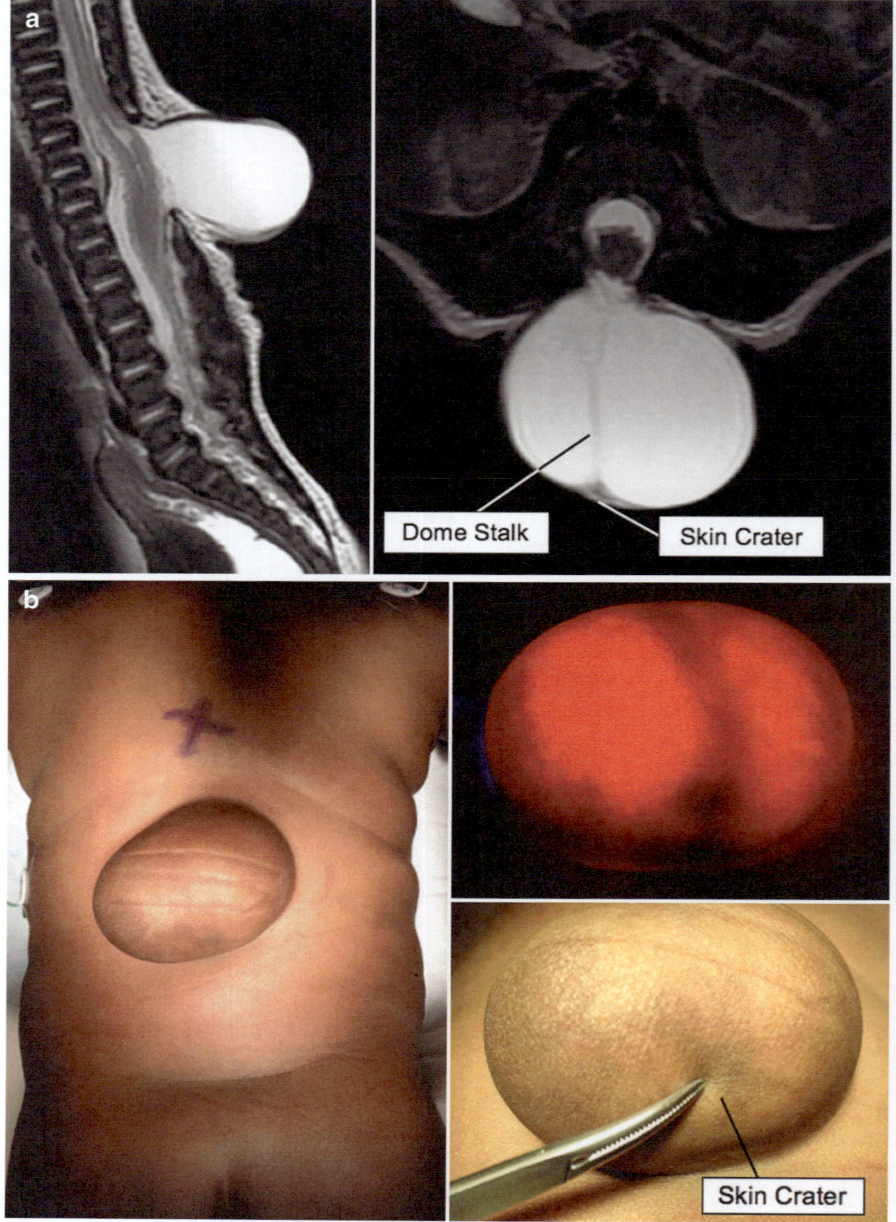

a
Dome Stalk
Skin Crater
b
Skin Crater

Fig. 61 Saccular LDM with the stalk-to-dome subtype of fibroneural stalk attachment. (**a**) T_2 MR shows slight tenting of the cord towards the sac on the sagittal image, and the fibroneural stalk (Dome stalk) traversing the sac to the cord from the base of the skin crater in the axial image. (**b**) The sac with the slightly darker irregular skin at the lower dome with a slightly thinner covering (skin crater, lower right) that may be thick squamous epithelium. The transilluminated picture (upper right) shows the small nubbin of (neural) tissue beneath the skin crater and the stream of bands traversing the middle of the sac. (**c**) Shows the wide neck of the dural fistula at the base of the sac, and its relationship with the cord dura. (**d**) Sac opened from the top, showing the white area where the LDM stalk attaches to the cord surface. (**e**) Close-up to show the strands of the LDM stalk inserting on the dorsal cord surface (upper). After resecting these strands (lower), the cord surface shows abnormal clusters of wiggly blood vessels and scar tissue

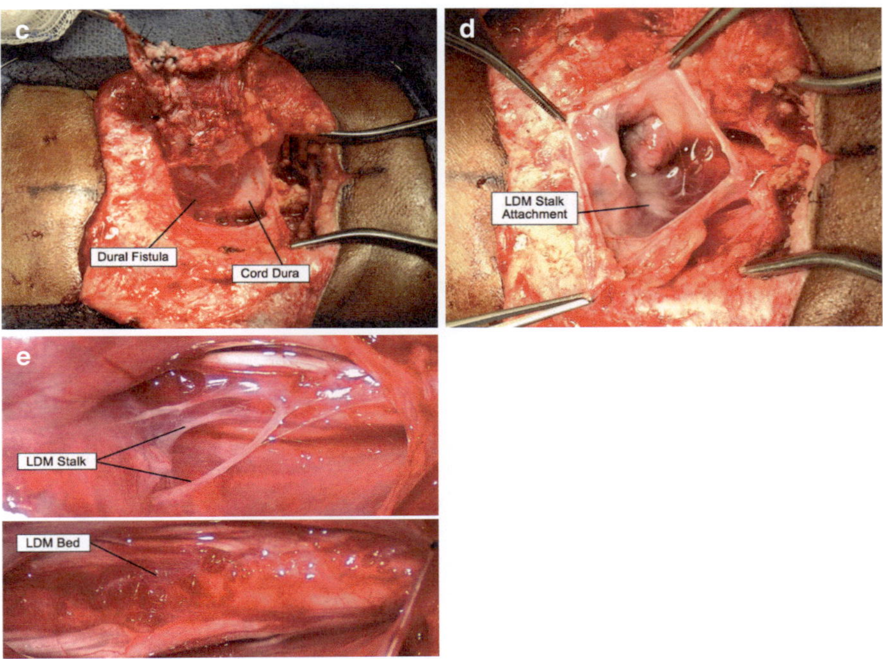

Fig. 61 (continued)

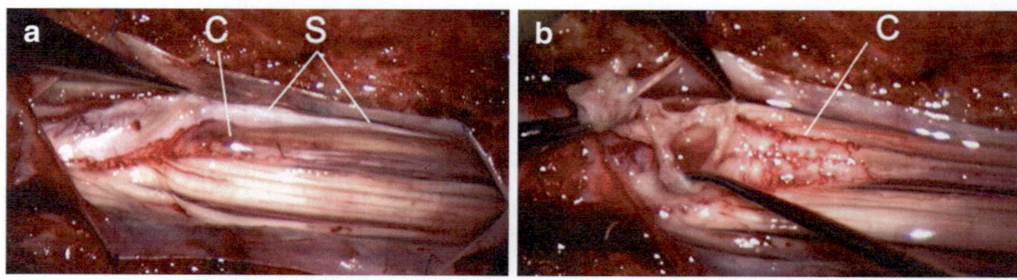

Fig. 62 Lumbar saccular LDM with segmental myelocystocele. (**a**) A long intradural stalk (S) picked up by micro-forceps. (**b**) Stalk traced to the hydromyelic portion of the cord after partial stalk resection. *C* conus

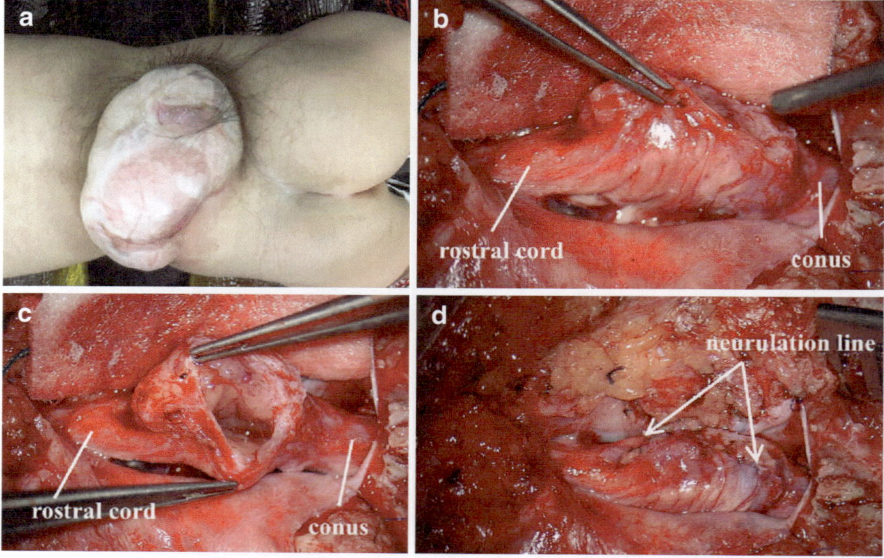

Fig. 63 Intraoperative photos of the case shown in Fig. 20. (**a**) A large skin-based sac with pearly epithelium, and hypertrichosis around the base of the sac. (**b**) The non-functional top of the cystocele has been cut off leaving the functional base with nerve roots. (**c**) Operative view looking through the neck of the cystocele into the hydromyelic cavity. (**d**) After neurulation closure of the myelocystocele neck

Surgical Technique for FSNDs Associated with Other Anomalies

The operative strategy for these composite lesions is predominately the specific techniques suitable for the associated malformations combined with the above techniques for FSNDs (Figs. 64 and 65) [1, 2, 65]. The most important point is to ensure total extirpation of any dermal elements in a lesion, complex or simple.

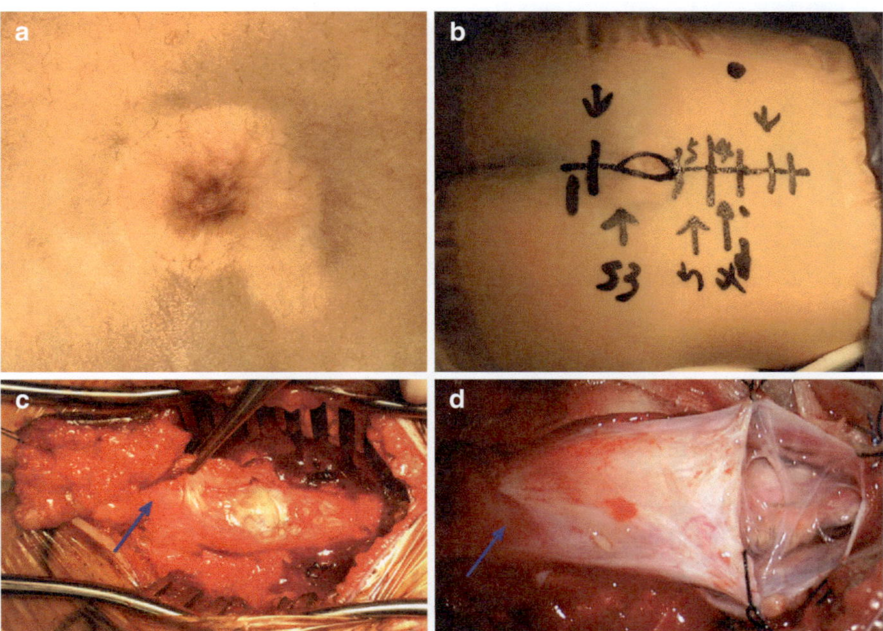

Fig. 64 Intra-operative photographs showing the excision of a LDM—lipoma complex (MRI images are shown in Fig. 46). (**a**) The skin lesion, a cigar burn crater with surrounding skin discoloration. (**b**) Markings for the skin incision. (**c**) Surgical exposure after L4–S2 laminectomies. (**d**) The dura has been opened. (**e**) Surgical exposure after completion of "crotch dissection". (**f**) Detaching the stout LDM stalk and lipoma from the spinal cord. (**g**) Residual fat on the placode before final trimming. (**h**) Appearance of the spinal cord after neurulation. The nerve roots at the end of the spinal cord were stimulation positive. Blue arrow = Extradural portion of the LDM. The patient has no neurological deficits before and after the untethering surgery

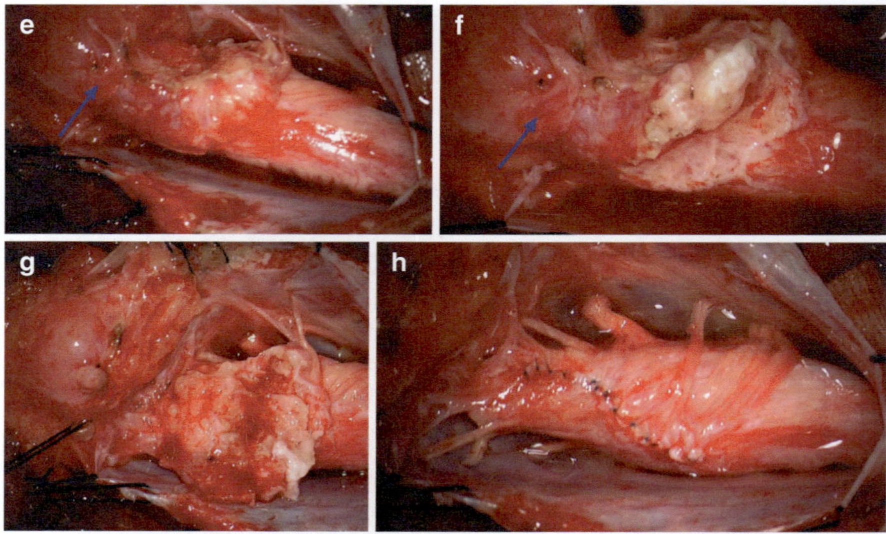

Fig. 4.64 (continued)

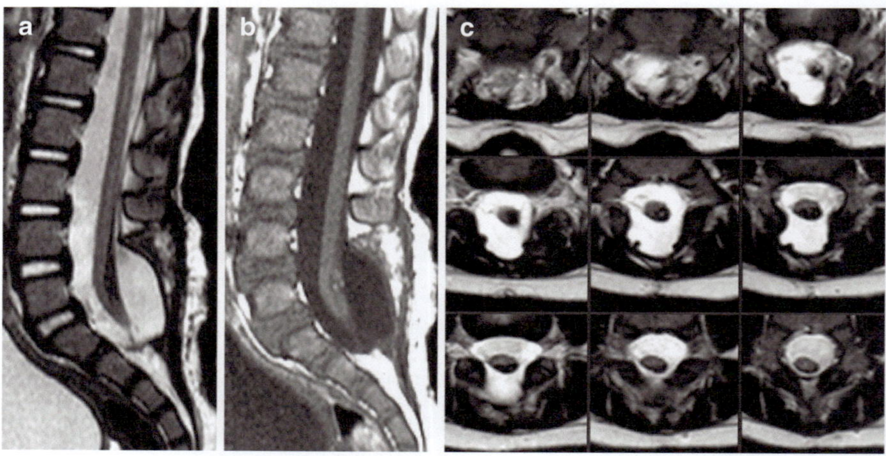

Fig. 65 Post-operative MRI images of the patient shown in Fig. 64. (**a**) T2-weighed sagittal MRI image showing a cord-sac ratio of 33%. (**b**) T1-weighted sagittal MRI image. (**c**) Serial T2-weighted axial MRI images showing the spinal cord completely surrounded by cerebrospinal fluid

Table 4 Pre-operative, 3-month post-operative, and 1-year post-operative neurological grades in LDM patients grouped against LDM location

LDM location	Pre-operative grade				Post-operative grade							
					3 months				1 year			
	0	1	2	3	0	1	2	3	0	1	2	3
Cervical (11)	4	4	3	0	4	5	2	0	7	4	0	0
Thoracic upper (9)	2	6	1	0	3	6	0	0	6	3	0	0
Thoracic lower (7)	4	2	0	1	4	2	1	0	4	2	1	0
Thoracolumbar (8)	4	3	0	1	4	3	1	0	5	3	0	0
Lumbar (28)	15	8	3	2	17	6	4	1	20	7	0	1
Total number of patients (63)	29	23	7	4	31	22	8	1	41	19	1	1

From Pang et al. (2013), [2]

Neurological grading system in LDM. **Grade 0**: No deficits or symptoms. **Grade 1**: Mild upper or lower extremity weakness, or pure sensory deficits +/− pain. **Grade 2**: Moderate to severe upper or lower extremity weakness ± sensory deficits, or neurogenic bladder without weakness. **Grade 3**: Upper or lower extremity weakness + neurogenic bladder

Clinical Outcomes of FSND

The clinical status at presentation dictates the clinical outcome of FSNDs. With proper surgical techniques, surgery for FSNDs without large intradural dermoid/epidermoid cysts is usually uncomplicated. Recurrence of dermal elements and re-tethering should be extremely rare; and most FSND patients without neurological deficits remain neurologically intact after surgery [1, 2, 12, 66]. Over two thirds of patients with pre-operative neurological deficits improve after surgery; about one third will not improve though remain stable (Table 4) [1, 17, 66]. In CSDST patients with large intradural dermoid/epidermoid cysts or active infections, the results are less salubrious [5, 51, 66]. These statistics thus highlight the importance of early detection and prompt surgical intervention in FSNDs.

Conclusion

Grasping the salient events in normal neuroembryology has enabled us to recognize and systematically categorize FND malformations, which can present with diverse clinico-radiological manifestations. Knowing the embryogenetic mechanisms of the subtypes of FND malformations helps us to unravel their complex pathological anatomy and visualize their basic configuration, thus allowing us to tackle them safely and effectively in the operating theatre.

Deeper knowledge about the molecular-genetic milieu of non-disjunctional malformations will almost certainly give us new insights into their biological behaviours, but carefully planned and executed surgery will remain the only appropriate remedy in the foreseeable future.

References

1. Pang D, Zovickian J, Oviedo A, Moes GS. Limited dorsal myeloschisis: a distinctive clinico-pathological entity. Neurosurgery. 2010;67:1555–80.
2. Pang D, Zovickian J, Wong ST, Hou YJ, Moes GS. Limited dorsal myeloschisis: a not-so-rare form of primary neurulation defect. Childs Nerv Syst. 2013;29:1459–84.
3. O'Rahilly R, Müller F. Neurulation in the normal human embryo. Ciba Found Symp. 1994;181:70–82.
4. Müller F, O'Rahilly R. The development of the human brain, the closure of the caudal neuropore, and the beginning of secondary neurulation at stage 12. Anat Embryol (Berl). 1987;176(4):413–30.
5. Wong ST, Kan A, Pang D. Limited dorsal spinal nondisjunctional disorders: limited dorsal myeloschisis, congenital spinal dermal sinus tract, and mixed lesions. In: Di Rocco C, Pang D, Rutka J, editors. Textbook of pediatric neurosurgery. Cham: Springer; 2019. https://doi.org/10.1007/978-3-319-31512-6_110-1.
6. Wong ST, Pang D. Focal spinal nondisjunction in primary neurulation. J Korean Neurosurg Soc. 2021;64(2):151–88.
7. Cornips EM, Weber JW, Vles JS, van Aalst J. Pseudo-dermal sinus tract or spinal dermal-sinus-like stalk? Childs Nerv Syst. 2011;27:1189–91.
8. Eibach S, Moes G, Zovickian J, Pang D. Limited dorsal myeloschisis associated with dermoid elements. Childs Nerv Syst. 2017;33:55–67.
9. Elton S, Oakes WJ. Dermal sinus tracts of the spine. Neurosurg Focus. 2001;10(1):e4.
10. Lee JY, Park SH, Chong S, Phi JH, Kim SK, Cho BK, Wang KC. Congenital dermal sinus and limited dorsal myeloschisis: "spectrum disorders" of incomplete disjunction between cutaneous and neural ectoderms. Neurosurgery. 2019;84:428–34.
11. van Aalst J, Beuls EA, Cornips EM, van Straaten HW, Boselie AF, Rijkers K, Weber JW, Vles JS. The spinal dermal-sinus-like stalk. Childs Nerv Syst. 2009;25:191–7.
12. Wang KC, Yang HJ, Oh CW, Kim HJ, Cho BK. Spinal congenital dermal sinus—experience of 5 cases over a period of 10 years. J Korean Med Sci. 1993;8:341–7.
13. Colas JF, Schoenwolf GC. Towards a cellular and molecular understanding of neurulation. Dev Dyn. 2001;221:117–45.
14. O'Rahilly R, Gardner E. The timing and sequence of events in the development of the human nervous system during the embryonic period proper. Z Anat Entwicklungsgesch. 1971;134(1):1–12.
15. Martins-Green M. Origin of the dorsal surface of the neural tube by progressive delamination of epidermal ectoderm and neuroepithelium: implications for neurulation and neural tube defects. Development. 1988;103:687–706.
16. Schoenwolf GC, Smith JL. Mechanisms of neurulation: traditional viewpoint and recent advances. Development. 1990;109:243–70.
17. van Straaten HW, Jaskoll T, Rousseau AM, et al. Raphe of the posterior neural tube in the chick embryo: its closure and reopening as studied in living embryos with a high definition light microscope. Dev Dyn. 1993;198:65–76.
18. Silver MH, Kerns JM. Ultrastructure of neural fold fusion in chick embryos. Scan Electron Microsc. 1978;2:209–15.
19. Schoenwolf GC. On the morphogenesis of the early rudiments of the developing central nervous system. Scan Electron Microsc. 1982;1:289–308.
20. Martins-Green M, Erickson CA. Basal lamina is not a barrier to neural crest cell emigration: documentation by TEM and by immunofluorescent and immunogold labelling. Development. 1987;101:517–33.
21. Wang S, Garcia MD, Lopez AL 3rd, Overbeek PA, Larin KV, Larina IV. Dynamic imaging and quantitative analysis of cranial neural tube closure in the mouse embryo using optical coherence tomography. Biomed Opt Express. 2016;8(1):407–19.

22. Müller F, O'Rahilly R. Somitic-vertebral correlation and vertebral levels in the human embryo. Am J Anat. 1986;177(1):3–19.

23. O'Rahilly R, Müller F. Somites, spinal ganglia, and centra. Enumeration and interrelationships in staged human embryos, and implications for neural tube defects. Cells Tissues Organs. 2003;173(2):75–92.

24. O'Rahilly R, Müller F. The two sites of fusion of the neural folds and the two neuropores in the human embryo. Teratology. 2002;65(4):162–70.

25. Dady A, Havis E, Escriou V, Catala M, Duband JL. Junctional neurulation: a unique developmental program shaping a discrete region of the spinal cord highly susceptible to neural tube defects. J Neurosci. 2014;34(39):13208–21.

26. Eibach S, Moes G, Hou YJ, Zovickian J, Pang D. Unjoined primary and secondary neural tubes: junctional neural tube defect, a new form of spinal dysraphism caused by disturbance of junctional neurulation. Childs Nerv Syst. 2017;33(10):1633–47.

27. O'Rahilly R, Müller F. Bidirectional closure of the rostral neuropore in the human embryo. Am J Anat. 1989;184(4):259–68.

28. Müller F, O'Rahilly R. Cerebral dysraphia (future anencephaly) in a human twin embryo at stage 13. Teratology. 1984;30(2):167–77.

29. O'Rahilly R, Müller F. The embryonic human brain. 3rd ed. Wiley; 2006. p. 337.

30. Hoving EW, Vermeij-Keers C, Mommaas-Kienhuis AM, Hartwig NG. Separation of neural and surface ectoderm after closure of the rostral neuropore. Anat Embryol (Berl). 1990;182(5):455–63.

31. Puelles L, Domenech-Ratto G, Martinez-de-la-Torre M. Location of the rostral end of the longitudinal brain axis: review of an old topic in the light of marking experiments on the closing rostral neuropore. J Morphol. 1987;194(2):163–71.

32. ten Donkelaar HJ, Bekker M, Renier WO, Hori A, Shiota K. Neurulation and neural tube defects. In: Clinical neuroembryology. Berlin: Springer; 2014. https://doi.org/10.1007/978-3-642-54687-7_4.

33. Barkovich AJ, Vandermarck P, Edwards MS, Cogen PH. Congenital nasal masses: CT and MR imaging features in 16 cases. AJNR Am J Neuroradiol. 1991;12(1):105–16.

34. Kim JW, Wang KC, Chong S, Kim SK, Lee JY. Limited dorsal myeloschisis: reconsideration of its embryological origin. Neurosurgery. 2020;86:93–100.

35. Müller F, O'Rahilly R. The prechordal plate, the rostral end of the notochord and nearby median features in staged human embryos. Cells Tissues Organs. 2003;173:1–20.

36. Müller F, O'Rahilly R. The primitive streak, the caudal eminence and related structures in staged human embryos. Cells Tissues Organs. 2004;177:2–20.

37. Quon JL, Grant GA. Commentary: Limited dorsal myeloschisis: reconsideration of its embryological origin. Neurosurgery. 2020;86:E13–4.

38. Selleck MA, Bronner-Fraser M. Origins of the avian neural crest: the role of neural plate–epidermal interactions. Development. 1995;121:525–38.

39. Theveneau E, Mayor R. Neural crest delamination and migration: from epithelium-to-mesenchyme transition to collective cell migration. Dev Biol. 2012;366:34–54.

40. Nikolopoulou E, Galea GL, Rolo A, Greene ND, Copp AJ. Neural tube closure: cellular, molecular and biomechanical mechanisms. Development. 2017;144:552–66.

41. Rolo A, Escuin S, Greene NDE, Copp AJ. Rho GTPases in mammalian spinal neural tube closure. Small GTPases. 2018;9:283–9.

42. Abdul-Aziz NM, Turmaine M, Greene ND, Copp AJ. EphrinA-EphA receptor interactions in mouse spinal neurulation: implications for neural fold fusion. Int J Dev Biol. 2009;53(4):559–68.

43. Yamaguchi Y, Shinotsuka N, Nonomura K, et al. Live imaging of apoptosis in a novel transgenic mouse highlights its role in neural tube closure. J Cell Biol. 2011;195:1047–60.

44. Pang D. Surgical management of spinal dysraphism. In: Fessler R, Sekhar L, editors. Atlas of neurosurgical techniques. New York: Thieme Medical and Scientific Publishers; 2006. p. 729–58.

45. Pang D, Dias M, Ahdab-Barmada M. Split cord malformation part I: a unified theory of embryogenesis for double spinal cord malformation. Neurosurgery. 1992;31:451–80.
46. Pang D, Devadass A, Thompson D. Limited dorsal myeloschisis involving one hemicord of a split cord malformation—a "hemi-LDM". Childs Nerv Syst. 2022;38(11):2223–30.
47. Wong ST, Moes GS, Yam KY, Fong D, Pang D. Intrinsic brainstem neurenteric cyst with extensive squamous metaplasia in a child. J Neurosurg Imaging Tech. 2016;1(1):26–37.
48. Hiraoka A, Morioka T, Murakami N, Suzuki SO, Mizoguchi M. Limited dorsal myeloschisis with no extradural stalk linking to a flat skin lesion: a case report. Childs Nerv Syst. 2018;34:2497–501.
49. Martínez-Lage JF, Almagro MJ, Ferri-Ñiguez B, et al. Spinal dermal sinus and pseudo-dermal sinus tracts: two different entities. Childs Nerv Syst. 2011;27:609–16.
50. van Aalst J, Beuls EA, Cornips EM, Vanormelingen L, Vandersteen M, et al. Anatomy and surgery of the infected dermal sinus of the lower spine. Childs Nerv Syst. 2006;22:1307–15.
51. Girishan S, Rajshekhar V. Rapid onset paraparesis and quadriparesis in patients with intramedullary spinal dermoid cysts: report of 10 cases. J Neurosurg Pediatr. 2016;17:86–93.
52. De Vloo P, Lagae L, Sciot R, Demaerel P, van Loon J, Van Calenbergh F. Spinal dermal sinuses and dermal sinus-like stalks analysis of 14 cases with suggestions for embryologic mechanisms resulting in dermal sinus-like stalks. Eur J Paediatr Neurol. 2013;17:575–84.
53. Tisdall MM, Hayward RD, Thompson DN. Congenital spinal dermal tract: how accurate is clinical and radiological evaluation? J Neurosurg Pediatr. 2015;15:651–6.
54. Pang D, Dias MS. Cervical myelomeningoceles. Neurosurgery. 1993;33:363–72.
55. Steinbok P. Dysraphic lesions of the cervical spinal cord. Neurosurg Clin N Am. 1995;6(2):367–76.
56. Steinbok P, Cochrane DD. The nature of congenital posterior cervical or cervicothoracic midline cutaneous mass lesions. Report of eight cases. J Neurosurg. 1991;75:206–12.
57. Rossi A, Piatelli G, Gandofolo C, Pavanello M, et al. Spectrum of nonterminal myelocystoceles. Neurosurgery. 2006;58:509–15.
58. Suneson A, Kalimo H. Myelocystocele with cerebellar heterotopia. J Neurosurg. 1979;51:392–6.
59. Schoenwolf GC. Observations on closure of the neuropores in the chick embryo. Am J Anat. 1979;155:445–66.
60. Morioka T, Suzuki SO, Murakami N, Mukae N, et al. Surgical histopathology of limited dorsal myeloschisis with flat skin lesion. Childs Nerv Syst. 2019;35:119–28.
61. Morioka T, Suzuki SO, Murakami N, Shimogawa T, et al. Neurosurgical pathology of limited dorsal myeloschisis. Childs Nerv Syst. 2018;34:293–303.
62. Lee JY, Chong S, Choi YH, Phi JH, Cheon JE, Kim SK, Park SH, Kim IO, Wang KC. Modification of surgical procedure for "probable" limited dorsal myeloschisis. J Neurosurg Pediatr. 2017;19:616–9.
63. Asiri A, Dimpudus F, Atcheson N, Al-Najjar A, McMahon K, Kurniawan ND. Comparison between 2D and 3D MEDIC for human cervical spinal cord MRI at 3T. J Med Radiat Sci. 2021;68(1):4–12.
64. Lee SM, Cheon JE, Choi YH, Kim IO, Kim WS, Cho HH, Lee JY, Wang KC. Limited dorsal myeloschisis and congenital dermal sinus: comparison of clinical and MR imaging features. AJNR. 2017;38:176–82.
65. Pang D, Zovickian J, Wong ST, Hou YJ, Moes GS. Surgical treatment of complex spinal cord lipomas. Childs Nerv Syst. 2013;29:1485–513.
66. Ackerman LL, Menezes AH. Spinal congenital dermal sinuses: a 30-year experience. Pediatrics. 2003;112(3 Pt 1):641–7.

Junctional Neural Tube Defect (JNTD): A Rare and Relatively New Spinal Dysraphic Malformation

Sebastian Eibach and Dachling Pang

Abbreviations

EMG	Electromyography
HH	Hamburger et Hamilton
JNTD	Junctional neural tube defect
mA	Milliampere
MET	Mesenchymal-epithelial transition
MRI	Magnetic resonance imaging
NSB	Node streak border
PCP	Planar cell polarity
SSD	Segmental spinal dysgenesis
TcMEP	Transcranial motor evoked potentials

S. Eibach
Department of Clinical Medicine, Faculty of Medicine, Health and Human Sciences, Macquarie University, Sydney, Australia

Paediatric Neurosurgery, Sydney Children's Hospital Randwick, Sydney, Australia

D. Pang (✉)
Great Ormond Street Hospital for Children, NHS Trust, London, UK

Department of Paediatric Neurosurgery, University of California, Davis, USA

© The Author(s), under exclusive license to Springer Nature Switzerland AG 2023
D. Pang, K.-C. Wang (eds.), *Spinal Dysraphic Malformations*, Advances and Technical Standards in Neurosurgery 47,
https://doi.org/10.1007/978-3-031-34981-2_5

Introduction

Junctional neurulation completes the sequential embryological processes of primary and secondary neurulation as the intermediary step linking the end of primary neurulation and the beginning of secondary neurulation. Its exact molecular process is a matter of ongoing scientific debate. Abnormality of junctional neurulation—junctional neural tube defect (JNTD)—was first described in 2017 based on a series of three patients who displayed a well-formed secondary neural tube, the conus, that is physically separated by a fair distance from its companion primary neural tube and functionally disconnected from rostral corticospinal control. Several other cases conforming to this bizarre neural tube arrangement have since appeared in the literature, reinforcing the validity of this entity. The clinical, neuroimaging, and electrophysiological features of JNTD, as well as the hypothesis of its embryogenetic mechanism, will be described in this chapter.

Neurulation

Three fundamentally different embryological processes, primary, secondary and junctional neurulation, form the central neuraxis. Their deficiency causes specific spinal dysraphic malformations, respectively.

Primary neurulation involves dorsal folding and midline fusion of a neuroepithelial plate derived from the ectoderm. Due to continuity of the primitive neural plate with the cutaneous ectoderm, fusion and closure of the neural tube also pre-empts successful closure of the skin and mesodermal tissues. Therefore, complete failure of neural plate closure results in an open neural tube defect. A very focal incomplete closure and spatially confined non-disjunction of the neural and cutaneous ectoderms result in limited dorsal myeloschisis as a diminutive variant within the open defect spectrum [1–3]. Primary neurulation ends with closure of the caudal neuropore, and secondary neurulation begins in chronological sequence with the process of mesenchymal-epithelial transition (MET), consisting of aggregation and transformation of a loosely cellular, pluripotent mesenchymal blastema into tightly adherent, apicobasally polarized epithelial cells [4–8]. The pluripotent mesenchymal blastema is called caudal cell mass in humans [9–11], and tail bud in avians [12–16], rodents [17] and amphibians [18]. Besides the secondary neural tube, the caudal notochord, caudal somites, most of the hind gut and urogenital tract are all derived from the caudal cell mass [9, 19, 20]. Following MET, secondary neurulation in chick and mouse consists of three phases – condensation of neuroprogenitor cells to form the medullary cord, cavitation of the medullary cord, and degenerative regression of most of the caudal medullary cord to form the conus (S_{2-5} spinal cord segments) and the filum terminale [16, 21, 22]. Secondary neurulation failure leads to closed neural tube defects without cutaneous opening, which include complete lack of medullary cord condensation in cases of absent conus and high grade caudal agenesis [23], or failure of regression as in retained medullary cord, terminal myelocystocele, terminal lipoma, and thickened filum terminale [24, 25]. Even though malformation of the conus is the main focus of most secondary neurulation defects, the conus itself is neither functionally nor anatomically disconnected from the primary neural tube.

Like most developmental anomalies, there are also mixed forms of spinal cord malformations that seem to straddle the classic types of primary and secondary neurulation defects and combine characteristics of both. Dorsal spinal cord lipomas, for example, with its normal skin covering unlike most primary neurulation defects, is thought to arise from premature rather than incomplete neural folds fusion and disjunction during primary neurulation. Transitional spinal lipomas consist of a rostral portion identical to a dorsal lipoma but also a conus clearly invaded by adipogenic mesenchyme during secondary neurulation [26].

Junctional Neurulation

The latest adjunct and yet least understood of the neurulation processes is junctional neurulation. During spinal cord development, junctional neurulation is responsible for the fusion and functional connectivity of the rostral primary neural tube with the emerging caudal secondary neural tube. Junctional neurulation therefore takes place chronologically at the end of primary neurulation and the beginning of caudal cell mass transformation.

The process of junctional neurulation varies significantly among species [5]. The chick model appears to be closest to the human spinal cord development. Morphological changes during junctional neurulation in chicks occur between Hamburger-Hamilton (HH) [21] stages 8 and 12 in a region of the neural plate known as the Node-Streak Border (NSB), that is, the area between the rostral Hensen's node and the caudal primitive streak [27, 28]. After HH stage 12, the transient NSB disappears simultaneous with caudal neuropore closure.

At HH stage 8, the NSB contains remnants of the primitive streak medially and Hensen's node laterally. As dorsal folding of the primary neural plate ends, Hensen's node regresses. The distribution of neuroprogenitor cells at the NSB can be traced with in situ hybridization for SOX-2 as an early neuronal marker normally found in cells of the neural plate in the primary neural tube. Within the NSB, SOX-2 positive cells are lined up dorsolaterally in continuity with the caudal tip of the primary neural tube, whereas immediately caudally, the ventromedially located SOX-2 negative cells represent remnants of the primitive streak. As junctional neurulation proceeds from HH 8 to 12, these ventromedial cells become SOX-2 positive, suggesting neuronal differentiation. DiI microcrystal fluorescence tracking of cells at the NSB shows the dorsolateral cell population undergo dorsal folding followed by midline fusion as expected for primary neural tube closure, whereas the ventromedial cells migrate caudally to give rise to the secondary neural tube [29]. The medial SOX-2 negative cell population initially expresses Snail-2, Bmp-4 and

N-cadherin instead of E-cadherin, indicative of mesodermal progenitor cells undergoing epithelium-to-mesenchyme transition [30–32], but soon these same cells migrate caudally and start expressing SOX-2, evidence of their final commitment to form neuroprogenitor cells which ultimately become the rostral-most portion of the secondary neural tube overlapped by the dorsally located tip of the primary neural tube at the junctional zone [29].

Multifactorial causes for neurulation defects are discussed in the literature, and specific gene mutations play a crucial role. For example, the Sonic Hedgehog signalling pathway is involved in the bending of the neural plate, and the Planar Cell Polarity (PCP) pathway in the initiation of neural tube closure [33, 34]. Genes within the PCP pathway like *Prickle-1*, *Flamingo*, *Scrib* and *Vangl-2* are essential for a process called convergent extension [35, 36], which involves morphological cellular changes along the medio-lateral and cranio-caudal axes in cell-to-cell intercalation. The *Prickle-1* gene may have a crucial role in junctional neurulation, since it is expressed mainly at the NSB and within the elongating caudal neural tube [37].

Junctional Neural Tube Defect

Since our first description of the entity junctional neural tube defect (JNTD) in 2017 [38] in three patients, more cases of JNTD appeared in the literature [39–41]. Detailed patient data of six published cases are summarized in Table 1. The common features of all six cases include the absence of an open skin defect, a well-formed and neurologically functioning primary neural tube at or above the L_5 spinal cord segment, complete urinary incontinence, a hypertonic bladder and anal sphincter, partial sacral agenesis and various other forms of caudal cell mass malformations. A perfectly formed conus is present but anatomically widely separated from the "primary" spinal cord and functionally unconnected to the rest of the central neuraxis derived from the primary neural tube including the cerebral cortex. Nevertheless, the conus locally shows active reflex circuits measurable by electrophysiology (see below).

Clinical Presentation

In our own series, none of the patients had any cutaneous stigmata typically seen with primary neurulation defects. The dominant symptom of two patients was club feet, one diagnosed in utero, the other postnatally. All three patients presented with delayed ability to walk at age 2 years due to lower extremity weakness and foot deformity. Two patients also had congenital scoliosis.

Motor functions corresponding to the L_5 and S_1 spinal cord segments (i.e. within the terminal primary spinal cord) were compromised to some degree but present in

Table 1 Published cases of junctional neural tube defect

Case	Author	Age [years]	sex	Cutaneous sign	Presenting symptom	"Primary spinal cord"/ conus level	Motor function	Sensation	External anal sphincter function	Kidney U/S or urodynamics	Spinal deformity/ malformation
1	Eibach et al.	8	M	None	Scoliosis, delayed walking, primary urinary incontinence	L_1/ $L_{3\text{-}4}$	L_5, S_1 weakness; absent toe flaring (S_2); positive BCR	Hypesthesia $L_5 + S_1$; anaesthesia $S_{2\text{-}4}$	Hypertonic sphincter, no voluntary contraction	Hydronephrosis	Hemivertebrae $T_{12} + L_3$, partial sacral agenesis scoliosis
2	Eibach et al.	13	F	None	Club feet in utero, primary urinary incontinence	$T_{12}\text{-}L_1$/ $S_{1\text{-}2}$	Weakness caudal to L_5, decreased hip abduction and flaccid feet; absent toe flaring (S_2)	Hypesthesia $L_5 + S_1$; anaesthesia $S_{2\text{-}4}$	Hypertonic sphincter, no voluntary contraction, clonic contractions of anal sphincter to perianal stimulation	Resolved hydronephrosis, Detrusor hyperreflexia, DSD, spastic, small capacity, heavily trabeculated bladder	Lumbo-sacral vertebral segmentation failure
3	Eibach et al.	30	F	None	Club feet, scoliosis, primary urinary incontinence	T_{11}/ $L_5\text{-}S_1$	L_5, S_1 weakness; absent toe flaring (S_2)	Hypesthesia $L_5 + S_1$; anaesthesia $S_{2\text{-}4}$	Hypertonic sphincter, no voluntary contraction	Detrusor hyperreflexia, DSD, spastic, small capacity, heavily trabeculated bladder	Partial sacral agenesis, scoliosis

(continued)

Table 1 (continued)

Case	Author	Age [years]	sex	Cutaneous sign	Presenting symptom	"Primary spinal cord"/ conus level	Motor function	Sensation	External anal sphincter function	Kidney U/S or urodynamics	Spinal deformity/ malformation
4	Schmidt et al.	Newborn	M	None	Anorectal atresia	T_{11}/ L_2	Normal newborn movements	Normal	Ano-rectal atresia	Normal U/S, no urodynamics	Partial sacral agenesis
5	Florea et al.	5	M	Not specified	Club feet, delayed walking, Uretero-rectal fistula, anteriorly displaced anus, primary urinary incontinence	T_{11}/ L_5-S_1	L_5, S_1 weakness and muscle atrophy	Not specified	Hypertonic sphincter	Urinary retention	Partial sacral agenesis, Filum lipoma
6	Ali et al.	28	M	Lumbo-sacral dimple	Planovalgus foot deformity b/l, lower extremity atrophy, urinary incontinence	T_{12}/ L_{4-5}	Weakness caudal to L5, decreased hip abduction, normal dorsiflexion, decreased plantarflexion	Partial L_5 hyper-sensitivity	Not specified	Normal U/S, no urodynamics	Sacral agenesis

Abbreviations: *BCR* Bulbocavernosus reflex, *b/l* Bilateral, *DSD* Detrusor-sphincter-dyssynergia, *F* Female, *M* Male, *U/S* Ultrasound

all three patients. There was complete atrophy and paralysis of intrinsic foot muscles suggesting non-functional S_2 spinal cord segment within the rostral conus in all patients.

All patients had sensory deficits with clearly diminished but discriminable L_5 and S_1 sensation and complete anaesthesia including and caudal to S_2.

All three patients had a hypertonic external anal sphincter without voluntary control, and all presented with primary urinary incontinence. Two patients had urodynamics study showing detrusor hyperreflexia with severe detrusor-sphincter-dyssynergia; and both also had hydronephrosis prior to starting clean intermittent catheterization.

Imaging

Pathognomonic features on magnetic resonance imaging (MRI) seen in all three patients are a rostral "primary" spinal cord ending in a blunt stump at the thoracolumbar (T_{11}–L_1) vertebral levels, and a separate caudal "secondary" spinal cord located three to five vertebral levels (at L_3–S_2) below the primary spinal cord, with MRI signal characteristic of spinal cord, and a tapering appearance resembling the normal conus, complete with exiting sacral nerve roots and a terminal filum. A slender non-neural looking band links the rostral with the caudal spinal cords (Fig. 1).

Associated spinal deformities are various degrees of sacral agenesis, alone or in combination with scoliosis and/or hemivertebrae.

Intraoperative Electrophysiology

Electrophysiological monitoring was performed intraoperatively during exploratory surgery of the first encountered patient initially thought to have a retained medullary cord [25].

The intraoperative findings were astonishing. The termination of the rostral spinal cord was abrupt and blunt. The structure connecting the upper "primary" to the lower "secondary" spinal cord was a white, thick band. The lower spinal cord showed a gradual conical taper at its caudal termination resembling the appearance of a normal conus (Fig. 2). It was richly endowed with bilateral nerve roots. In fact, the number of rootlets (7 or 8 pairs) exceeded the usual number expected from the S_{2-5} cord segments. The most caudal nerve roots were very puny and small, suggesting they were vestigial coccygeal roots.

Stimulating the individual ventral rootlets of the upper spinal cord segment with 0.5 milliampere (mA) current activated the rectus femoris, anterior tibialis, and gastrocnemius muscle, generating compound action potentials of equal amplitudes on each side. Bilateral anal sphincter response was absent. These findings suggest

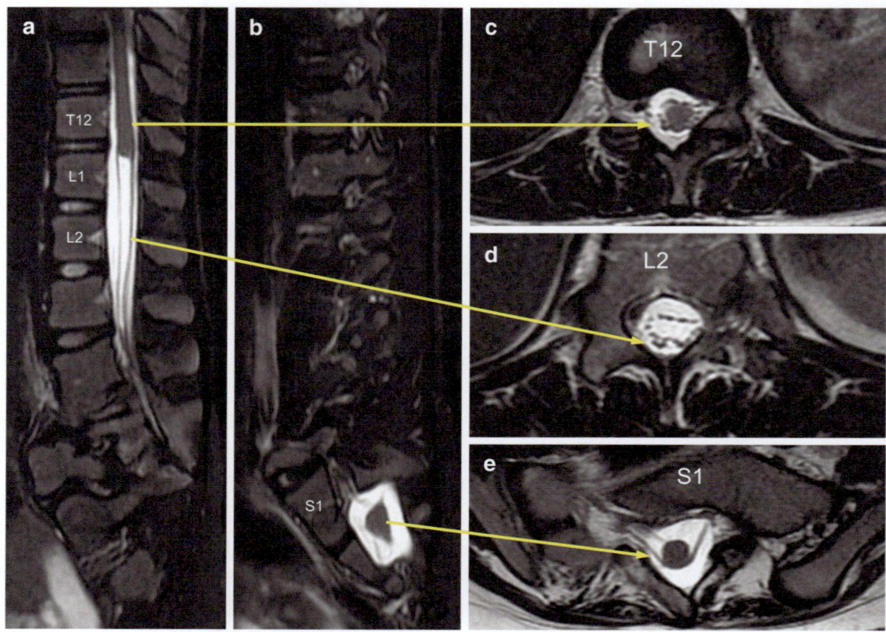

Fig. 1 T2-weighted MRI of JNTD. (**a**) Sagittal view shows the rostral spinal cord formed by primary neurulation ending abruptly at T_{12}/L_1 with the appearance of a blunt stump instead of the usual taper. (**b**) Sagittal view at $S_{1/2}$ shows the caudal spinal cord formed by secondary neurulation tapering as usual into the filum, resembling a true conus. (**c**) Axial view at T_{12} shows the rostral spinal cord. (**d**) Axial view at L_2 shows the bridging band linking the two spinal cords. (**e**) Axial view at S_1 demonstrates the caudal spinal cord with bilateral ventral and dorsal roots

that the rostral spinal cord was derived from the primary neural tube "normally" terminating at the L_5 to S_1 cord segments.

Equivalent stimulation of the proximal three to four pairs of nerve roots from the lower spinal cord activated strong external anal sphincter contractions on the corresponding side. Distally, the effect dwindled and stimulating the last few pairs of nerve rootlets elicited no response. Direct stimulation of the lower spinal cord surface with a current of 5 mA activated both sides of the external anal sphincter, but no response in any lower extremity muscles (Fig. 3). Stimulation of the sensory domain of the pudendal nerve (S_2-S_5) generated bilateral robust bulbocavernosus reflexes with strong anal sphincter contractions having normal latencies.

Stimulating the connecting whitish band between the upper and lower spinal cords with currents as high as 6 mA did not elicit any muscle response (Fig. 4).

Transcranial motor evoked potentials (TcMEP) stimulation elicited symmetric bilateral responses from the rectus femoris, anterior tibialis, and gastrocnemius, but nothing from the abductor hallucis (S2) or external anal sphincter (S2-S4), strongly suggesting that only the rostral spinal cord, formed by primary neurulation, but not the conus, formed by secondary neurulation, was under cortical control (Fig. 5).

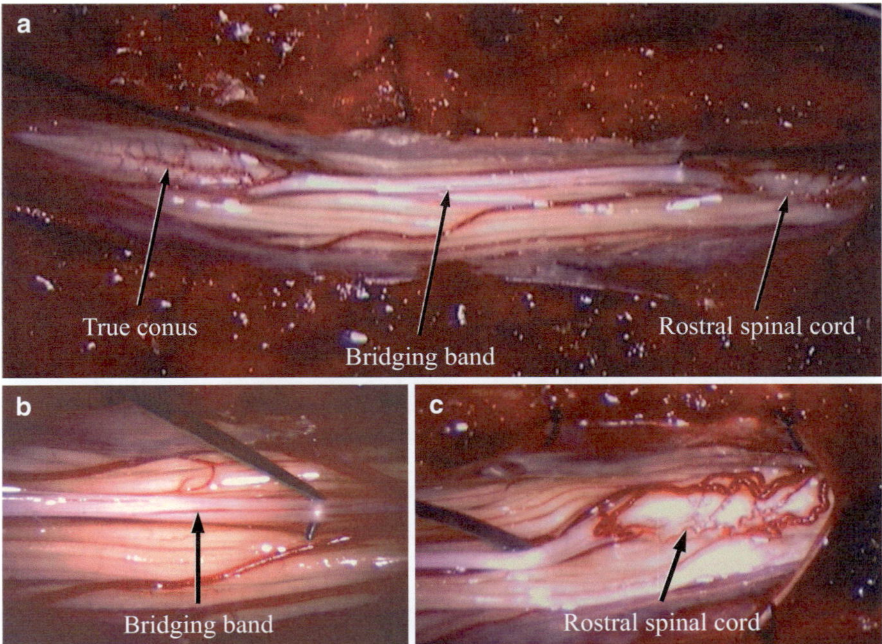

Fig. 2 Intraoperative pictures during exploratory surgery of JNTD. (**a**) The rostral spinal cord is joined to the well-formed conus by a bridging band. (**b**) Close-up view of the whitish, connective tissue bridging band. (**c**) Close-up view of the rostral spinal cord formed by primary neurulation shows a dense leash of nerve roots

These electrophysiological findings confirmed that the anatomically and functionally fully formed conus is completely isolated and physiologically unconnected to the upper primary spinal cord or to the cerebral motor cortex.

Discussion

The remarkable feature of JNTD is complete disruption of structural and functional connectivity between the primary and secondary neural tubes, while in loco secondary neurulation has succeeded to form a locally functioning but isolated conus with proper innervation to the bladder and external anal sphincter, albeit totally disconnected from corticospinal control. According to recent understanding of junctional neurulation, at least some ventromedial cells of the NSB express *SOX-2* and migrate as neuroprogenitor cells caudally and initialize secondary neurulation. Despite their intended fate, these neuroprogenitor cells fail to maintain functional and physical continuity with the dorsolateral cells of the NSB, which form the terminal primary neural tube. Other ventromedial, primitive streak-derived

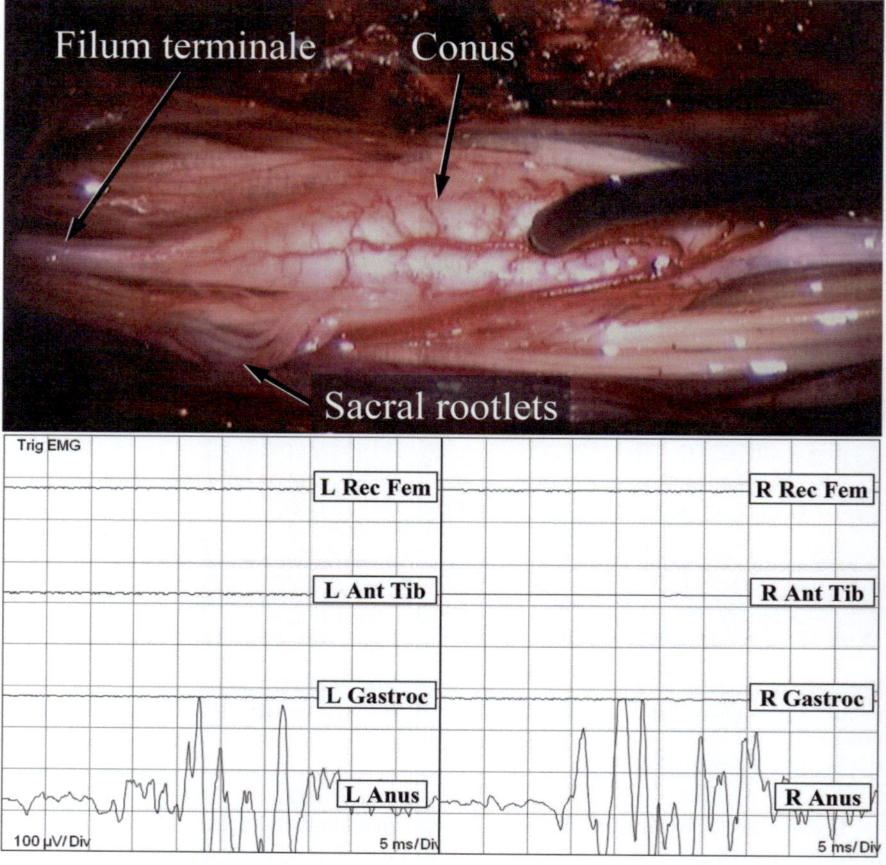

Fig. 3 Direct stimulation of the caudal spinal cord in JNTD elicits strong bilateral EMG responses in the external anal sphincter, indicating it is in fact a functioning conus

cells, however, presumably remain SOX-2 negative and undergo epithelium-to-mesenchyme transition to form a dense mesodermal, connective tissue stalk, which is without neuronal cell properties and therefore electrophysiologically inert.

Prickle-1, as a member gene of the PCP pathway, also regulates polarised deposition of the cell adhesion molecule fibronectin on the surface of cells undergoing convergent extension during mouse gastrulation [42–44]. In the chick embryo, fibronectin deposition in the basement membrane of the junctional neural tube accurately matches *Prickle-1* expression in the NSB. In *Prickle-1* knockdown chick embryo, fibronectin distribution becomes unpolarized and haphazardly scattered [29]. Thus, impairment of neural progenitor cell adhesions in the NSB can theoretically prevent proper coupling between the dorsal and ventral cell populations, leaving them unconnected. The discordant growth rates between the neural and mesodermal components of the craniocaudal axis of the embryo subsequently lead

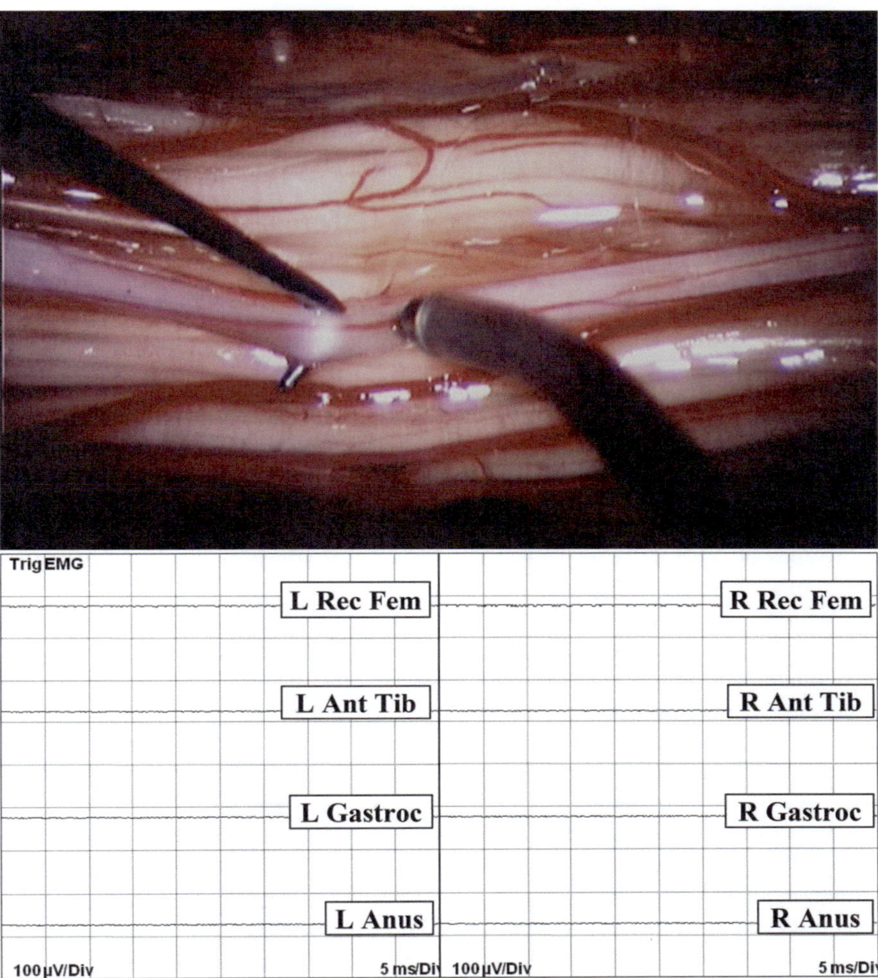

Fig. 4 Bipolar stimulation of the non-functional bridging band in JNTD between the rostral and caudal spinal cords shows no EMG response

to rising of the primary neural tube rostrally towards the thoracolumbar vertebrae, leaving behind the secondary neural tube within its embryonic location in the sacral region.

Interestingly, in all reported JNTD patients, the L_5 and S_1 spinal cord segments corresponding to the caudal tip of the primary neural tube were formed but functionally abnormal, with various degrees of paresis of ankle dorsi- and plantarflexion. Similarly, all patients had severe wasting of the intrinsic foot muscles, suggesting absence of S_2 motor neurons and defective formation of the upper portion of the secondary neural tube. This picture of impaired formation of the opposing

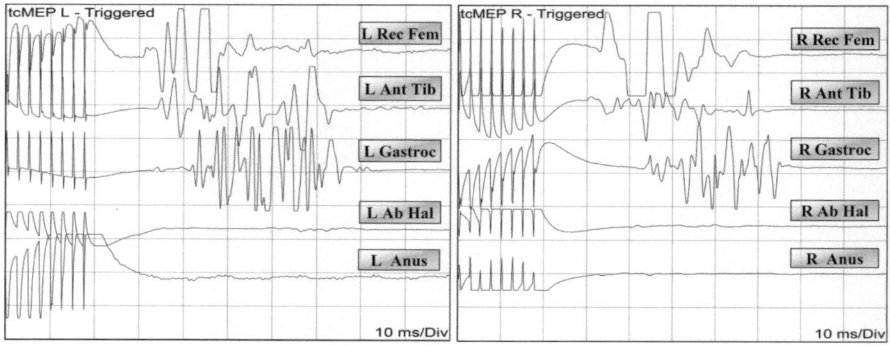

Fig. 5 TcMEP in JNTD showing motor responses in bilateral rectus femoris, anterior tibialis, and gastrocnemius muscles. There is no motor response of the abductor hallucis or sphincter ani muscles bilaterally, indicating no functional connection between the conus (S_2-S_5 segments) and the motor cortex

tips of the primary and secondary spinal cords suggests defective development of both types of NSB cells located at the transitional zones of the two developing neural tubes during junctional neurulation.

Contrary to segmental spinal dysgenesis (SSD) where any spinal segment including the cervical ones may be affected, JNTD is a specific disturbance of junctional neurulation and therefore impacts only the NSB zone between the opposing extremities of the primary and secondary neural tubes. Thus, in JNTD, only the neural segments caudal to L_5 are clinically affected, as shown throughout all published cases [38–41], and not the more rostral segments as commonly seen in SSD. As primary neurulation is almost completed when junctional neurulation begins, most of the primary neural tube is already formed when the embryogenic insult occurs during the temporospatial events of JNTD formation. As well, local formation of the secondary neural tube is primarily unaffected, though other caudal cell mass derivatives may be defective as seen in the association with sacral agenesis. Also, in JNTD, the whitish connecting band between primary and secondary neural tube is floating within a wide cerebrospinal fluid space without any bony compression, unlike most cases of segmental spinal dysgenesis. It has been posited that in SSD, an initial neurulation defect also results in concurrent bony malformation at the corresponding levels, and that these latter malformations in turn cause bony compression and myelopathy [45], but the levels of myelopathy in reported cases of SSD do not usually correspond to the embryological junction between the primary and secondary neural tubes, as in JNTD. Like most developmental anomalies, there are always mixed forms of phenotypes that seem to implicate more than one neurulation mechanism, as in dorsal and transitional spinal cord lipomas [26]. Though JNTD and SSD may share some common features and malfunctioning pathways, JNTD nevertheless represents a very specific temporospatial neurulation defect with pathognomonic clinical and electrophysiological signatures.

Conclusion

Junctional neural tube defect is caused by genetic mutation(s) within the narrow temporospatial interlude between the termination of primary and commencement of secondary neurulation, resulting in successful formation of the secondary neural tube which nevertheless lacks anatomical and functional connection with the rest of the central neuraxis. This rare and unique neurulation defect leads to a locally functional but isolated and unintegrated conus without corticospinal inhibition or control. The handful of cases described in the literature all share common clinical features of hypertonic bladder and bowel dysfunction lacking central control, and variable loss of sensory-motor function below the L_5–S_1 level. The complex embryology and metabolic pathways determining complete and integrative neurulation will continue to raise controversies, encouraging critical appraisal of new scientific data as well as challenges of old paradigms, which should ultimately improve our current understanding of neurulation.

References

1. Eibach S, Moes G, Zovickian J, Pang D. Limited dorsal myeloschisis associated with dermoid elements. Childs Nerv Syst. 2017;33:55–67.
2. Pang D, Zovickian J, Oviedo A, Moes GS. Limited dorsal myeloschisis: a distinctive clinicopathological entity. Neurosurgery. 2010;67:1555–79.; discussion 1579-1580,.
3. Pang D, Zovickian J, Wong ST, Hou YJ, Moes GS. Limited dorsal myeloschisis: a not-so-rare form of primary neurulation defect. Childs Nerv Syst. 2013;29:1459–84.
4. Colas JF, Schoenwolf GC. Towards a cellular and molecular understanding of neurulation. Dev Dyn. 2001;221:117–45.
5. Hughes AF, Freeman RB. Comparative remarks on the development of the tail cord among higher vertebrates. J Embryol Exp Morphol. 1974;32:355–63.
6. Lowery LA, Sive H. Strategies of vertebrate neurulation and a re-evaluation of teleost neural tube formation. Mech Dev. 2004;121:1189–97.
7. Nievelstein RAJ, Hartwig NG, Vermeij-Keers C, Valk J. Embryonic development of the mammalian caudal neural tube. Teratology. 1993;48:21–31.
8. Schoenwolf GC, Smith JL. Mechanisms of neurulation. Methods Mol Biol. 2000;136:125–34.
9. Müller F, O'Rahilly R. The primitive streak, the caudal eminence and related structures in staged human embryos. Cells Tissues Organs. 2004;177:2–20.
10. Saitsu H, Yamada S, Uwabe C, Ishibashi M, Shiota K. Development of the posterior neural tube in human embryos. Anat Embryol (Berl). 2004;209:107–17.
11. Saraga-Babic M, Krolo M, Sapunar D, Terzic J, Biocic M. Differences in origin and fate between the cranial and caudal spinal cord during normal and disturbed human development. Acta Neuropathol. 1996;91:194–9.
12. Criley BB. Analysis of the embryonic sources and mechanisms of development of posterior levels of chick neural tubes. J Morphol. 1969;128:465–501.
13. Griffith CM, Wiley MJ, Sanders EJ. The vertebrate tail bud: three germ layers from one tissue. Anat Embryol. 1992;185:101–13.
14. Mills CL, Bellairs R. Mitosis and cell death in the tail of the chick embryo. Anat Embryol. 1989;180:301–8.

15. Schoenwolf GC, Delongo J. Ultrastructure of secondary neurulation in the chick embryo. Am J Anat. 1980;158:43–63.

16. Yang HJ, Wang KC, Chi JG, Lee MS, Lee YJ, Kim SK, et al. Cytokinetics of secondary neurulation in chick embryos: Hamburger and Hamilton stages 16-45. Childs Nerv Syst. 2006;22:567–71.

17. Kostovic-Knezevic L, Gajovic S, Svajger A. Morphogenetic features in the tail region of the rat embryo. Int J Dev Biol. 1991;35:191–5.

18. Beck CW, Slack JMW. A developmental pathway controlling outgrowth of the Xenopus tail bud. Development. 1999;126:1611–20.

19. O'Rahilly R, Müller F. Somites, spinal ganglia, and centra: enumeration and interrelationships in staged human embryos, and implications for neural tube defects. Cells Tissues Organs. 2003;173:75–92.

20. Tam PPL. The histogenetic capacity of tissues in the caudal end of the embryonic axis of the mouse. J Embryol Exp Morphol. 1984;82:253–66.

21. Hamburger V, Hamilton HL. A series of normal stages in the development of the chick embryo. J Morphol. 1951;88:49–92.

22. Schoenwolf GC. Histological and ultrastructural studies of secondary neurulation in mouse embryos. Am J Anat. 1984;169:361–76.

23. Pang D. Sacral agenesis and caudal spinal cord malformations. Neurosurgery. 1993;32:755–79.

24. Pang D, Zovickian J, Lee JY, Moes GS, Wang KC. Terminal myelocystocele: surgical observations and theory of embryogenesis. Neurosurgery. 2012;70:1383–404.

25. Pang D, Zovickian J, Moes GS. Retained medullary cord in humans: late arrest of secondary neurulation. Neurosurgery. 2011;68:1500–19.

26. Pang D, Zovickian J, Oviedo A. Long-term outcome of total and near-total resection of spinal cord lipomas and radical reconstruction of the neural placode: part I-surgical technique. Neurosurgery. 2009;65:511–28; discussion 528-519.

27. Catala M, Teillet MA, De Robertis EM, Le Douarin NM. A spinal cord fate map in the avian embryo: while regressing, Hensen's node lays down the notochord and floor plate thus joining the spinal cord lateral walls. Development. 1996;122:2599–610.

28. Shimokita E, Takahashi Y. Secondary neurulation: fate-mapping and gene manipulation of the neural tube in tail bud. Dev Growth Differ. 2011;53:401–10.

29. Dady A, Havis E, Escriou V, Catala M, Duband JL. Junctional neurulation: a unique developmental program shaping a discrete region of the spinal cord highly susceptible to neural tube defects. J Neurosci. 2014;34:13,208–21.

30. Dady A, Blavet C, Duband JL. Timing and kinetics of E- to N-cadherin switch during neurulation in the avian embryo. Dev Dyn. 2012;241:1333–49.

31. Nakaya Y, Kuroda S, Katagiri YT, Kaibuchi K, Takahashi Y. Mesenchymal-epithelial transition during somitic segmentation is regulated by differential roles of Cdc42 and Rac1. Dev Cell. 2004;7:425–38.

32. Thiery JP, Sleeman JP. Complex networks orchestrate epithelial-mesenchymal transitions. Nat Rev Mol Cell Biol. 2006;7:131–42.

33. Copp AJ, Greene ND. Genetics and development of neural tube defects. J Pathol. 2010;220:217–30.

34. Copp AJ, Greene ND, Murdoch JN. The genetic basis of mammalian neurulation. Nat Rev Genet. 2003;4:784–93.

35. Doudney K, Ybot-Gonzalez P, Paternotte C, Stevenson RE, Greene ND, Moore GE, et al. Analysis of the planar cell polarity gene Vangl2 and its co-expressed paralogue Vangl1 in neural tube defect patients. Am J Med Genet A. 2005;136:90–2.

36. Ybot-Gonzalez P, Savery D, Gerrelli D, Signore M, Mitchell CE, Faux CH, et al. Convergent extension, planar-cell-polarity signalling and initiation of mouse neural tube closure. Development. 2007;134:789–99.

37. Cooper O, Sweetman D, Wagstaff L, Munsterberg A. Expression of avian prickle genes during early development and organogenesis. Dev Dyn. 2008;237:1442–8.

38. Eibach S, Moes G, Hou YJ, Zovickian J, Pang D. Unjoined primary and secondary neural tubes: junctional neural tube defect, a new form of spinal dysraphism caused by disturbance of junctional neurulation. Childs Nerv Syst. 2017;33:1633–47.
39. Ali M, McNeely PD. Junctional neural tube defect: a supporting case report. Childs Nerv Syst. 2018;34:1447–8.
40. Florea SM, Faure A, Brunel H, Girard N, Scavarda D. A case of junctional neural tube defect associated with a lipoma of the filum terminale: a new subtype of junctional neural tube defect? J Neurosurg Pediatr. 2018;21:601–5.
41. Schmidt C, Voin V, Iwanaga J, Alonso F, Oskouian RJ, Topale N, et al. Junctional neural tube defect in a newborn: report of a fourth case. Childs Nerv Syst. 2017;33:873–5.
42. Dzamba BJ, Jakab KR, Marsden M, Schwartz MA, DeSimone DW. Cadherin adhesion, tissue tension, and noncanonical Wnt signaling regulate fibronectin matrix organization. Dev Cell. 2009;16:421–32.
43. Goto T, Davidson L, Asashima M, Keller R. Planar cell polarity genes regulate polarized extracellular matrix deposition during frog gastrulation. Curr Biol. 2005;15:787–93.
44. Tao H, Suzuki M, Kiyonari H, Abe T, Sasaoka T, Ueno N. Mouse prickle1, the homolog of a PCP gene, is essential for epiblast apical-basal polarity. Proc Natl Acad Sci U S A. 2009;106:14426–31.
45. Wang KC, Lee JS, Kim K, Im YJ, Park K, Kim KH, et al. Do junctional neural tube defect and segmental spinal dysgenesis have the same pathoembryological background? Childs Nerv Syst. 2019;36:241.

The Current Status of the Surgical Management of Complex Spinal Cord Lipomas: Still Navigating the Labyrinth?

Dachling Pang and Dominic N. P. Thompson

Introduction

In our recent reviews of the subject of surgical management of complex spinal cord lipomas [1, 2], we have posed two debated issues regarding the indications and techniques of surgery. The first issue was whether surgery should be reserved for only symptomatic cases or endorsed for both symptomatic and asymptomatic ones. Our tentative conclusion was that all dorsal and transitional lipomas (not chaotic lipomas; more later) should be operated on regardless of the presence or absence of symptoms. This was based on solid evidence that spinal lipomas are undisputedly a progressive disease and that ours and others' experience also showed that once deficits have arisen, especially those involving bladder function, surgery will unlikely reverse the disability. And for the urinary bladder, this could be life-changing. As quoted, in 2004, Kulkarni et al. [3], from L'Hopital Necker-Enfants Malades, Paris, published a prospective study of a relatively large cohort of children with lipomas that were followed without surgery and concluded that *asymptomatic* lipomas have a 33% chance of deterioration over 9 years. A comparable though retrospective study from London in 2012 [4] similarly reported a 40% 10-year deterioration rate in unoperated asymptomatic lipomas. The London study also

D. Pang (✉)
Department of Paediatric Neurosurgery, University of California, Davis, USA

Great Ormond Street Hospital for Children, NHS Trust, London, UK

D. N. P. Thompson
Great Ormond Street Hospital for Children, NHS Trust, London, UK

Department of Developmental Neuroscience, University College London-Institute of Child Health, London, UK
e-mail: dominic.thompson@gosh.nhs.uk

© The Author(s), under exclusive license to Springer Nature Switzerland AG 2023
D. Pang, K.-C. Wang (eds.), *Spinal Dysraphic Malformations*, Advances and Technical Standards in Neurosurgery 47,
https://doi.org/10.1007/978-3-031-34981-2_6

showed that females with transitional lipomas, especially those harbouring a terminal syrinx, fared even worse. Thus, since half of their cohort were females and approximately 70% of their lipomas were of the transitional type, the poor outcome rate of the group, when projected to a larger cohort size and longer follow-up, may well exceed 40%. Such dire statistics for untreated lipomas in children with presumably long actuarial survival seem to demand some type of intervention, which led to our recommendation that both symptomatic and asymptomatic dorsal and transitional lipomas should be treated with total resection.

With deeper thinking, however, like all "full-proof" statistics, the above straight recommendation may, in fact, be inflected by some irksome reconsiderations. The progression-free survival (PFS) curves of both the Paris [3] and London [4] series of non-surgical management of lipomas appear at first glance to be relentlessly regressive, i.e. if the cases were followed *ad nauseam* beyond the series' 9 or 10 years and the curves were drawn over many more years, they will both eventually reach zero on the vertical axis, implying all patients will develop symptoms. But in constructing statistical trends, assuming the future without hard data is, at base, "anti-scientific", as there may, in fact, be a small subset of patients with lipomas that will never develop deficits, and if they could be identified and set aside without radical surgery, their post-operative complication, albeit rare but potentially serious, could be avoided. The trick of all these lofty arguments is, of course, how to predict which patient with lipomas will be spared of future deficits and thus of unnecessary surgery.

The second debated issue posed in our previous reviews concerns the question of what is the safest and most effective surgery that offers long-term benefits over the natural history of the disease. Data from most large series [5–11] do not support the opinion that partial resection offers adequate long-term protection against disease progression. For example, Dorward et al. [12] reported a symptomatic recurrence rate of 48% over merely 2.2 years. Colak et al. [13] reported a 52% recurrence rate over 10 years with partial resection, but their series comprised 37% terminal lipomas, which are known to have much better prognosis than dorsal and transitional lipomas, implying that the progression rate if calculated just for the latter lipoma types must be even higher than 52%. Pierre-Kahn [14] documented a 10-year recurrence of 46%, but again their series contains many terminal and filar lipomas; and Cochrane, et al. [15] and Xenos et al. [16] similarly recorded early recurrence. These results pose the obvious question whether leaving behind a large amount of residual fat on the neural placode[1] with its broad, raw, and sticky abraded surface actually provokes new adhesions to the adjacent dura and consequently incurs earlier and firmer retethering than if the lipoma had been left untouched.

---

[1] The term neural placode in lipoma is borrowed from the main neural core of an open neural tube defect or ONTD, to emphasise its similar "neural" nature once the lipoma is removed. The synonymous usage of the term in lipoma and ONTD is logical if one compares the embryogenesis of the two entities (see below): the "placode" in each case represents the original embryonic neural plate blighted in its final completing stage: having been invaded by paraxial mesenchyme in lipoma, and thwarted in its midline dorsal fusion in ONTD.

The obvious need for a different procedure other than partial resection occurred to the senior author in 1991, when his own series of 116 partial resections following conventional teaching [7, 10, 17–21] showed an alarming 65% symptomatic recurrence rate. His subsequent development of the technique of total resection of dorsal and transitional lipomas and radical reconstruction of the neural placode [22] is founded on three almost intuitive premises: (1) the high recurrence rate after partial resection is due to re-tethering at the resection site; (2) re-tethering is in turn promoted by three conditions, a tight content-container relationship between the affected placode and its adjacent intradural space, a broad "sticky" nidus of remaining fat, and incomplete separation of the terminal placode from the caudal fat (see below); and (3) total resection eliminates these conditions contributory to re-tethering and thus reduces the probability of late deterioration. The object of total resection is therefore to create a milieu least conducive to re-sticking of the neural placode. It is known that the spinal cord normally shows considerable intradural motion to gravity and postural changes demonstrable on dynamic imaging [23, 24]. Lowering the content-container ratio and amplifying the amount of free placode movements within the dural sac should therefore reduce sustained contacts between placode and dura, hence also the probability of adhesion. In a "virgin" (previously untouched) lipoma, the bulk of the lipoma-cord composite must first be severely trimmed by resecting all or most of the engorging fat down to the thin, supple neural placode; for "redo" lesions that have had previous surgery, the stiff fibrous scar must also be resected. The goal is to render the thinnest, most malleable neural placode so that through tensionless pia-to-pia neurulation (see below), a slender but unstrangled, pia-covered neural tube can be created. The sticky lipoma bed is thus concealed within this tube, and the dural sac is then made capacious by a generous graft.

In 2009 and 2010 [19, 22], the senior author and colleagues published their early series of 238 patients who had total / near-total resection of complex lipomas and compared their short and long-term outcomes with our prior series of 116 patients with partial resection. In 2013, we updated our series of total resection to 315 cases [25], and recently, our number has risen to over 500 cases [2]. Our ever enlarging data pool unfailingly shows an overwhelming advantage of total over partial resection in almost all respects.

Despite accusations, or perhaps for the sake of didacticism, we will, in this review, include sections on practical anatomy and embryology, helpful information concerning intraoperative neurophysiology monitoring (IONM), and a rather detailed exposition of the technique of total lipoma resection as a sort of surgical *vade mecum*. Besides reiterating the obvious merits of total resection over partial resection, we will revisit the question of whether total resection should be done for ALL dorsal and transitional lipomas regardless of symptoms and attempt to wrestle with the idea of predicting the probability of clinical deterioration of a certain subclass of lipomas segregable by magnetic resonance imaging (MRI) appearance.

We will also put in record our present preoccupation with the question whether measuring the bulbocavernosus reflex (BCR) as part of our routine IONM practice has predictive value for post-operative micturition. Against initial intuition, our very preliminary assessment unexpectedly shows that the intraoperative BCR may not be as tightly correlated with post-operative bladder function as hoped.

Anatomy and Classification

In the literature, the nomenclature and classification of spinal cord lipomas are imprecise and inconsistent. Here, we are defining the types of lipomas as follows:

Dorsal Lipoma

A dorsal lipoma perches entirely on the dorsal surface of the lumbar spinal cord and does not involve the conus (Fig. 1). The junction between lipoma, spinal cord, and pia, the *fusion line* (see below), is usually traceable along a roughly oval track, demarcating fat from the more lateral dorsal root entry zone (DREZ) and nerve roots (Fig. 2a, b), which means the nerve roots and DREZ are never mixed up with

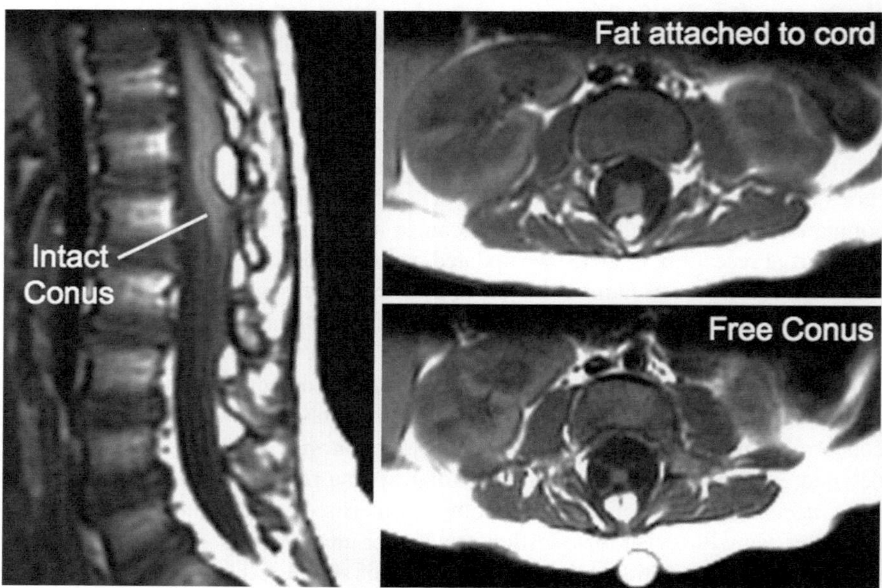

Fig. 1 Dorsal lipoma on MRI. Sagittal image shows intact conus caudal to lipoma stalk. Axial images: upper shows site of lipoma attachment to cord; lower shows free conus just caudal to the level of lipoma attachment. (Reprinted from: Pang D, Zovickian J, Wong ST, Hou YJ, and Moes GS. Surgical treatment of complex spinal cord lipomas. Childs Nerv Syst (2013) 29:1485–1513; with Permission from Springer Nature)

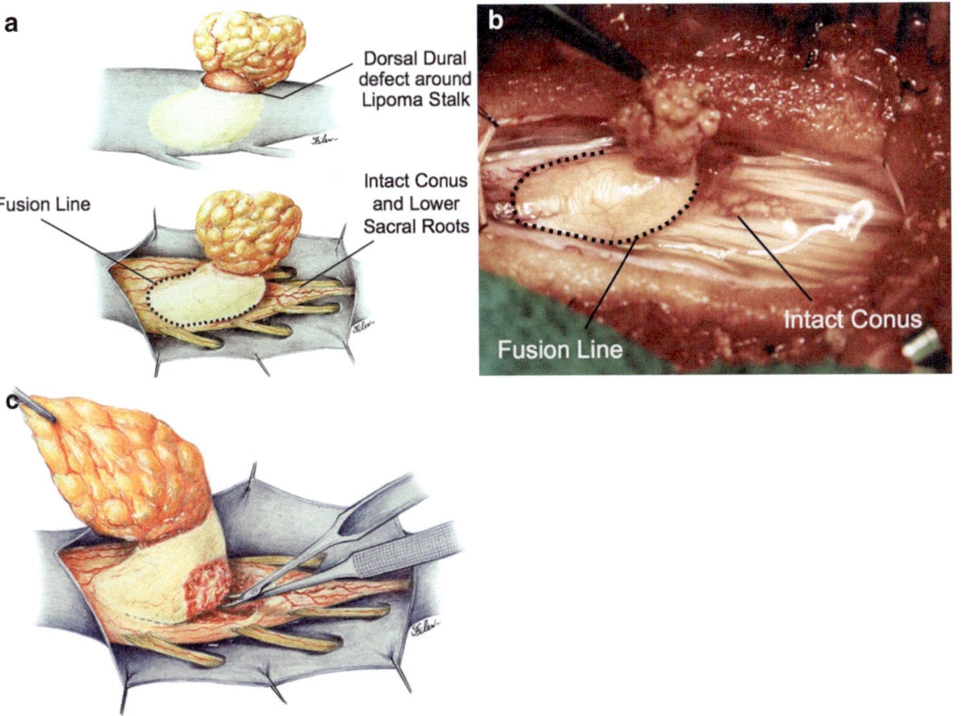

Fig. 2 Dorsal lipoma. (**a**) Intraoperative drawings: upper shows neat dorsal dural defect through which lipoma stalk goes. Lower shows circumferential fusion line and intact conus. (Reprinted from: Pang D, Zovickian J, Wong ST, Hou YJ, and Moes GS. Surgical treatment of complex spinal cord lipomas. Childs Nerv Syst (2013) 29:1485–1513; with Permission from Springer Nature). (**b**) Intraoperative picture shows neat oval fusion line around lipoma-cord interface on a horizontal plane. Note intact conus and caudal sacral roots. (**c**) Resection of dorsal lipoma can be executed with a completely circumscribed perspective from all sides of the fusion line, impossible with transitional lipoma. (Reprinted from: Pang D, Zovickian J, Wong ST, Hou YJ, and Moes GS. Surgical treatment of complex spinal cord lipomas. Childs Nerv Syst (2013) 29:1485–1513; with Permission from Springer Nature)

the lipoma. The lipomatous stalk usually traverses a fairly discrete defect in the dorsal dura to blend with the subcutaneous fat. The uninvolved conus often ends in a thickened filum terminale. An idealised depiction of the resection of a typical dorsal lipoma is shown in Fig. 2c, which illustrates a clear view of the entire circumference of the fusion line, and how the surgeon can command a full 360° approach to the lipoma-cord interface.

Transitional Lipoma

The rostral part of a transitional lipoma resembles a dorsal lipoma in that it features a discrete fusion line and a reasonably organized array of nerve roots and DREZ, but unlike the dorsal type, the fat plane of a transitional lipoma then cuts ventro-caudally to involve the entire conus likened to making an oblique, bevelled knife-cut across the end of a rod (Fig. 3a). Also, unlike the dorsal type, its lipoma-cord interface is often not horizontally levelled, and the neural placode may be so rotated in its longitudinal axis that it literally spins into a parasagittal orientation, but the neural tissue is always recognisable "ventral" to this interface, so that the DREZ and nerve roots are lateral and ventral to the fusion line and therefore also do not usually traverse the lipoma (Fig. 3b). An idealised depiction of total resection of a transitional lipoma thus shows a ventrally-slanting oblique plane of resection set by the fusion line (Fig. 3c). A filum may or may not be present and the dural defect often extend way past the neural placode to involve the caudal dural sac.

In general, dorsal lipomas conform to the "standard" architecture described above and are mostly horizontal and symmetrical. Transitional lipomas, on the other hand, tend more to be "irregular" and unpredictable: many are not symmetrical or flat as some are rotated 90° as mentioned; the larger ones often overhang the nerve roots and will require special handling; congenitally defunct nerve roots do sometimes run through the lipoma and must be correctly recognized and dispensed with; and monstrous transitional lipomas have been known to overwhelm any earnest attempt to sort out the "good" anatomy.

Terminal Lipoma

All terminal lipomas are sharply attached across the base of the conus without ever involving the dorsal parts of the spinal cord or nerve roots. Thus the lipoma-cord interface lies entirely below all the functional sacral roots and conus, which essentially looks normal except for being a bit more blunted than conical, and for the attached fat at the end. The dural sac and the overlying myofascial layers are intact. The lipoma either replaces the filum entirely or is embedded within a portion of the filum, in which case it is often called a filar lipoma.

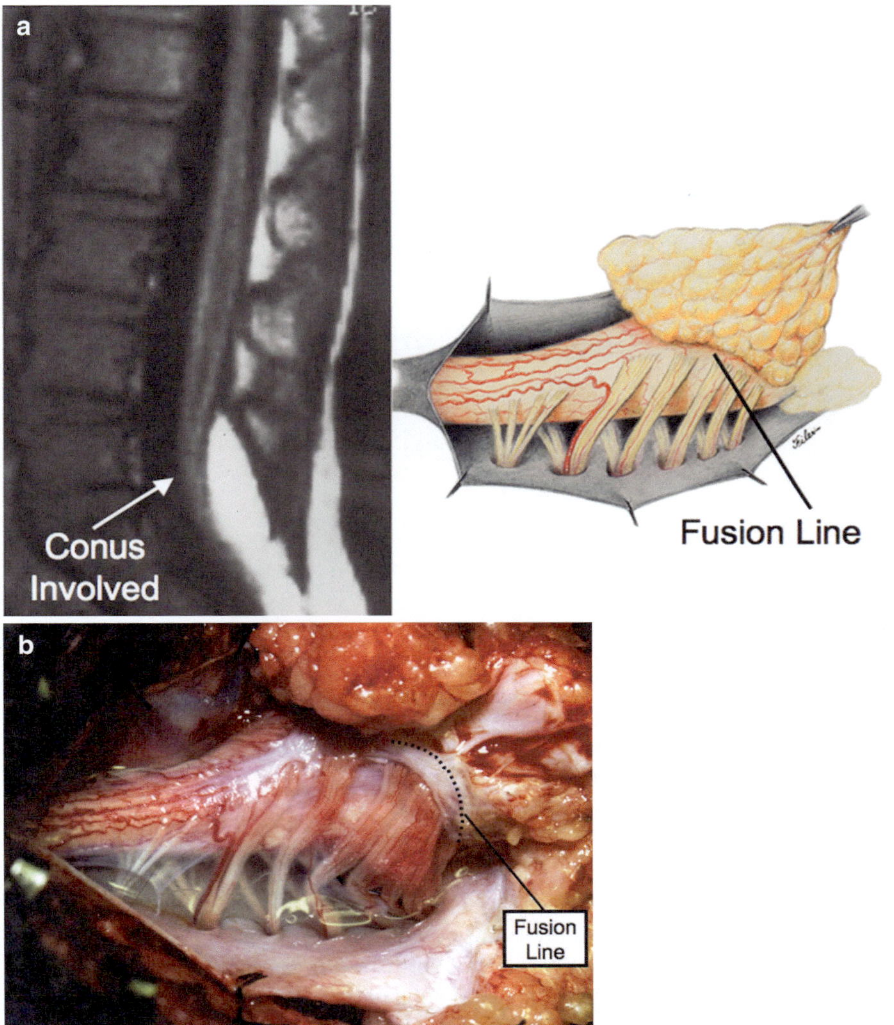

Fig. 3 Transitional lipoma. (**a**) Left: Sagittal MRI shows lipoma begins dorsally but involves entire conus. Ventral side of neural placode is free of fat. Right: The plane of the fusion line begins dorsally then cuts obliquely towards the tip of the conus. The array of DREZ and dorsal roots is also forced to slant dorso-ventrally. (Reprinted from: Pang D, Zovickian J, Wong ST, Hou YJ, and Moes GS. Surgical treatment of complex spinal cord lipomas. Childs Nerv Syst (2013) 29:1485–1513; with Permission from Springer Nature). (**b**) Intraoperative picture showing massive lipoma but very distinct dorso-ventral fusion line separating fat from the DREZ and dorsal roots, which always lie lateral and ventral to the fusion line. The ventral side of the placode is always free of fat in a regular transitional lipoma. (**c**) Top: Idealised drawings of pre- and post-resection of a relatively "standard" transitional lipoma, along an asymmetrical and oblique plane bound by the fusion line on each side, over an occasionally undulating lipoma-cord interface. Bottom shows pre- and post-resection intraoperative pictures. (Reprinted from: Pang D, Zovickian J, Wong ST, Hou YJ, and Moes GS. Surgical treatment of complex spinal cord lipomas. Childs Nerv Syst (2013) 29:1485–1513; with Permission from Springer Nature)

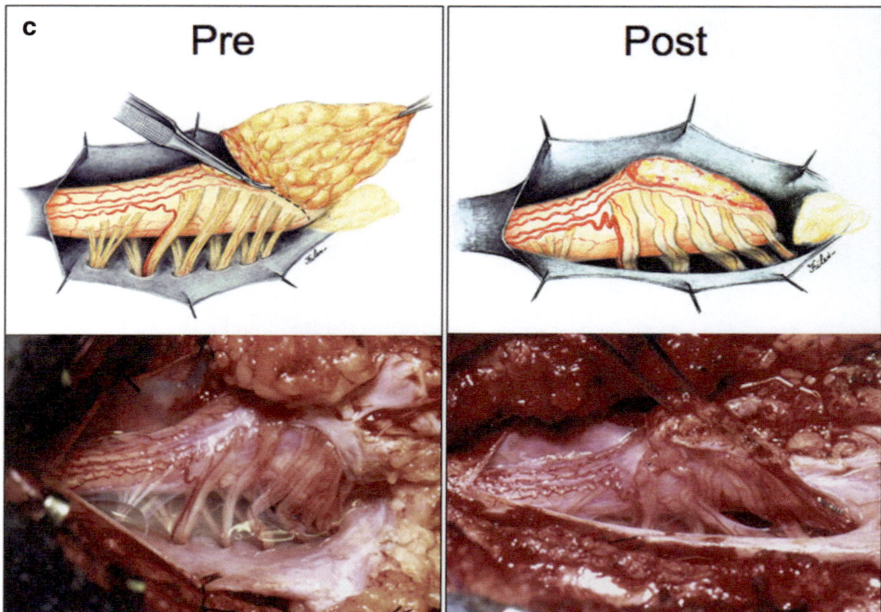

Fig. 3 (continued)

The excision of terminal lipoma is relatively simple, and its prognosis is far better than the other types; both are beyond the scope of this review.

Chaotic Lipoma

This novel type the senior author and colleagues introduced in 2009 [22] is so named because neither its embryogenesis nor its anatomy "follows the rules" of the other lipoma types. Its rostral portion may look disarmingly orthodox like the dorsal or transitional lipoma, but the fat of its caudal portion percolates through the neural placode to its *ventral* side and always engulfs neural tissue and nerve roots to some degree (Fig. 4a, b). The fusion line may be visible in its rostrodorsal portion but becomes undefinable caudally as it vanishes behind the ventral fat, where the DREZ and nerve roots are no longer easily identifiable. The moniker "chaotic" depicts the confusing blend of ventral fat and neural placode and the often impossible task of differentiating the wandering fat from the invisible neural tissue and nerve roots at surgery (Fig. 4b). Chaotic lipomas are uncommon but are typically associated with sacral agenesis [22].

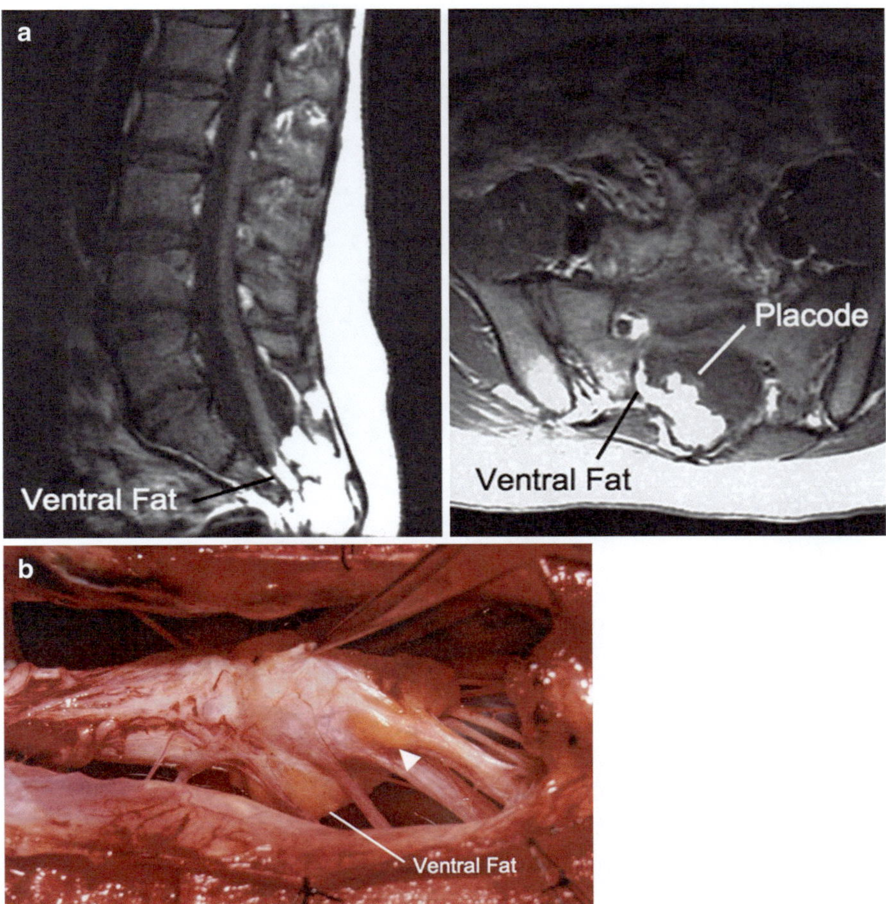

Fig. 4 Chaotic lipoma. (**a**) Left: Sagittal MRI shows ventral as well as dorsal fat in relation to the neural placode. Note sacral agenesis with only 2 visible sacral segments. Right: Axial image shows ventral fat and extremely irregular lipoma-fat interface. (**b**) Intraoperative picture showing fat ventral to placode and on one of the sacral roots (arrowhead). Note absence of discrete fusion line. (Reprinted from: Pang D, Zovickian J, Wong ST, Hou YJ, and Moes GS. Surgical treatment of complex spinal cord lipomas. Childs Nerv Syst (2013) 29:1485–1513; with Permission from Springer Nature)

The literature [5, 26] mentions one other lipoma type, the lipomyelomeningo-cele, in which the caudal spinal cord and parts of the lipoma extrude dorsally out of the spinal canal, together with an outpouching of the cerebrospinal fluid (CSF) sac (Fig. 5). The basic configuration of the lipoma is not different from that of a conventional transitional or dorsal lesion. Accordingly, we choose to include this variant subtype as either a transitional or dorsal lipoma with a descriptive qualifier of "extraspinal extension".

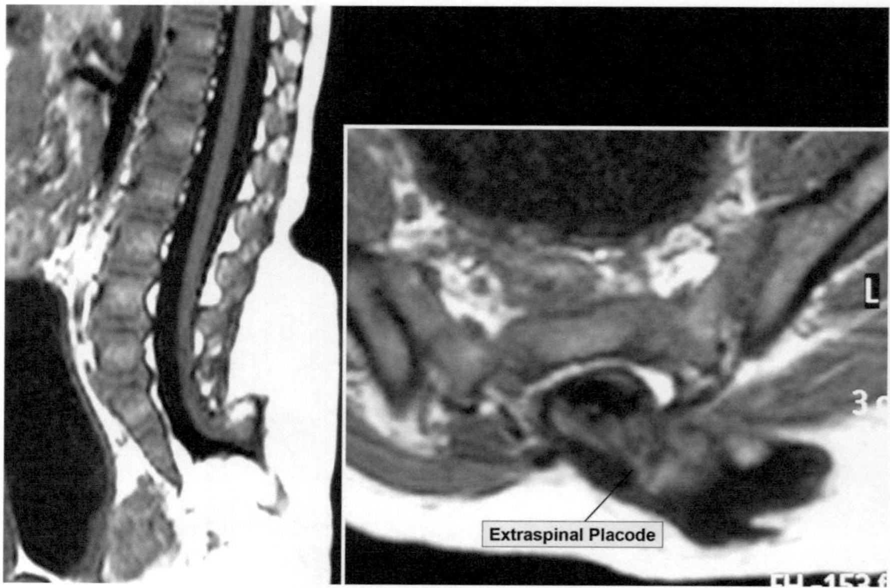

Fig. 5 Transitional lipoma with extraspinal extension ("lipomyelomeningocele"), with the lipoma, CSF sac, and part of the neural placode extending out of the spinal canal through a dorsal defect. (Reprinted from: Pang D, Zovickian J, Wong ST, Hou YJ, and Moes GS. Surgical treatment of complex spinal cord lipomas. Childs Nerv Syst (2013) 29:1485–1513; with Permission from Springer Nature)

Surgically Relevant Embryology

An understanding of the embryogenesis of lipomas is helpful in appreciating the surgical nuances.

Embryogenesis of Dorsal and Transitional Lipomas

In the human embryo, a progressive longitudinal disparity develops between the spinal cord and vertebral column because of their unequal growth rates [27–30]. Allowing for some shortening of the caudal neural tube by programmed apoptosis during secondary neurulation, the tip of the cord is still noted to have ascended a fair distance from opposite the coccyx in the 30-mm embryo to approximately the L_2 level at birth [29–32]. Smooth upward movement requires a well-constructed neural tube within a smooth dural tunnel. If during the ascent a dorsal defect develops in the dura and neural tube, the surrounding mesenchyme will invade through the defect and form a fibrofatty stalk that attaches to the sliding neural tube to cause its entrapment. This embryogenetic sequence implies a focal failure in neural tube closure during primary neurulation (secondary neurulation does not involve neural folds fusion) and thus applies only to the dorsal and transitional lipomas (see below). It also explains why these two lipoma types are always associated with adjacent bifid neural arches.

Before completion of primary neurulation, the cutaneous and neural ectoderms must first separate from each other, but this process, called disjunction, does not occur until *after* the midline fusion of the dorsal neural folds. This time sequence is important because it guarantees exclusion of the extraneural mesenchyme from ever entering the neural tube to make contact with its inner (ependymal) surface. The embryologic error leading to the mesenchymal invasion of the sliding neural tube probably lies in *premature disjunction* between the two ectoderms [33, 34]; i.e. ectodermal separation occurs *before* fusion of the converging neural folds, leaving a small gap next to the open neural tube through which paraxial mesenchyme can migrate into the central canal. Once such a mesenchymal stalk forms through this gap, further closure of the neural tube is prevented and a segmental dorsal myeloschisis is created (Fig. 6a, b). Alternatively, the inversion of the

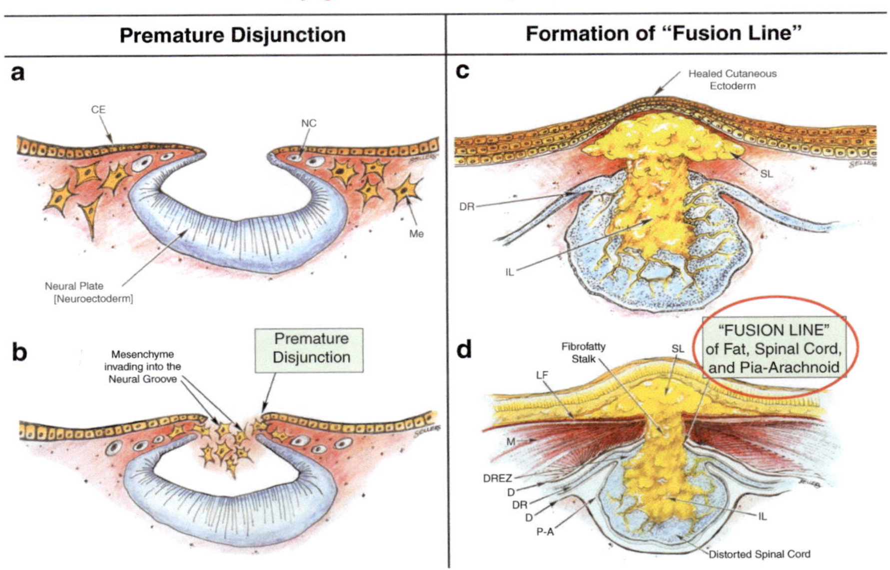

Fig. 6 Embryogenesis of dorsal lipoma, a pure primary neurulation defect. (**a**, **b**) Premature disjunction before complete closure of neural plates allows migration of mesenchymal cells into neural groove to establish contact with the ependymal surface. (**c**, **d**) Formation of fusion line between lipoma, cord, and pia-arachnoid. DREZ and dorsal root are always lateral to the fusion line and thus not entangled in fat. *CE* Cutaneous ectoderm, *NC* Neural crest, *Me* Mesenchyme, *SL* Subcutaneous lipoma, *DR* Dorsal root, *IL* Intramedullary lipoma, *DREZ* Dorsal root entry zone, *D* Dura, *P-A* Pia-arachnoid, *M* Muscle, *LF* Lumbodorsal fascia. (Reprinted from Pang D. Total resection of complex spinal cord lipomas: how, why, and when to operate. Neuro Med Chir (Tokyo) 55: 695–721, 2015; with permission from the Japanese Neurosurgical Society. CC-BY-NC-ND (https://creativecommons.org/licenses/by-nc-nd/4.0/deed.ja)

fusion-disjunction sequence can also be caused by incompetence of the paraxial mesoderm in forcing timely convergence of the opposing neural folds, delaying their fusion and allowing disjunction to happen first [35–41]. Lastly, metabolic disturbance of the cell membrane-bound glycosaminoglycans at the edges of the neural folds, which are vital to cell-cell recognition and adhesion [42–45], could likewise delay neural folds fusion and reverse the sequence of fusion-disjunction.

Pluripotential mesenchyme has been shown to form diverse derivatives depending on the kind of inductors secreted by the adjacent neuroectoderm [46, 47] (Fig. 6c). Once exposed to the invading mesenchyme, the ependymal lining of the neural tube has the inherent propensity to induce it to form fat, muscles, collagen, and even bone and cartilage (Fig. 7). In contrast, the outer surface of the neural tube normally initiates the production of meninges [48]. However, new meninges cannot now form across the dorsal midline because of the impeding lipoma stalk in-evolution, which ultimately tethers the neural tube to the subcutaneous fat. Similarly, defects in the developing myofascial structures (from myotomal mesoderm) and neural arches (from sclero mesoderm) also neatly surround the lipoma stalk (Fig. 6d).

Once formed, the mesenchyme-derived fat and collagen within the neural tube fuse with the developing alar and basal plates. Because the dorsal root ganglions descend from neural crest cells pinched from the external surface of the neural folds

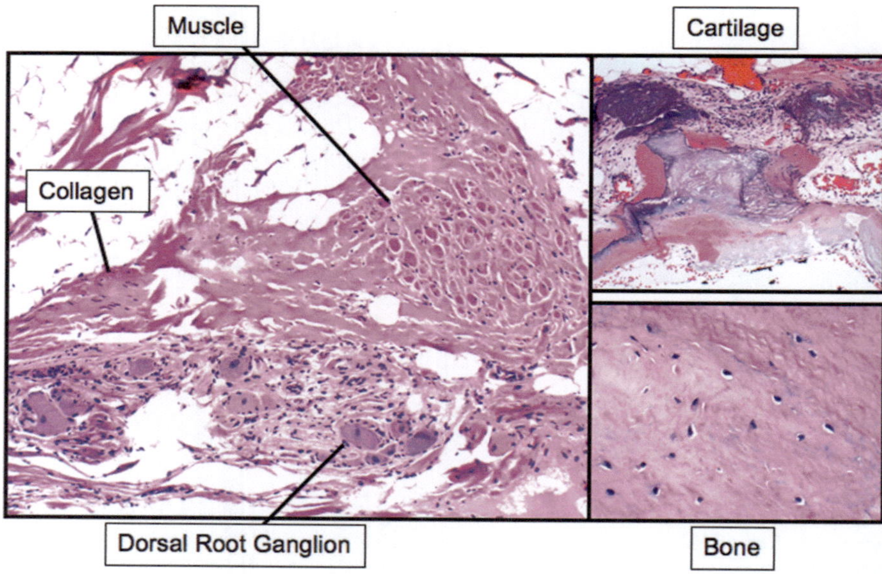

Fig. 7 Mesenchymal derivatives in a dorsal lipoma, including muscle, collagen, cartilage, and bone. Doral root ganglion is from entrapped neural crest cells. (Reprinted from: Pang D, Zovickian J, Wong ST, Hou YJ, and Moes GS. Surgical treatment of complex spinal cord lipomas. Childs Nerv Syst (2013) 29:1485–1513; with Permission from Springer Nature)

just lateral to their site of failed fusion, their central processes, the dorsal nerve roots, also enter the spinal cord lateral to, *but never traversing*, the lipoma stalk. Their entry zone (DREZ) must correspondingly lie very near, *but always lateral,* to the exact junctional boundary between lipoma and spinal cord. Recognising and understanding this boundary, called *fusion line*, is essential before undertaking the actual resection of the lipoma [22, 49, 50] (Fig. 6d). Meanwhile, the "disjoined" cutaneous ectoderm crosses over the chaos underneath to form wholesome skin above, although minor perturbation in the process may produce subtle signatures such as a dimple, crater, or capillary haemangioma overlying the subcutaneous lipoma.

The embryogenesis of dorsal lipoma perfectly exemplifies mistimed disjunction during *primary* neurulation. Its fatty stalk only involves cord segments above the conus, the latter being product of secondary neurulation. Furthermore, premature disjunction of the converging neural folds is always *segmental*, meaning proper disjunction and closure take place "business-as-usual" both immediately rostral and caudal to the faulty focus. This "square pulse" time-line of the abnormal event in dorsal lipoma therefore results in a sharply demarcated fusion line both rostral and caudal to the lipomatous stalk [1, 2, 22, 49–52] (Fig. 2a, b). Dorsal lipomas thus exist only on parts of the matured spinal cord *formed from the primary neural tube* and represent only 15% of lipomas in our series [19, 22, 25].

In transitional lipoma, faulty development involves much more than simple mistimed disjunction in an isolated segment of the primary neural tube. Even though its rostral part resembles the dorsal lipoma, the fatty invasion of the whole of the conus means that not only primary but also secondary neurulation have been profoundly disturbed. This is evidenced by the frequent incorporation of the filum, an undisputed remnant of late secondary neurulation, into the transitional lipoma, and that vacuoles resembling the cavitary spaces typically seen in the medullary cord during mid-secondary neurulation are found in abundance within the core of the transitional lipoma (see below). Also, while the rostral part of the transitional lipoma only affects the dorsal surface of the lumbar cord, the distal part involves the entire core of the conus, strongly suggestive of aberrant inclusion of wayward mesenchyme into the developing conus during the condensation phase of secondary neurulation. Intramedullary mesenchyme may then migrate up and down the neural tube within the conjoint primary and secondary neural canals [53]. The hypothesis that the rostral half of the transitional lipoma comes from faulty primary neural tube fusion affecting only the superficial layers of the lumbar cord, and its caudal half from abnormal condensation within the deeper core of the secondary neural tube may well explain the oblique ventral-caudal slant of its lipoma-cord interface. The far less confined and "non-square pulse" nature of its embryogenetic error also explains why the fusion line of a transitional lesion is never as well-defined and levelled as that of the dorsal lipoma, often has no caudal demarcation, and its fatty acreage is a great deal more sprawling. In spite of the latter, the lipoma-cord interface remains relatively distinct in most transitional lipomas.

Embryogenesis of Chaotic Lipomas

Chaotic lipoma does not quite fit into the scheme for either the dorsal or transitional type. It may have a rostral part half-resembling a dorsal lipoma, but caudally there is no definable lipoma-cord interface, and the fat percolates through the whole thickness of the neural placode to its ventral surface in large and unruly measures. The confusing interplay between fat and cord in this type of lipoma seems to be in constant chaos.

Embryologically, the obvious dissimilarities between the features of a chaotic lipoma and the familiar consequences of mistimed disjunction, as well as its strong association with sacral agenesis (82% in our 2009 series [22]), suggest that its origin may be part of a general failure of the caudal cell mass during early secondary neurulation (Fig. 8) [54, 55]. Secondary neurulation comprises three distinct stages: (1) condensation and transformation of pluripotential stem cells from the caudal cell mass into committed neuro-progenitor cells to form the solid medullary cord; (2)

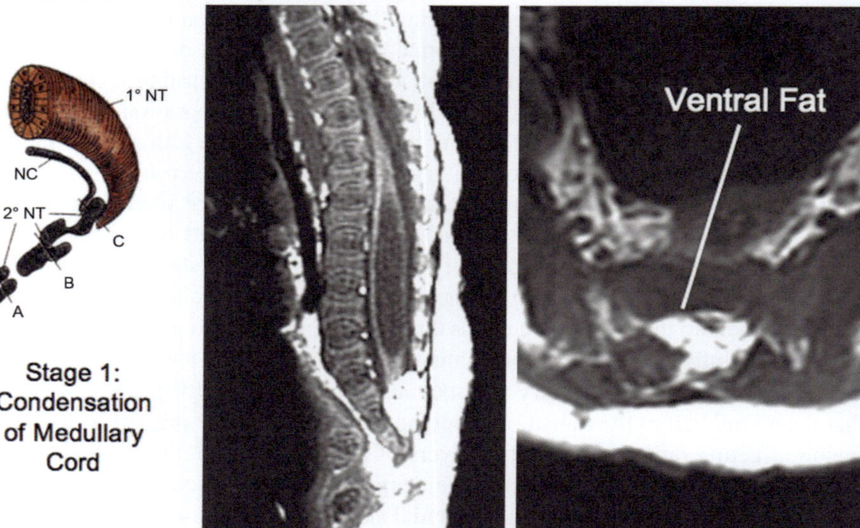

Fig. 8 Embryogenesis of chaotic lipomas. Left: Basic error probably occurs with accelerated differentiation of lipogenic mesenchymal cells within the caudal cord during condensation stage (Stage 1) of secondary neurulation and formation of the medullary cord, thereby incorporating fat tissue in the substance of the mature neural placode. Middle and right show dorsal and ventral fat and associated sacral agenesis. *1° NT* Primary neural tube, *2° NT* Secondary neural tube, *NC* Notochord. (Reprinted from: Pang D, Zovickian J, Wong ST, Hou YJ, and Moes GS. Surgical treatment of complex spinal cord lipomas. Childs Nerv Syst (2013) 29:1485–1513; with Permission from Springer Nature)

intrachordal cavitation of the medullary cord [20, 53, 55] followed by its integration with the primary neural tube; and (3) partial dissolution of the cavitary medullary cord by programmed apoptosis to form the filum terminale [29, 53]. In this context, chaotic lipoma probably results from an aberrant preponderance and accelerated differentiation of lipogenic stem cells from the caudal cell mass during early medullary cord condensation, leading to inclusion of lipoid cells within the neuro-progenitor cell pool, destined to beget a distorted conus permeated with fat through and through [22].

Embryogenesis of Terminal Lipoma

Terminal lipomas involve only the conus and never the lumbar or upper sacral cord, strong evidence that they arise from faulty *secondary* rather than primary neurulation. Furthermore, defects in the lumbodorsal fascia, dura, and dorsal spinal cord, all hallmarks of failed primary neural tube closure, are never seen with terminal lipomas. Lastly, terminal lipomas either replace or are embedded in portions of the filum, which temporally and topographically places their pathogenesis within the period of secondary neural tube formation. The fact that their distal conus always appears well-formed argues against disrupted condensation of the medullary cord in early secondary neurulation. Rather, the almost obligatory presence of disorganized neuroglial and ependymal tubules within terminal lipomas [56] suggests instead an incompetent apoptotic machinery during the late degenerative stage of secondary neurulation as the basic pathogenetic mechanism [57].

Intraoperative Neurophysiological Monitoring (IONM)

Intraoperative neurophysiological monitoring is sine qua non in lipoma surgery [1, 22, 25, 52, 58–60].

Electromyographic Needle Placements

A comprehensive electromyography (EMG) system is set up to capture triggered responses from muscles supplied by the lumbosacral nerve roots. Standard 27-gauge EMG needle electrodes are inserted into the rectus femorus (L_4), anterior tibialis (L_4-L_5), gastrocnemius (S_1), and abductor hallucis (S_2). A pair of smaller gauge (No. 29) EMG needles is inserted obliquely into the external anal sphincter at the anal verge on each side. A plug of dry muslin gauze is pushed half way into the anal canal to isolate the sphincter contractions of one side from the other [58]. In addition, EMG measurements are made from the abductor policis brevis in each hand as a monitor for equipment malfunction. All stimulations and EMG recordings in the authors' unit are done with the Cadwell Cascade Intraoperative Monitoring System (Cadwell Laboratories, Inc., Kennewick, WA 99336) using the Cascade Software Version 2.5, but several other system brands on the market are equally proficient.

Bulbocavernosus Reflex (BCR)

This is the "electrical" version of the reflexive contraction of the external anal sphincter when the glans penis is firmly squeezed and quickly released. For the afferent sensory arm of the reflex, pairs of pad or needle electrodes are placed on the sides of the penile shaft in males and between the labia minora and the periclitoral skin in females. Stimulation of the somatic sensory domain of the pudendal nerve via these electrodes generates a reflexive contraction of the external anal sphincter measurable by EMG. BCR is therefore a form of H reflex within the conus useful in monitoring the integrity of the central sensorimotor connections of the sacral cord segments [58, 59].

Special comments need to be made about BCR, which is still very much a work-in-progress. The pudendal somatic sensory—pudendal somatic motor arc, i.e. the basic BCR circuit, is bilateral, meaning that stimulation on one side will generate sphincter contractions on both sides. The response is highly stimulation-parameter dependent. We use a train of 4 stimuli to capitalise on the powerful principle of post-tetanic potentiation and fairly reliably obtain motor responses from the anus. However, BCR is highly sensitive to inhalation anaesthetic concentrations, so that a sevoflurane level of higher than 0.5 Mac may disrupt it. The BCR is also uncertain in infants younger than 6 months so that allowances must be made for its inconstancy in newborn cases. But most of all, it must be clearly stipulated that the actual neuroelectrical circuit responsible for the BCR involves *somatic* sensory inputs from the perineal skin corresponding to the dermatomes of S_2 to S_4 via the pudendal sensory fibres and *somatic* motor neurons within the anterior horn (Onuf's nucleus) projecting out via the pudendal motor fibres to the external anal sphincter. On the other hand, the sacral bladder circuit involves afferent *visceral* sensory fibres from the bladder wall stretch receptors via the pelvic nerve, and the efferent *visceral* motor neurons to the bladder detrusor muscles that reside within the autonomic (*visceral*) intermediolateral column of the central grey core of the sacral spinal cord, projecting out via the parasympathetic pelvic nerve. Thus, the anatomical pathways for the BCR and for the bladder voiding reflex are located in different, albeit neighbouring, parts of the spinal cord, though both are within the S_2-S_4 cord segments. Theoretically, a disrupted BCR during surgery does not necessarily imply damage to the bladder wall tension-detrusor reflex function, although frequently the prediction is true. A correlative study of the two is needed to sort out BCR's true value (see later).

Nerve Root Stimulation and Direct Spinal Cord Stimulation

Triggered EMG is obtained from direct stimulation of the motor roots and spinal cord using the concentric coaxial bipolar stimulation probe with a small tip diameter of 1.75 mm (Medtronic Xomed, Inc., Jacksonville, Fl, USA) (Fig. 9). The concentric configuration and small sizes of the anode-cathode rings permit delivery of extremely focused current to a very small target volume, ideal for selective activation of small and crowded electroresponsive units such as the delicate sacral rootlets and the compact anterior horn of the conus [60]. Stimulating currents from 0.3 to 5.0 miliamperes (mA) are used depending on target impedance. Most functional motor roots can be triggered by currents of 0.3–1.0 mA, though sometimes needing 1.5 mA if the roots are partially fibrotic or wrapped up in arachnoid adhesions. Stimulation of sensory roots is less reliable, although a functional sensory root should trigger a corresponding motor response using a current of 3–3.5 mA. Direct spinal cord stimulation will require a current of 3.0 mA or higher, but seldom more than 6 mA. Both sides will be recruited if the probe is placed on the midline, but biased ipsilateral response can be elicited if the probe is shifted to a point ventral to the equatorial plane of the cord's coronal aspect. The stimulation frequency is usually

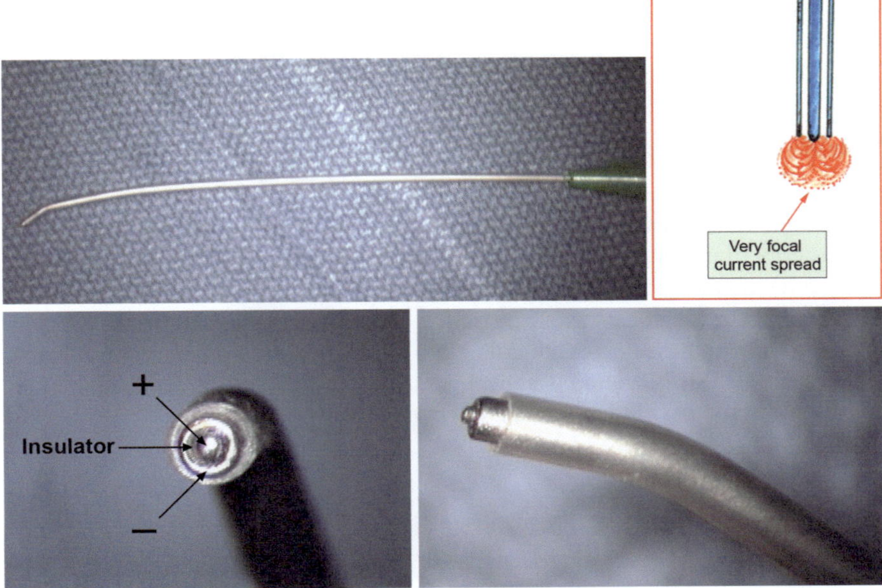

Fig. 9 Concentric coaxial bipolar microprobe stimulator, in which the concentric cathode and anode are separated by a coaxial insulator. Tip diameter is approximately 1.75 mm. The microprobe delivers very focal current spread (Inset). (Reprinted from Pang D. Total resection of complex spinal cord lipomas: how, why, and when to operate. Neuro Med Chir (Tokyo) 55: 695–721, 2015; with permission from the Japanese Neurosurgical Society. CC-BY-NC-ND (https://creativecommons.org/licenses/by-nc-nd/4.0/deed.ja))

10 per second. Noting the rythmic nature of the triggered contractions will distinguish them from the random spontaneous firing caused by surgical manipulation. Clearance of arachnoid bands and efficient suctioning of cerebrospinal fluid (CSF) at the stimulation site will enhance the likelihood of motor response.

Transcortical Motor Evoked Potentials (TcMEP)

In recent years, we have been able to reliably obtain continuous monitoring of TcMEP from the external anal sphincter [1, 2]. The stimulation parameters are the same as for the lower limbs: a train of 8 pulses, each with a duration of 75 µs and intensity of 100–300 volts. In adults and children older than 2 years of age, 150–225 volts are generally adequate but in infants, the stimulation intensity may have to be raised to 350 volts, presumably because of the poorly myelinated motor cortex and its higher impedance, only partially compensated for by the thin cranium. The inhalation anaesthetic concentration, e.g. of sevoflurane, is usually set no higher than 0.5 Mac to ensure a high response rate or, failing that, abandoned completely for total intravenous anaesthesia (TIVA) in some infants and young children. Given that the BCR can be variable or even unobtainable in infants, TcMEP is an important modality for assessing the integrity of the central motor circuits of the sacral spinal cord.

Somatosensory Evoked Potentials (SSEPs)

Stimulating electrodes either of the pad or needle type are placed over the course of the posterior tibial nerve behind the medial malleolus and over the common peroneal nerve at the fibular neck to provide the somatic sensory inputs for SSEP monitoring of the spinal cord segments above S_2 [58]. It should be emphasized that the sensory inputs from both these nerves are going into the L_5-S_1 cord segments, considerably higher than the usual location of most lipomas, so disturbance of conduction in the S_2-S_4 sensory roots will therefore not affect the SSEPs.

Surgical Technique of Total/Near-Total Lipoma Resection

The surgical technique described below concerns the case of an unusually large and rambling dorsal lipoma that illustrates most of the key technical points of total resection applicable to both dorsal and transitional lipomas. The case is a 12-month-old girl who was neurological normal at birth but had magnetic resonance imaging (MRI) because of a lumbosacral fatty lump. The MRI showed a moderate-sized

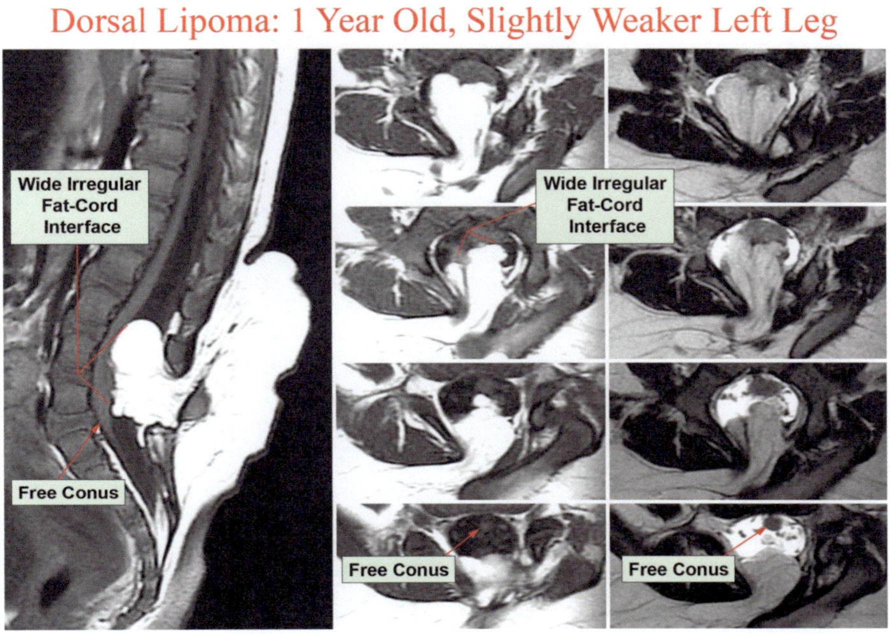

Dorsal Lipoma: 1 Year Old, Slightly Weaker Left Leg

Fig. 10 MRI of a 12 month old girl with left leg weakness shows a large dorsal lipoma. The sagittal image shows a long stretch of lipoma-cord interface, but the conus is clearly free of fat. The axial images reveal the irregular nature of the lipoma-cord interface, but the neural placode is not excessively tilted to one side. (Reprinted from Pang D. Total resection of complex spinal cord lipomas: how, why, and when to operate. Neuro Med Chir (Tokyo) 55: 695–721, 2015; with permission from the Japanese Neurosurgical Society. CC-BY-NC-ND (https://creativecommons.org/licenses/by-nc-nd/4.0/deed.ja))

dorsal lipoma involving the lower lumbar cord. At 1 year, she began showing left leg weakness, and repeat MRI showed massive enlargement of the lipoma (Fig. 10).

Step 1. Exposure and Dealing with the Extraspinal Lipoma Stalk

The upper extent of the skin incision should be about 2 cm above the rostral end of the lipoma. The lower extent ideally includes at least 1 cm beyond the tip of the conus in a dorsal lipoma or of the neural placode in a transitional lipoma. Two metal skin markers are used to mark the longitudinal span of the planned laminectomies for a lateral X-Ray, which is then matched up with the sagittal MRI to finalise the skin incision (Fig. 11).

During the soft tissue exposure, temptation to remove the subcutaneous lipoma must be resisted to avoid creating a tense fluid-filled dead space afterwards which

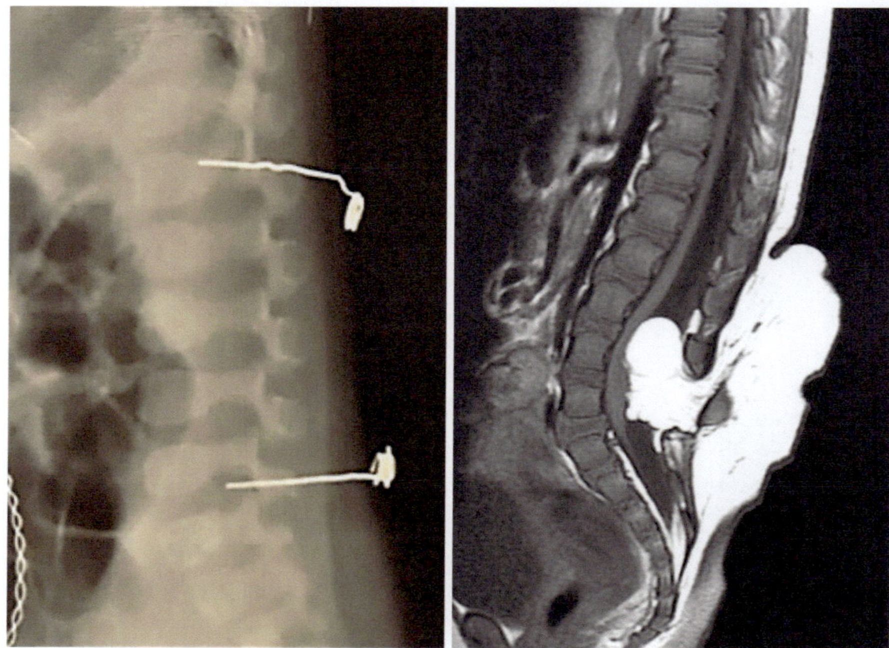

Fig. 11 The lateral radiograph showing the localising markers is matched to the sagittal MRI to finalise the top and bottom extent of the exposure. (Reprinted from Pang D. Total resection of complex spinal cord lipomas: how, why, and when to operate. Neuro Med Chir (Tokyo) 55: 695–721, 2015; with permission from the Japanese Neurosurgical Society. CC-BY-NC-ND (https://creativecommons.org/licenses/by-nc-nd/4.0/deed.ja))

may compromise wound healing. Frequently, a relatively robust fatty stalk slightly more compact than the loose subcutaneous adiposity can be discretely traced through a defect in the lumbodorsal fascia with minimal dissection (Fig. 12). This fatty stalk is a signpost to the lipoma's attachment on the spinal cord below and must therefore be handled with care during fascial exposure.

The amount of proximal bone removal must be adequate to allow for an unencumbered view of the upper tip of the lipoma where the "last" set of normal nerve roots and DREZ are used as anatomical landmarks, but more importantly, wide bilateral laminectomy down to the pedicles must be done to gain access to the far lateral corners of the dural tube (see below). Exposure of some normal dura proximal to the lipoma also provides a visual perspective of how much the neural placode had protruded beyond the spinal canal in lipomas with extraspinal extension. The heavy mound of fat attached to the fatty stalk can now be removed to avoid inadvertent tugging on the spinal cord (Fig. 12).

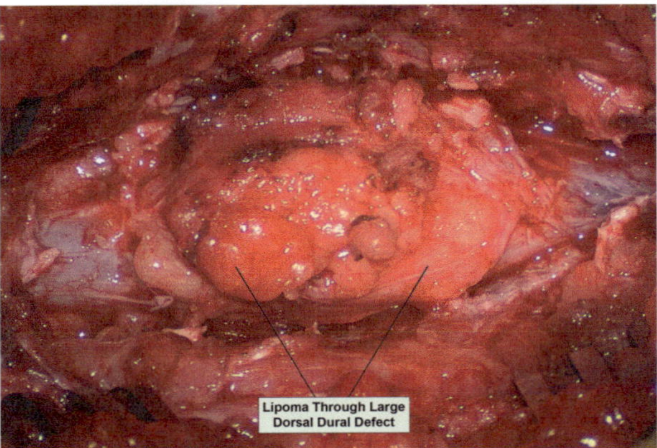

Fig. 12 Large extradural portion of the lipoma before dural opening. Note huge dural defect through which the extradural lipoma extends. Rostral exposure is to the right. Note the essential wide bony exposure. (Reprinted from Pang D. Total resection of complex spinal cord lipomas: how, why, and when to operate. Neuro Med Chir (Tokyo) 55: 695–721, 2015; with permission from the Japanese Neurosurgical Society. CC-BY-NC-ND (https://creativecommons.org/licenses/by-nc-nd/4.0/deed.ja))

Step 2. Detachment of Lipoma from Dura: Unhinging the Hammock

The dura is opened in the midline about 1 cm rostral to the upper end of the lipoma, identified by its slight yellow tinge below the pia. Tight and closely spaced dural tagging sutures are placed to gain maximum exposure of the far lateral alcoves of the dural tube afforded by the wide laminectomy. This is a crucial but often neglected manoeuvre, because tagging the dural edge helps to reveal the "crotch" at the embryological fusion line where the lateral fringe of the lipoma is attached to the inner edges of the dural defect. The critical importance of adequately exposing the "crotch" is shown best by examining any given axial slice of the lesion, in which the lipoma is roughly divided by a transverse line joining the site of lipoma-dura attachment, i.e. the "crotch", on each side. The entire lipoma-cord assembly is, in effect, suspended from the dural ceiling like a hammock at these two "crotches". From a dorsal perspective, the surgeon thus has no visualisation whatsoever of any meaningful anatomy ventral to this transverse line, such as the dorsal roots, DREZ, neural placode, or CSF pool (Fig. 13 Upper), until this hammock can be unsuspended by releasing the two crotch hinges. The lateral edges of the neural placode and nerve roots can then be folded inward enough to be identified and preserved. (Fig. 13 Lower).

Safe unhinging of the hammock must begin at the rostral extent of the crotch line where there is at least a semblance of normal anatomy. The "crotch" is kept under tension by pulling the fat firmly away from the dura, and its attachment to the inner dural lining minutely cut literally millimetre at a time to avoid injuring the dorsal roots on the DREZ, which are very close to the "crotch" only millimetres below the

Lipoma Suspended at Dural Adhesion Points Like a Hammock

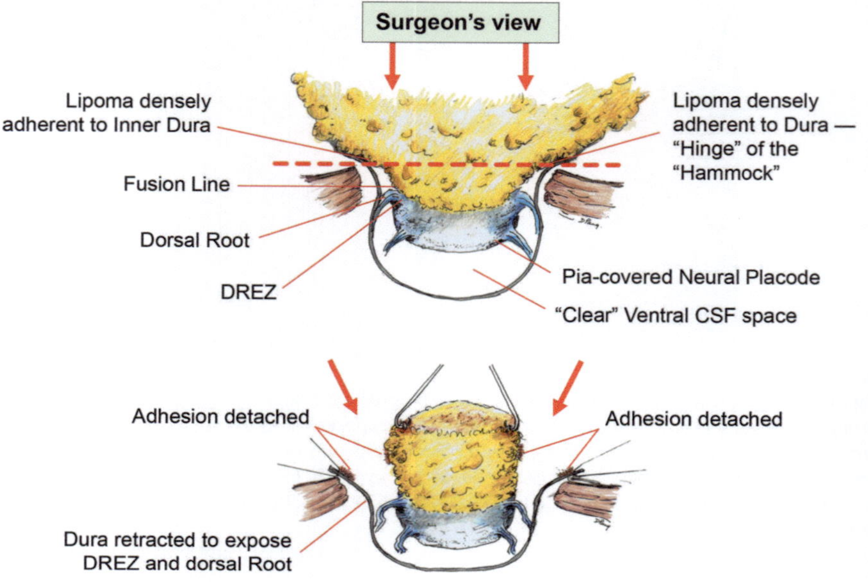

Fig. 13 Drawing depicting the relationship between the lipoma, neural placode, nerve roots and dural sac in an axial slice. Upper: The lipoma-cord assembly is suspended at the dural edges at far lateral adhesion points like a hammock against side hinges. The dotted transverse line that joins the two side hinges divides the assembly into a dorsal disorderly, fibrofatty half that completely blocks the surgeon's view to a much more orderly ventral half, containing the important anatomical landmarks of fusion line, DREZ, dorsal roots, fat-free ventral placode, and pristine ventral CSF space. Lower: After detaching the far lateral adhesion points (the hinges) by careful "crotch dissection", and folding-in the fatty mass, the ventral anatomical landmarks can now be visualized. (Reprinted from Pang D. Total resection of complex spinal cord lipomas: how, why, and when to operate. Neuro Med Chir (Tokyo) 55: 695–721, 2015; with permission from the Japanese Neurosurgical Society. CC-BY-NC-ND (https://creativecommons.org/licenses/by-nc-nd/4.0/deed.ja))

fat (Fig. 14). These initially hidden roots should "pop" into view as more of the fatty hammock is peeled back (Fig. 15a, b), and any binding adhesions to the arachnoid can be gently dissected away (Fig. 16). The clean ventral surface of the neural placode is now seen to advantage. (Fig. 17). This laborious but indispensable and ultimately rewarding step of "crotch dissection" is carried caudally until all the functioning nerve roots are revealed, and the entire lipoma-neural placode assembly is completely unsuspended and freed from the dura (Fig. 18).

Preparing the "crotch" for dissection is sometimes difficult. If the dura is so attenuated that it clings to the side of the lipoma and spinal cord like pia mater, as on the left side here, the surgeon can lose perspective and mistakenly stray into the extradural space, where the nerve roots are entangled in stringy extradural fat and can be accidentally injured. When caught in this predicament, it is best to abandon

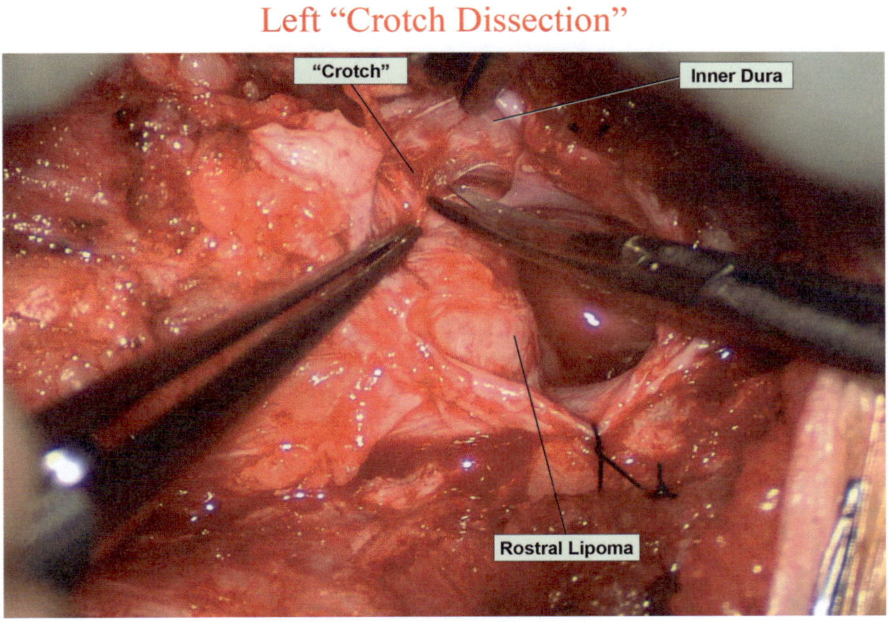

Left "Crotch Dissection"

Fig. 14 Left crotch dissection in the large dorsal lipoma shown in Fig. 10. The lipoma is grasped firmly and pulled gently away from the adherent points on the inner dura, stretching the adhesion bands and thick arachnoid, creating the "crotch" and making the adhesions safe to be cut. (Reprinted from Pang D. Total resection of complex spinal cord lipomas: how, why, and when to operate. Neuro Med Chir (Tokyo) 55: 695–721, 2015; with permission from the Japanese Neurosurgical Society. CC-BY-NC-ND (https://creativecommons.org/licenses/by-nc-nd/4.0/deed.ja))

further dissection on the "bad" left side and pick up brisker pace by opening the crotch on the less problematic right side. After the crotch adhesions here are dispatched with and the free ventral subarachnoid space is entered, the collapsed left subarachnoid space can now be confidently accessed by navigating under the neural placode, and the left crotch dissection can finally be accomplished (Fig. 19).

Step 3. Lipoma Resection

Before the actual lipoma resection, the fusion line must first be clearly identified because a good amount of sharp dissection of fat will fall on this line where the lateral edge of the lipoma is attached to the cord just medial to the DREZ. In most dorsal lipomas, the fusion line is traceable as a neat complete oval or circle from side to side, often outlining a flat horizontal plane, and is usually bilaterally symmetrical. This circular line ends short of the conus which is never involved in the dorsal lipoma (Fig. 2b, c). In a transitional lipoma, the more distinct rostral

Fig. 15 Right crotch dissection. (**a**) Cutting of the "crotch" on the right side as in Fig. 14. (**b**) Lysing the crotch exposes the hidden nerve roots, the ventral neural placode, and the ventral free subarachnoid space. (Reprinted from Pang D. Total resection of complex spinal cord lipomas: how, why, and when to operate. Neuro Med Chir (Tokyo) 55: 695–721, 2015; with permission from the Japanese Neurosurgical Society. CC-BY-NC-ND (https://creativecommons. org/licenses/by-nc-nd/4.0/ deed.ja))

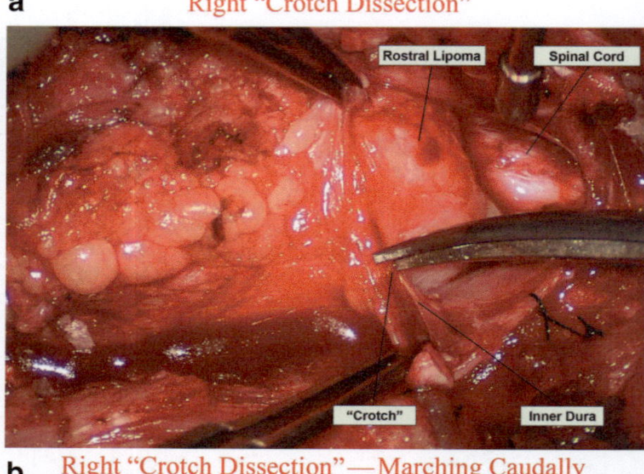

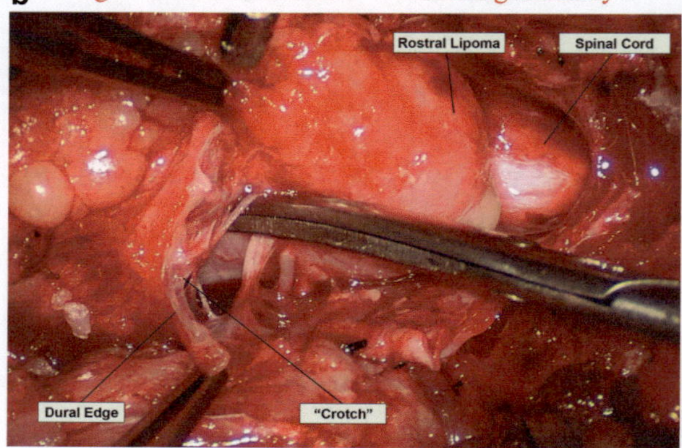

fusion line resembles that of a dorsal lipoma but distally it becomes blurry and cuts towards the ventral surface of the conus and never joins its mate from the other side at the bottom of the spinal cord (Fig. 3a–c). For a large lipoma of either type, as in the monstrous dorsal lipoma shown in Figs. 10 and 18, exuberant fat may hang over the fusion line and cover up the upper portion of the emergent dorsal roots (the "thighs" of the roots) to give the false impression that the roots *run through* and are not separate from the lipoma (Fig. 20). In reality, these festoons of overhanging fat can quite easily be sharply dissected off the "thighs" of the roots to expose the "knees" of the roots (Fig. 21), the DREZ (Fig. 22), and the elusive fusion line above (Fig. 23). We call this manoeuvre "knee dissection".

Actual lipoma resection may commence only after the fusion lines from both sides have been clearly identified (Fig. 24). Without exception, resection begins at the rostral tip of the lipoma where the anatomical relationships between fat, nerve roots and DREZ are clearly decipherable (Fig. 25). First order of business is to use the micro-scissors to locate a thin but distinct silvery *white plane* between fat and cord at the demi-lune of the rostral fusion line (Fig. 26a, b). The white plane is in

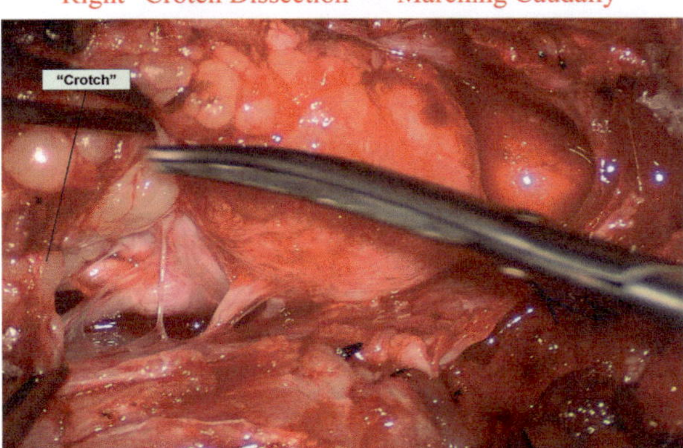

Fig. 16 Marching caudally with the right crotch dissection, the surgeon exposes the ventral surface of the placode, the free ventral subarachnoid space, and more nerve roots that can be traced all the way to their exit foramina. (Reprinted from Pang D. Total resection of complex spinal cord lipomas: how, why, and when to operate. Neuro Med Chir (Tokyo) 55: 695–721, 2015; with permission from the Japanese Neurosurgical Society. CC-BY-NC-ND (https://creativecommons. org/licenses/by-nc-nd/4.0/deed.ja))

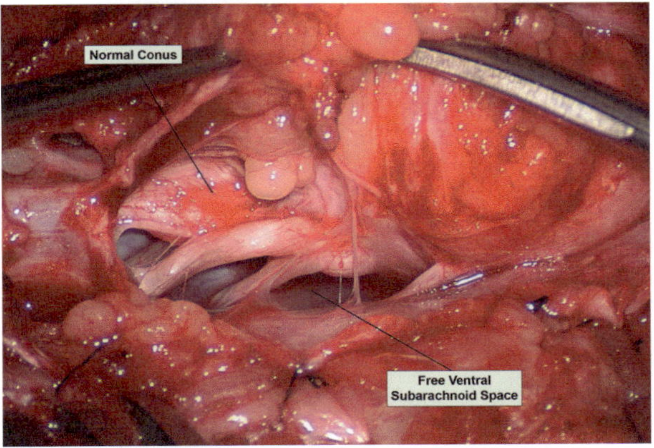

Fig. 17 After crotch dissection on the right side and complete detachment of the lipoma (hammock) from the right inner dural lining, the fat-free ventral subarachnoid space, caudal nerve roots, and conus are well seen. (Reprinted from Pang D. Total resection of complex spinal cord lipomas: how, why, and when to operate. Neuro Med Chir (Tokyo) 55: 695–721, 2015; with permission from the Japanese Neurosurgical Society. CC-BY-NC-ND (https://creativecommons. org/licenses/by-nc-nd/4.0/deed.ja))

essence a thin net of collagen fibres that is distinguishable from yellow fat by its glistening white colour and from soft spinal cord by its tough and gritty feel when cut. It can become convoluted and uneven within the main bulk of the lipoma, but its rostral end is almost always distinct and flat (Fig. 26c and Fig. 27a–c). The initial

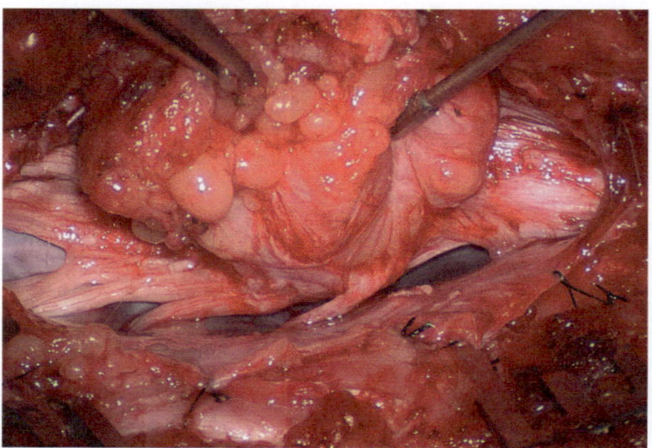

Fig. 18 Crotch dissection is complete on both sides. The entire right array of nerve roots are seen, but not the DREZ or the fusion line, which are covered by the lateral overhang of the large lipoma. The entire hammock is now unsuspended from the dura. (Reprinted from Pang D. Total resection of complex spinal cord lipomas: how, why, and when to operate. Neuro Med Chir (Tokyo) 55: 695–721, 2015; with permission from the Japanese Neurosurgical Society. CC-BY-NC-ND (https://creativecommons.org/licenses/by-nc-nd/4.0/deed.ja))

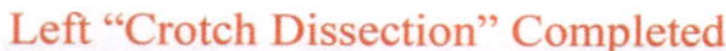

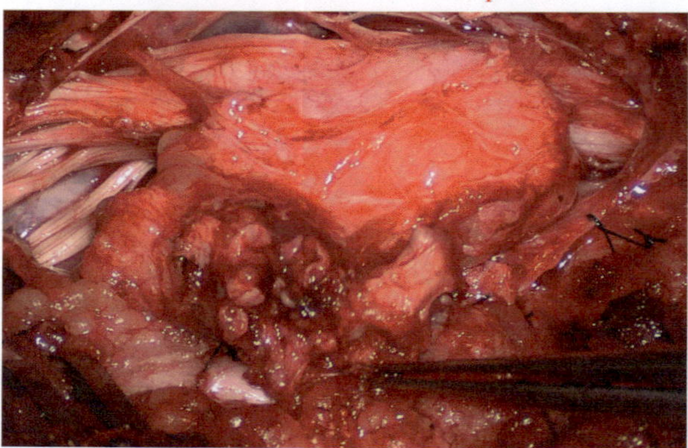

Fig. 19 Completed crotch dissection on the left side, showing left nerve roots and ventral placode surface. Anatomy here is not as distinct and normal as on the right. (Reprinted from Pang D. Total resection of complex spinal cord lipomas: how, why, and when to operate. Neuro Med Chir (Tokyo) 55: 695–721, 2015; with permission from the Japanese Neurosurgical Society. CC-BY-NC-ND (https://creativecommons.org/licenses/by-nc-nd/4.0/deed.ja))

sharp cut to locate the plane has to be directed seemingly straight into the spinal cord, but after neatly cutting through the tongue of yellow fat at the rostral tip of the lipoma, the gritty white plane can always be safely located here (Fig. 28a, b) and once found can then be followed by constantly sensing the grittiness through the micro-scissors and by noting the white glint between yellow globular fat and the

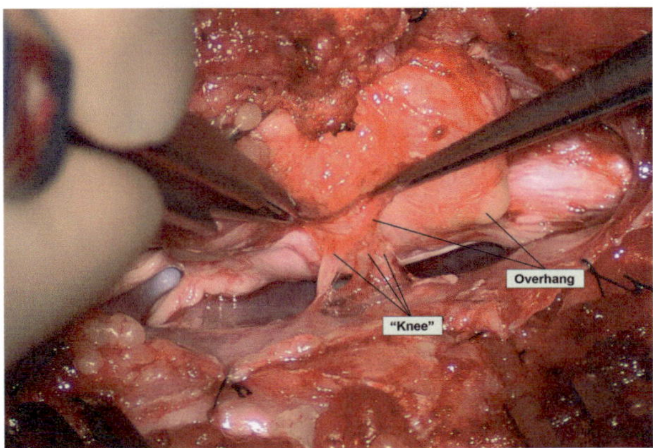

Fig. 20 The lateral overhang of the lipoma is well appreciated. Only the "knees" of the dorsal roots are seen. The "thighs", or the most proximal portions of the roots, are hidden by and adherent to the overhanging fat. (Reprinted from Pang D. Total resection of complex spinal cord lipomas: how, why, and when to operate. Neuro Med Chir (Tokyo) 55: 695–721, 2015; with permission from the Japanese Neurosurgical Society. CC-BY-NC-ND (https://creativecommons.org/licenses/by-nc-nd/4.0/deed.ja))

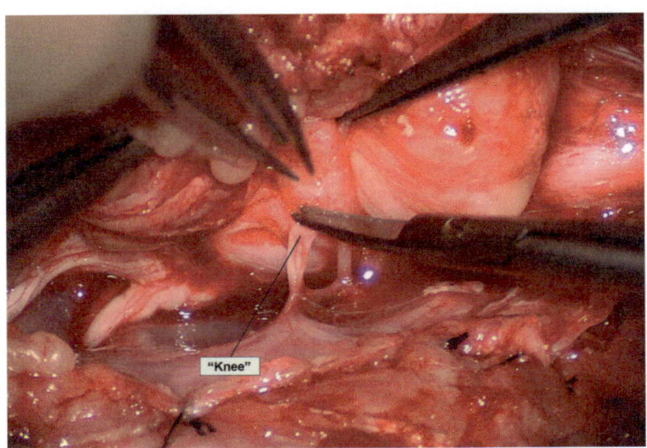

Fig. 21 "Knee dissection": the adhesions covering the "thigh" of the dorsal roots are sharply taken down. (Reprinted from Pang D. Total resection of complex spinal cord lipomas: how, why, and when to operate. Neuro Med Chir (Tokyo) 55: 695–721, 2015; with permission from the Japanese Neurosurgical Society. CC-BY-NC-ND (https://creativecommons.org/licenses/by-nc-nd/4.0/deed.ja))

dull, pasty pink spinal cord (Fig. 29). The CO_2 laser should never be used to vaporise the fat because it chars the surface and thus blots out the signature white colour of the white plane and also casts out the valuable tactile feedback from the micro-scissors which unerringly spots the characteristic gritty toughness of the fibrous plane from the softer semi-liquid fat. The Nd-YAG laser has less charring effect on

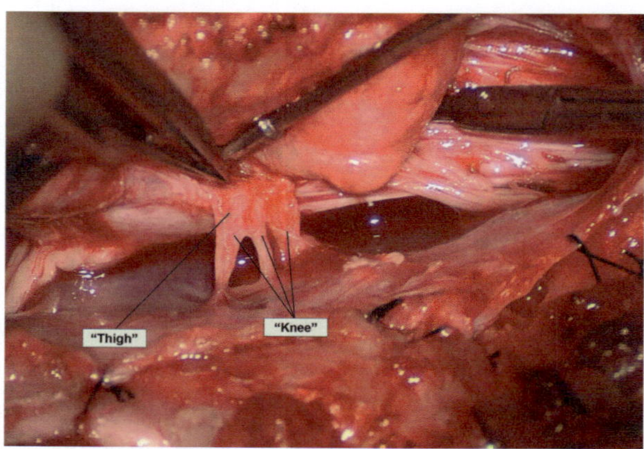

Fig. 22 After ridding the adhesions, the proximal "thigh" portions of the dorsal roots are exposed. (Reprinted from Pang D. Total resection of complex spinal cord lipomas: how, why, and when to operate. Neuro Med Chir (Tokyo) 55: 695–721, 2015; with permission from the Japanese Neurosurgical Society. CC-BY-NC-ND (https://creativecommons.org/licenses/by-nc-nd/4.0/deed.ja))

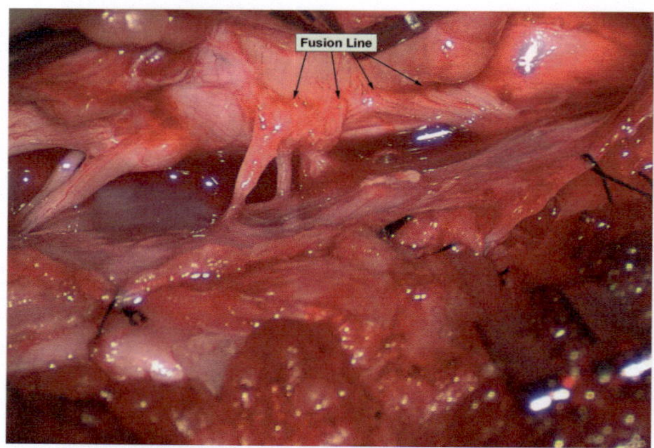

Fig. 23 The "true" fusion line on the right is revealed. Resection of lipoma on the lateral margin of the placode is now made safe. (Reprinted from Pang D. Total resection of complex spinal cord lipomas: how, why, and when to operate. Neuro Med Chir (Tokyo) 55: 695–721, 2015; with permission from the Japanese Neurosurgical Society. CC-BY-NC-ND (https://creativecommons.org/licenses/by-nc-nd/4.0/deed.ja))

the fat but, without the tactile feedback, is no better in finding or surfing the white plane.

Bleeding on the white plane, which is essentially bleeding on the cord, must be handled delicately. Instead of hastily digging with the sparking bipolar cautery, or worse, scrambling with the suction tip, the exact bleeding spot is accurately and atraumatically located by intermittent gentle jets of irrigation from a small hand

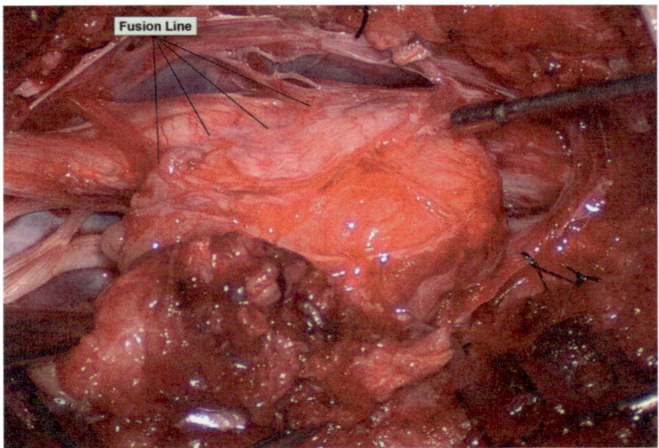

Fig. 24 The fusion line on the left is not as distinct as the right side and not on an even level. (Reprinted from Pang D. Total resection of complex spinal cord lipomas: how, why, and when to operate. Neuro Med Chir (Tokyo) 55: 695–721, 2015; with permission from the Japanese Neurosurgical Society. CC-BY-NC-ND (https://creativecommons.org/licenses/by-nc-nd/4.0/deed.ja))

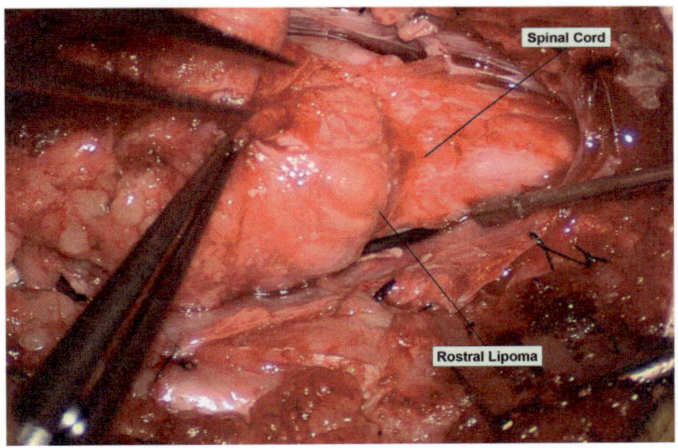

Fig. 25 Preparing for lipoma resection commencing on the rostral end of the fat where the lipoma-cord junction, the rostral dorsal roots, and beginning of the fusion lines are most distinct. (Reprinted from Pang D. Total resection of complex spinal cord lipomas: how, why, and when to operate. Neuro Med Chir (Tokyo) 55: 695–721, 2015; with permission from the Japanese Neurosurgical Society. CC-BY-NC-ND (https://creativecommons.org/licenses/by-nc-nd/4.0/deed.ja))

bubble-squeezer fitted with a fine blunt needle. Once precisely located by the irrigation, the bleeding can be deftly handled with the ultra-fine irrigating bipolar cautery (0.2 mm tips, Fig. 30) set at a low current. The cold irrigation prevents sticking but more importantly it dissipates heat rapidly from the cord. .

While resecting lipoma along the fusion lines (Fig. 31), strong diathermy and sharp gouging must be avoided at the DREZ to avert disturbing sensory symptoms

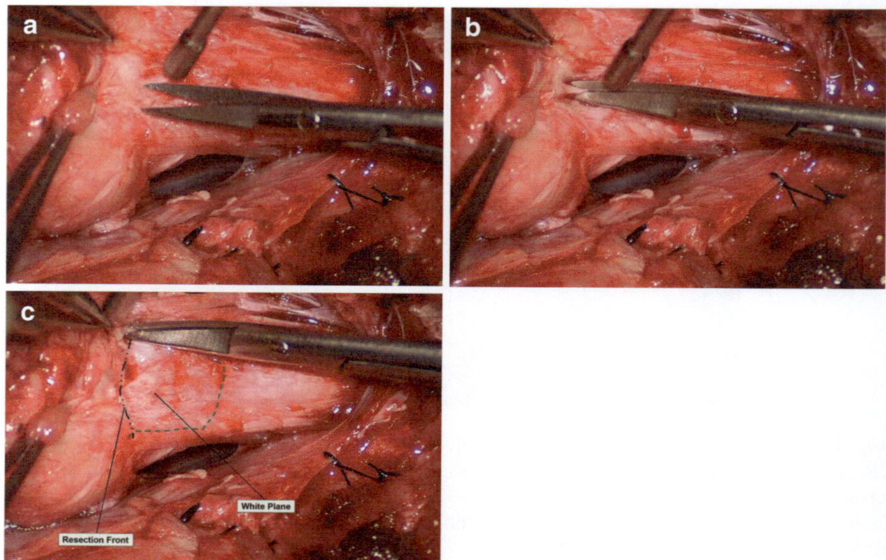

Fig. 26 Finding the white plane: (**a**) Beginning resection at the rostral extremity of the lipoma. (**b**) Boldly cutting sharply into the gritty fibrofatty base of the fat lump to locate the thin white plane. (**c**) White plane located, which is a discrete though thin layer of whitish fibrous netting separating fat from spinal cord. (Reprinted from Pang D. Total resection of complex spinal cord lipomas: how, why, and when to operate. Neuro Med Chir (Tokyo) 55: 695–721, 2015; with permission from the Japanese Neurosurgical Society. CC-BY-NC-ND (https://creativecommons.org/licenses/by-nc-nd/4.0/deed.ja))

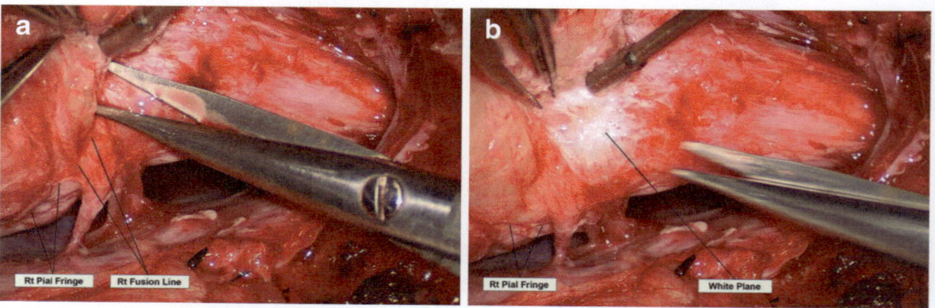

Fig. 27 Resection of lipoma along the right fusion line. (**a**) Cutting sharply on the white plane near the right fusion line. (**b**) Note the pial fringe, carefully preserved for neurulation. (Reprinted from Pang D. Total resection of complex spinal cord lipomas: how, why, and when to operate. Neuro Med Chir (Tokyo) 55: 695–721, 2015; with permission from the Japanese Neurosurgical Society. CC-BY-NC-ND (https://creativecommons.org/licenses/by-nc-nd/4.0/deed.ja))

[1]. Just medial to the DREZ at the fusion line, a robust cuff of pia mater must be preserved to provide sturdy stitch-hold for the neurulation sutures (see below) (Figs. 27a, b and 28b). As long as the sharp dissection is kept strictly on the white

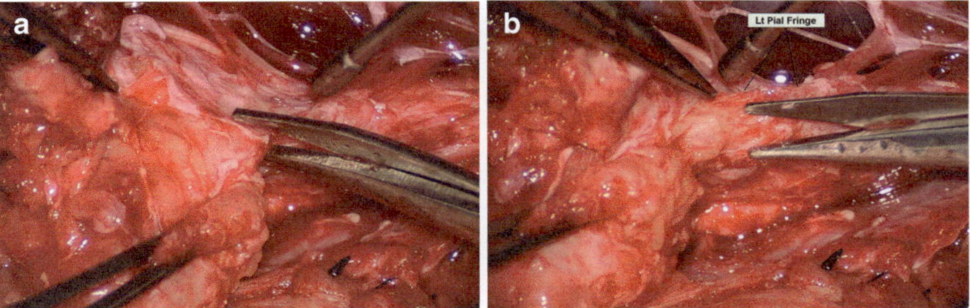

Fig. 28 Resection of lipoma along the left fusion line. (**a**) Cutting lipoma from fusion line. (**b**) Note white plane and left pial fringe. (Reprinted from Pang D. Total resection of complex spinal cord lipomas: how, why, and when to operate. Neuro Med Chir (Tokyo) 55: 695–721, 2015; with permission from the Japanese Neurosurgical Society. CC-BY-NC-ND (https://creativecommons.org/licenses/by-nc-nd/4.0/deed.ja))

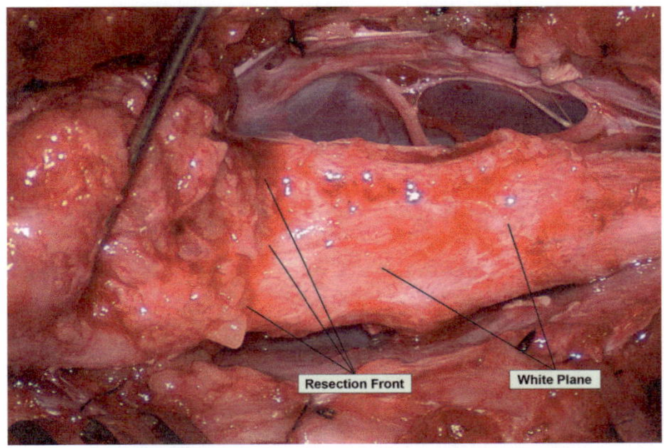

Fig. 29 The white plane, with the unresected portion of the lipoma on the left lifted up to show the resection front as a well-defined transverse line across the body of the neural placode. (Reprinted from Pang D. Total resection of complex spinal cord lipomas: how, why, and when to operate. Neuro Med Chir (Tokyo) 55: 695–721, 2015; with permission from the Japanese Neurosurgical Society. CC-BY-NC-ND (https://creativecommons.org/licenses/by-nc-nd/4.0/deed.ja))

plane medial to the fusion line and DREZ, complete lipoma resection can be carried out without injury to neural tissues. This is much easier to achieve in most dorsal lipomas because the white plane is usually predictably flat and levelle and because the entire fusion line can be readily charted and circumferentially approached from all 360° (Fig. 32a–c). In a particularly large and rambling dorsal lipoma, the white plane may undulate and ripple considerably so that the corresponding fusion line and its neighbouring DREZ will accordingly situate at uneven heights on the side of the cord (Fig. 24). Finding this safe zone of dissection may require systematic stimulation of the adjacent nerve roots for functional localization.

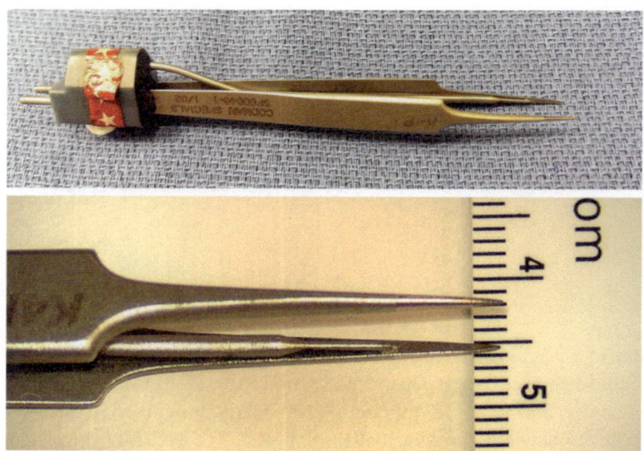

Fig. 30 Micro-irrigating bipolar cautery with super-fine tips measuring less than 0.2 mm. (Reprinted from Pang D. Total resection of complex spinal cord lipomas: how, why, and when to operate. Neuro Med Chir (Tokyo) 55: 695–721, 2015; with permission from the Japanese Neurosurgical Society. CC-BY-NC-ND (https://creativecommons.org/licenses/by-nc-nd/4.0/deed.ja))

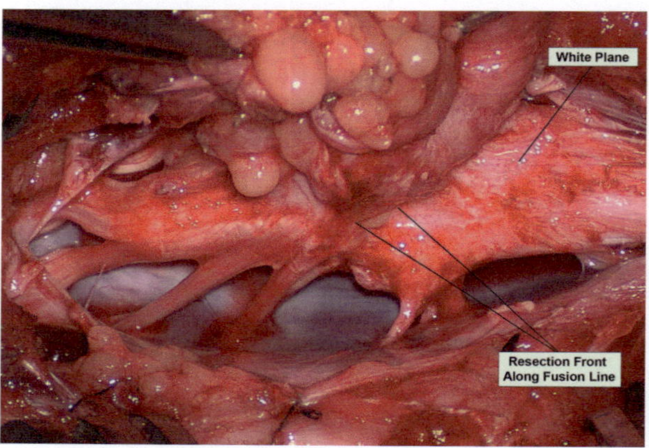

Fig. 31 Lateral white plane dissection along the right fusion line is almost complete. (Reprinted from Pang D. Total resection of complex spinal cord lipomas: how, why, and when to operate. Neuro Med Chir (Tokyo) 55: 695–721, 2015; with permission from the Japanese Neurosurgical Society. CC-BY-NC-ND (https://creativecommons.org/licenses/by-nc-nd/4.0/deed.ja))

Navigating the white plane in most transitional lipomas is considerably more challenging because the plane is never horizontal, usually undulates, and the corresponding fusion line is thus very jagged. One side of the white plane with the DREZ and nerve roots may even be tilted completely away from the surgeon when the entire neural placode is rotated 90° into the sagittal plane. In such extreme cases, the neural placode now faces one side of the canal and the lipoma the opposite side and the white plane is now vertical. Not uncommonly, the caudal portion of the

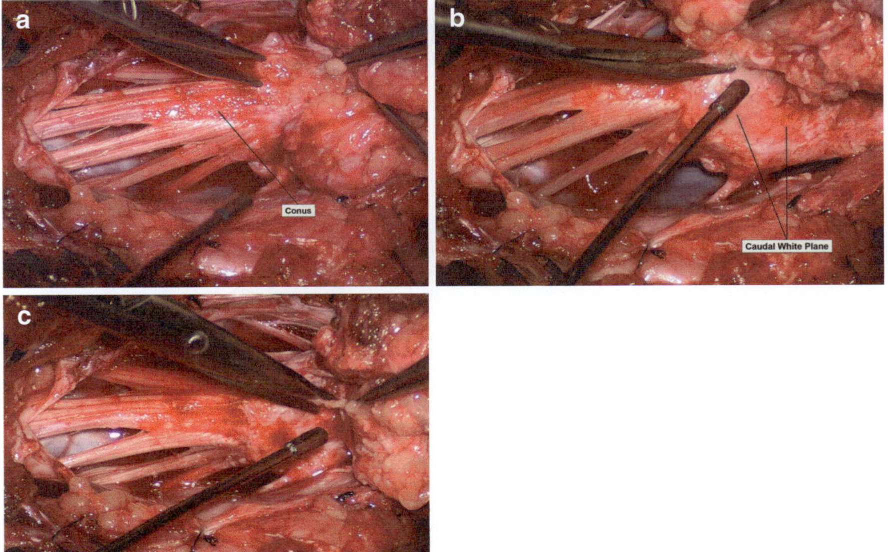

Fig. 32 Resection of the most caudal portion of the lipoma in the caudal to rostral direction, possible because this is a dorsal lipoma. The caudal white plane thus created will eventually merge with the proximal white plane resulting from the previous rostral-to-caudal dissection. (**a**) Beginning white plane dissection from the conus side. (**b**) More caudal white plane exposed. (**c**) Last cut before completing white plane dissection. (Reprinted from Pang D. Total resection of complex spinal cord lipomas: how, why, and when to operate. Neuro Med Chir (Tokyo) 55: 695–721, 2015; with permission from the Japanese Neurosurgical Society. CC-BY-NC-ND (https://creativecommons.org/licenses/by-nc-nd/4.0/deed.ja))

lipoma is so large as to obscure all edges of the caudal dural sac, and the white plane dissection feels endless, often amidst white bands that could be vestigial or functional nerves. Here, electrophysiological identification of the ventral nerve roots is the only way to determine where *functional* conus joins the fibrofatty muck of the caudal lipoma. The S_2 is the only motor root that activates both the anal sphincter and the abductor hallucis, and the next two sets of puny and adhesion-laden rootlets with "pure" sphincter response must therefore be the S_3 and S_4 roots. Any suspicious tissue or bands distal to the last "live" sphincter roots can now be considered non-functional and be freely discarded to consummate the final emancipation of the neural placode (Fig. 33b).

The same principle of using electrical identification of the caudal roots and placode may well be the only way to sort out the true termination of the functional conus in chaotic lipomas. With placode stimulation, the current is lifted up to 4–6 mA, but the drill is the same as for the motor roots. For the rostro-dorsal portion of the chaotic lipoma, dissection of the white plane is as described for dorsal lipomas, but the billows of fat ventral to the placode should be left alone and their pristine pial surfaces left unviolated (Fig. 33a–d). It is always the dorsal and never the ventral surface of an untouched lipoma that actually tethers the spinal cord [22].

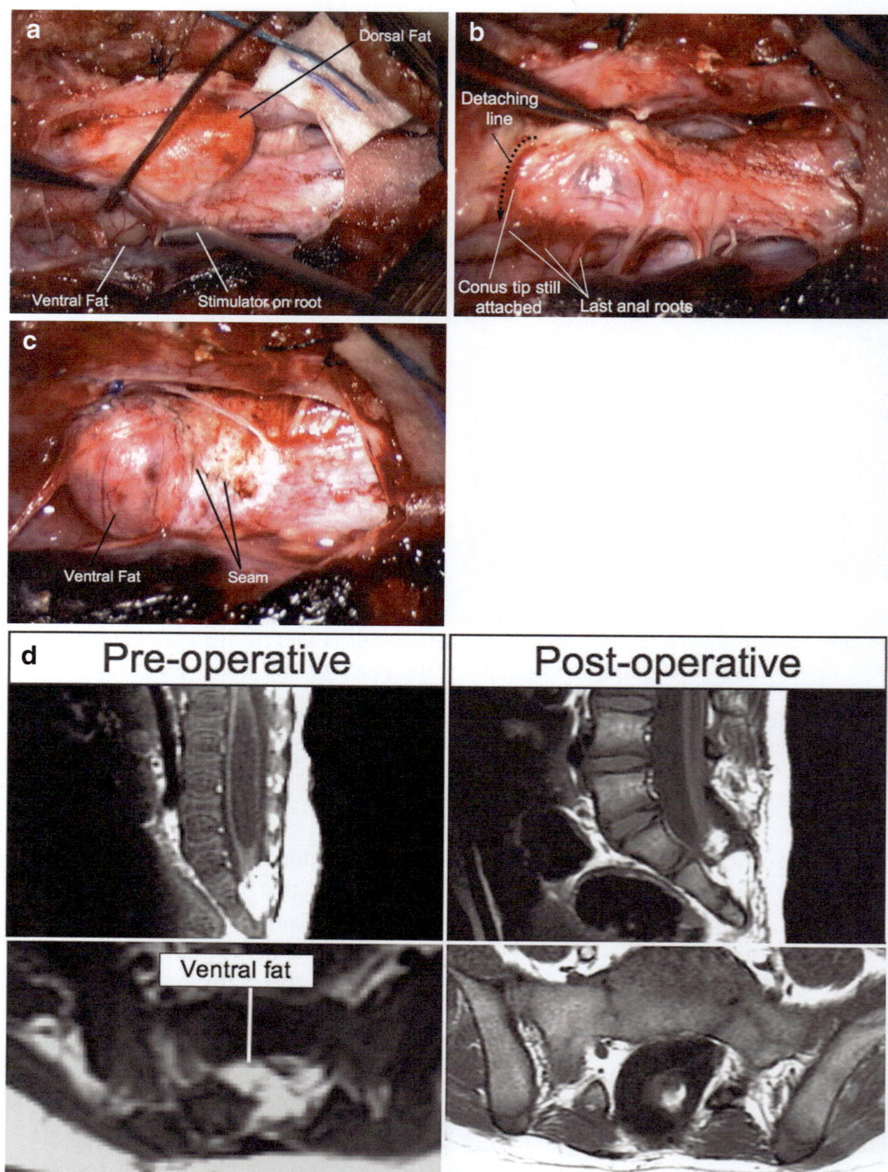

a
Dorsal Fat
Ventral Fat
Stimulator on root
b
Detaching line
Conus tip still attached
Last anal roots
c
Ventral Fat
Seam
d
Pre-operative
Post-operative
Ventral fat

Fig. 33 Surgery for chaotic lipoma. (**a**) Note ventral pia-covered fat medial to ventral nerve roots (being stimulated by concentric microprobe stimulator), and dorsal fat perched on the dorsal side of the placode. (Reprinted from Pang D. Total resection of complex spinal cord lipomas: how, why, and when to operate. Neuro Med Chir (Tokyo) 55: 695–721, 2015; with permission from the Japanese Neurosurgical Society. CC-BY-NC-ND (https://creativecommons.org/licenses/by-nc-nd/4.0/deed.ja)). (**b**) Terminal disconnection of neural placode from residual caudal lipoma stump after identification of 3 healthy pairs of anal sphincter motor roots. (Reprinted from Pang D. Total resection of complex spinal cord lipomas: how, why, and when to operate. Neuro Med Chir (Tokyo) 55: 695–721, 2015; with permission from the Japanese Neurosurgical Society. CC-BY-NC-ND (https://creativecommons.org/licenses/by-nc-nd/4.0/deed.ja)). (**c**) Caudal placode pulled up dorsally width-wise to be neurulated with the more proximal pial edge to form the seam, displaying the unviolated pia-covered ventral fat as a blunt stump. (Reprinted from Pang D. Total resection of complex spinal cord lipomas: how, why, and when to operate. Neuro Med Chir (Tokyo) 55: 695–721, 2015; with permission from the Japanese Neurosurgical Society. CC-BY-NC-ND (https://creativecommons.org/licenses/by-nc-nd/4.0/deed.ja)). (**d**) Pre- and postoperative MRI shows residual fat on the detached cord stump. The cord is untethered, the thecal sac is augmented, and the syrinx has collapsed. (Reprinted from: Pang D, Zovickian J, Wong ST, Hou YJ, and Moes GS. Surgical treatment of complex spinal cord lipomas. Childs Nerv Syst (2013) 29:1485–1513; with Permission from Springer Nature)

For ease of handling, we always try not to cut into the lipoma during the resection because lacerated fat tends to be weepy and fragile and its altered colour and texture may confound the dissection front on the white plane. Also, it is more secure to grasp on to firm, encapsulated fat than pulling on dripping, stringy grease. However, for the truly massive lipoma that completely obscures all anatomical landscapes, its central bulk has to be first reduced using the ultrasonic aspirator before its sides can be collapsed inward to locate the crotch hinges.

After the entire lipoma has been resected (Fig. 34), it is advisable to systematically stimulate each pair of motor roots on the "naked" placode and to run a few sets of transcortical motor potentials to ensure all baseline functions have been preserved. Functional deterioration has been known to occur during neurulation due to tight strangling of the placode.

Step 4. Pia-to-Pia Neurulation of the Neural Placode

Thorough resection of fat and fibrous scar converts a stiff, rotund, fat-engorged spinal cord to a supple, slender, and infinitely more manoeuvrable neural placode suited for tensionless pia-to-pia neurulation (Fig. 34). Well-executed neurulation in turn transforms the resection bed from a broad, wafery, sticky flat surface to a single seam on a trim and tidy pia-covered tube, duly minimising the likelihood of its adhering to the dura.

A few technical tips concerning neurulation deserve special mention. While folding up the neural placode to appose the pial edges, the surgeon may encounter a

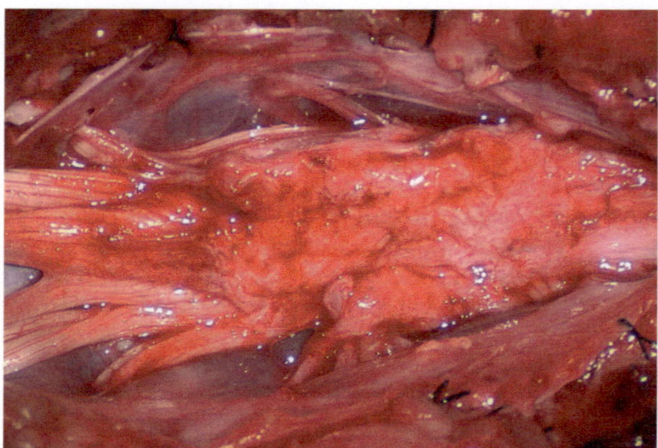

Fig. 34 Continuing from Fig. 32, the "naked" neural placode after complete resection of the dorsal lipoma. (Reprinted from Pang D. Total resection of complex spinal cord lipomas: how, why, and when to operate. Neuro Med Chir (Tokyo) 55: 695–721, 2015; with permission from the Japanese Neurosurgical Society. CC-BY-NC-ND (https://creativecommons.org/licenses/by-nc-nd/4.0/deed.ja))

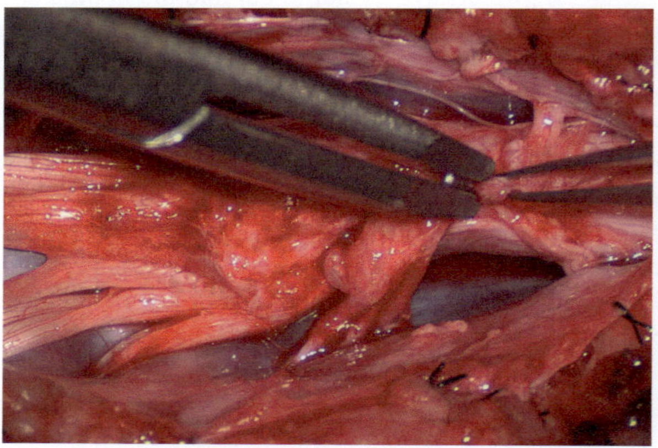

Fig. 35 Temporary small Weck Clips are applied to the apposed pial fringes to absorb the tissue torque tending to unfurl the dorsal bending of the placode. (Reprinted from Pang D. Total resection of complex spinal cord lipomas: how, why, and when to operate. Neuro Med Chir (Tokyo) 55: 695–721, 2015; with permission from the Japanese Neurosurgical Society. CC-BY-NC-ND (https://creativecommons.org/licenses/by-nc-nd/4.0/deed.ja))

substantial torque tending to unfurl the folding due to the natural inelastic property of neural tissue. This can be mitigated by applying small Weck clips on the apposed pial cuffs at short intervals along the seam (Fig. 35), before sewing in the 8-0 nylon pial sutures in between the clips and with buried knots. The Weck clips are then removed after enough sutures have been put in.

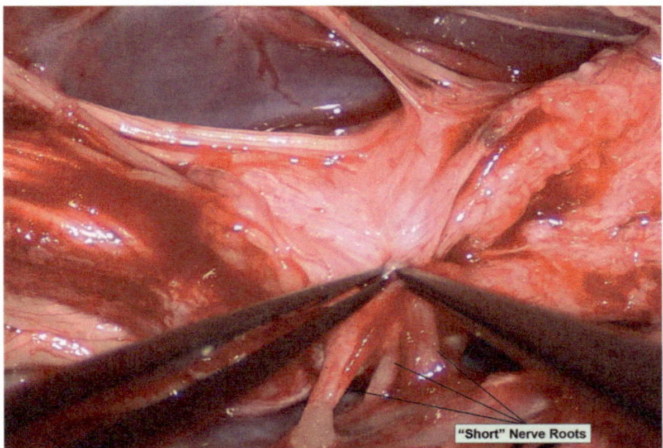

Fig. 36 On pulling the pial fringes together to check the ease of the dorsal neurulation, considerable lateral tugging is felt on the right, due to the "short" nerve roots. (Reprinted from Pang D. Total resection of complex spinal cord lipomas: how, why, and when to operate. Neuro Med Chir (Tokyo) 55: 695–721, 2015; with permission from the Japanese Neurosurgical Society. CC-BY-NC-ND (https://creativecommons.org/licenses/by-nc-nd/4.0/deed.ja))

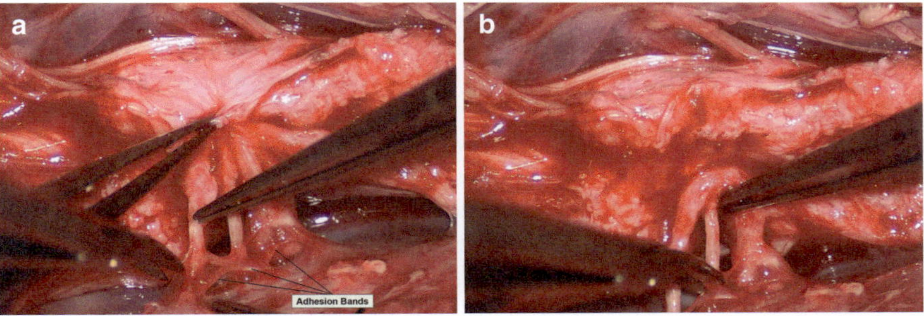

Fig. 37 Dealing with "short" nerve roots: (**a**) The impression of shortness is spurious; these functional and supple roots appear short because they were bound tightly to the inner lining of the dura by adhesion bands that are being cut. (**b**) More adhesion bands being cut. (Reprinted from Pang D. Total resection of complex spinal cord lipomas: how, why, and when to operate. Neuro Med Chir (Tokyo) 55: 695–721, 2015; with permission from the Japanese Neurosurgical Society. CC-B-Y-NC-ND (https://creativecommons.org/licenses/by-nc-nd/4.0/deed.ja))

Occasionally, strong tugging on the inbending folds prevents their easy coaptation, caused by "short" nerve roots on their underside (Fig. 36). These "short" and presumed to be non-functional and "fibrotic" roots have historically been blamed for unsuccessful untethering of the cord. In fact, on electrical stimulation, these roots are often found to be perfectly functional and pliant and have merely been made to appear short and unyielding by stiff adhesion bands to the dura. Cutting these bands releases the roots from the dura (Fig. 37a, b) and magically "lengthens" them (Fig. 38) to give a comfortable neurulation (Figs. 39a–f and 40).

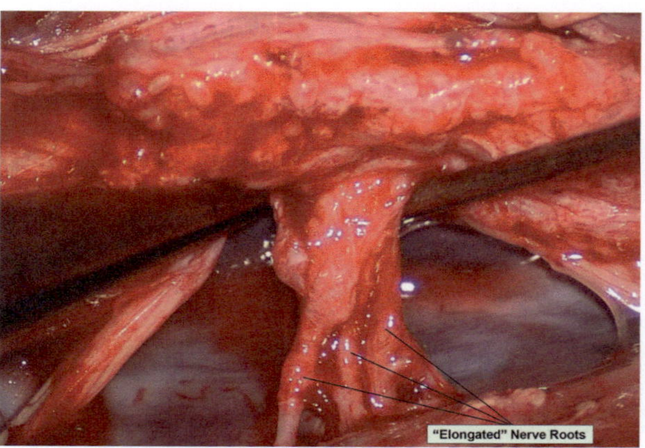

Fig. 38 After having been detached from the inner lining of the dura, these "short" nerve roots become magically "lengthened". (Reprinted from Pang D. Total resection of complex spinal cord lipomas: how, why, and when to operate. Neuro Med Chir (Tokyo) 55: 695–721, 2015; with permission from the Japanese Neurosurgical Society. CC-BY-NC-ND (https://creativecommons. org/licenses/by-nc-nd/4.0/deed.ja))

We cannot over-emphasise the importance of preserving a healthy width of pial cuff on each edge of the placode while resecting fat along the fusion line, not just for providing sturdy stitch-holds for the micro-sutures, but a generous pial fringe also imparts a certain resilience to the folded structure. Very rarely, the neural placode appears "pressed" into a narrow-based triangle resembling a tall steep pyramid by flanking fat buttresses (Fig. 41a). The pial cuffs in such cases are also exceedingly narrow, and suturing together short pial cuffs while forcefully folding up a squat, thick pyramid of unyielding neural tissue could result in a strangulated and ischaemic heap. The surgeon should recognize the potential hazard of the pyramidal placode on the pre-surgical MRI and be ready to exercise judgment while reconstructing the placode (Fig. 41b–d), which may mean abandoning neurulation especially when there are adverse changes in the MEP during infolding and suturing of the placode edges [25, 52].

If a filum is encountered after neurulation, it is usually also resected for completeness.

Step 5. Expansile Graft Duraplasty

Countless MRI images of loosely floating placodes and the undisputed salutary benefits of a small cord-sac ratio (see below) convinced the authors that a generous dural graft ensures free movement of the placode in CSF, thereby lessening its

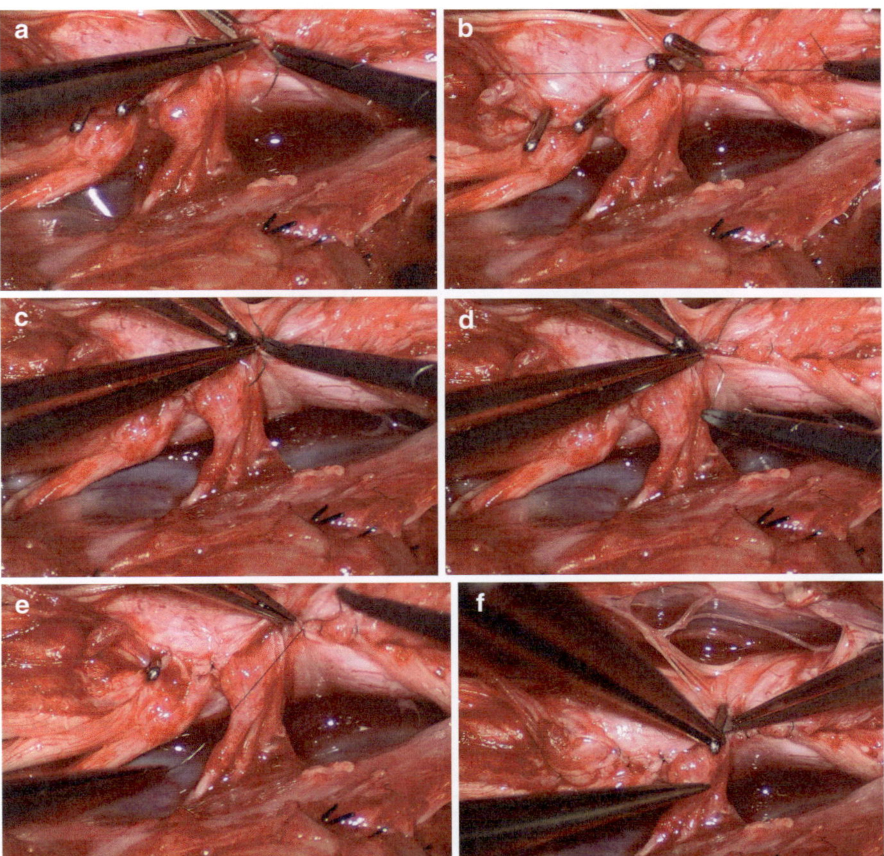

Fig. 39 Pia-to-pia neurulation of the neural placode. (**a**) Pia-to-pia suturing with 8–0 nylon sutures with knots buried. (**b**) Tying of micro sutures, apposing the pial fringes from each side of the placode. (**c**) More 8–0 nylon suture. (**d**) Yet more sutures. (**e**) Burying the nylon knot. (**f**) Removing the last Weck clip. (Reprinted from Pang D. Total resection of complex spinal cord lipomas: how, why, and when to operate. Neuro Med Chir (Tokyo) 55: 695–721, 2015; with permission from the Japanese Neurosurgical Society. CC-BY-NC-ND (https://creativecommons.org/licenses/by-nc-nd/4.0/deed.ja))

chances of adhering to the dura. The ideal graft material must satisfy two requirements: textural compatibility with juvenile dura and a low incidence of CSF leakage through the suture holes. Gortex is too stiff for young dura and leaks CSF profusely, as does Duragen. Both materials were discarded in our early trials. Autologous fascia lata is too soft and pliant so that it collapses on to the spinal cord even during normal inspiration and is only used when there is infection negating

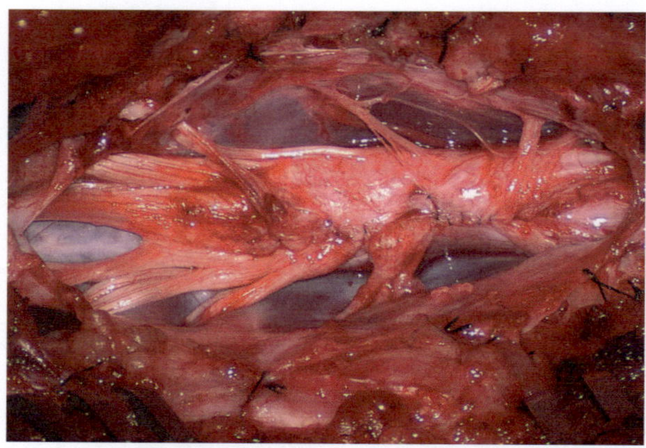

Fig. 40 Pia-to-pia neurulation completed with interrupted 8–0 nylon micro-sutures. The reconstituted neural tube is entirely pia-covered, with an unobtrusive dorsal seam. Note intact conus. (Reprinted from Pang D. Total resection of complex spinal cord lipomas: how, why, and when to operate. Neuro Med Chir (Tokyo) 55: 695–721, 2015; with permission from the Japanese Neurosurgical Society. CC-BY-NC-ND (https://creativecommons.org/licenses/by-nc-nd/4.0/deed.ja))

foreign graft materials. Our preferred graft material is the full-bodied yet texturally pliable bovine pericardium (Dura-Guard, by Synovis, St. Paul, MN) that can maintain a "puffed-up" scaffold in all phases of respiration and postures and shows minimal CSF leak. A close second choice is Durepair (Medtronic Neurologic Technologies, Goleta, CA), composed of reconstituted bovine collagen; it is slightly stiffer than bovine pericardium but does not leak. The graft is accurately shaped and sized to the dural opening to avoid creating infolds that may touch on the underlying placode (Fig. 42). The edge of the graft is then carefully matched up with the dural opening and anchored with judiciously spaced 4-0 sutures. Final water-tight closure is achieved with several running 5-0 prolene sutures, followed by challenges with Valsalva manoeuvres using pressures between 20 and 30 cm of water depending on the patient's size and age (Fig. 43). An inadvertent pseudomeningocele presses the dura against the neural placode and negates any intended perquisite of capacious grafting.

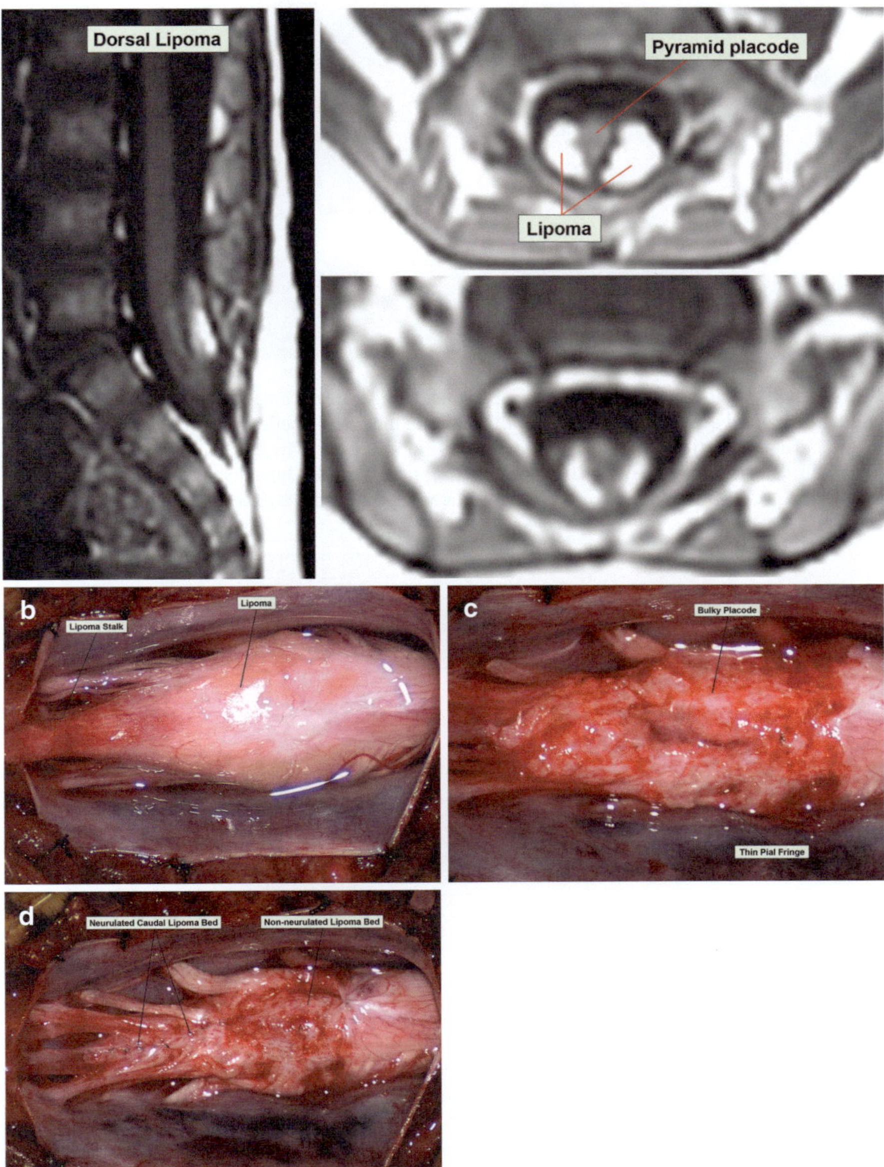

Fig. 41 Dorsal lipoma with bulky pyramid placode – lesson learned. (**a**) Note tall pyramid-shaped neural placode on axial profile, with steep side slopes interfacing with the lipoma. (**b**) Lipoma stalk and dorsal lipoma. (**c**) After lipoma resection, the placode is bulky in the middle and has thin pial fringes. (**d**) Only the loose caudal part of the placode was neurulated. Rostral bulky part is left open because of TcMEP deterioration on forced attempts to suture. (Reprinted from Pang D. Total resection of complex spinal cord lipomas: how, why, and when to operate. Neuro Med Chir (Tokyo) 55: 695–721, 2015; with permission from the Japanese Neurosurgical Society. CC-BY-NC-ND (https://creativecommons.org/licenses/by-nc-nd/4.0/deed.ja))

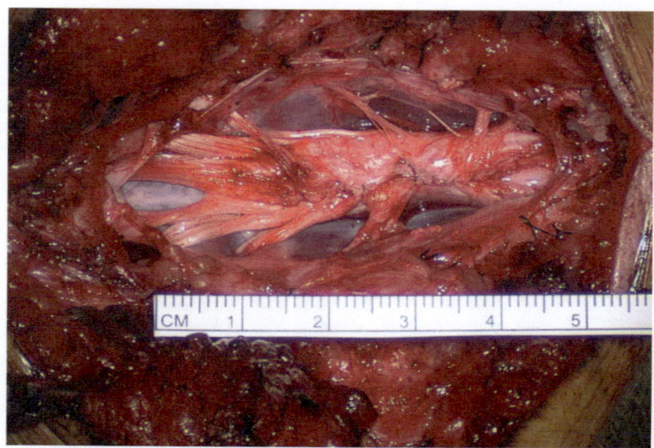

Fig. 42 Back to the dorsal lipoma in Fig. 10, showing careful measurement of the length and width of the dural defect in preparation for fashioning the bovine pericardial graft. (Reprinted from Pang D. Total resection of complex spinal cord lipomas: how, why, and when to operate. Neuro Med Chir (Tokyo) 55: 695–721, 2015; with permission from the Japanese Neurosurgical Society. CC-BY-NC-ND (https://creativecommons.org/licenses/by-nc-nd/4.0/deed.ja))

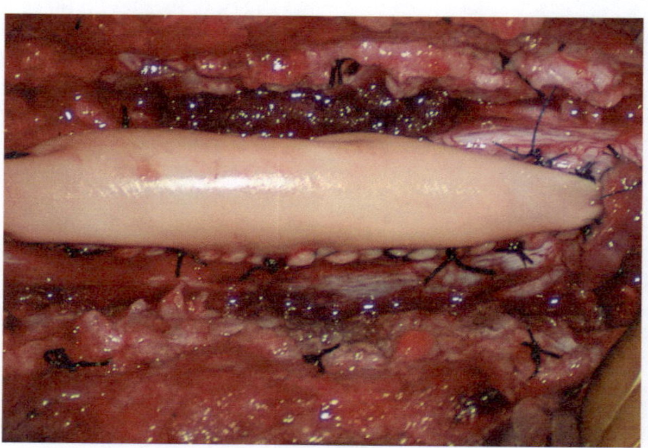

Fig. 43 After graft sutures are in place, water-tightness of the suture line is tested by several Valsalva manoeuvres. An optimal graft is one that does not leak, puffs up with expiration, and registers no inward folding, as this one. (Reprinted from Pang D. Total resection of complex spinal cord lipomas: how, why, and when to operate. Neuro Med Chir (Tokyo) 55: 695–721, 2015; with permission from the Japanese Neurosurgical Society. CC-BY-NC-ND (https://creativecommons. org/licenses/by-nc-nd/4.0/deed.ja))

Surgical Epilogue: Sundry Additional Comments

The senior author's data show that total or near-total resection of spinal cord lipomas can be achieved in over 90% of cases [1, 2, 19, 22, 25] (Fig. 44). In cases where small bits of fat were left on the DREZ for fear of gouging, they have been wrapped

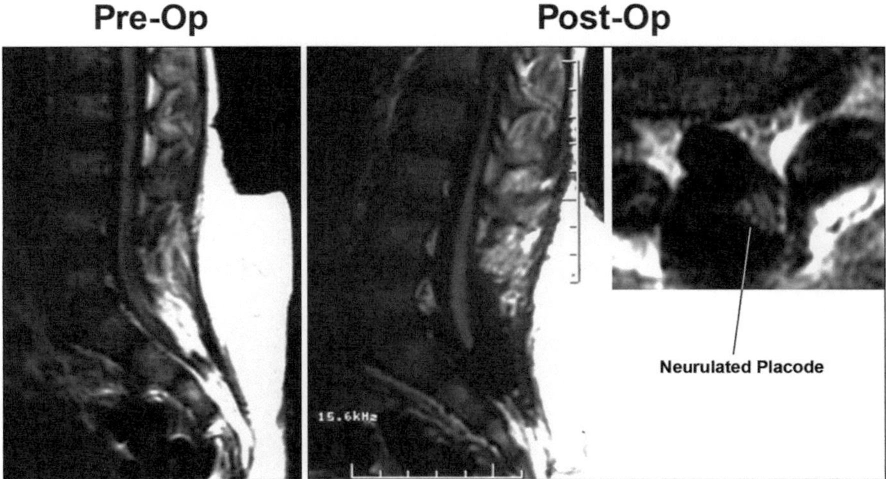

Fig. 44 Pre- and post-operative MRI of a case of transitional lipoma with no residual fat after total lipoma resection. Note neurulated oblong-shaped fat-free neural placode within a large dural sac. (Reprinted from Pang D. Total resection of complex spinal cord lipomas: how, why, and when to operate. Neuro Med Chir (Tokyo) 55: 695–721, 2015; with permission from the Japanese Neurosurgical Society. CC-BY-NC-ND (https://creativecommons.org/licenses/by-nc-nd/4.0/deed.ja))

up within the neurulation folds "out of mischief" (Fig. 45). In 8% of patients, the residual fat represents the ventral component of a chaotic lipoma that had been intentionally left untouched and pia-covered and presumably harmless.

To estimate the "looseness" or degree of freedom of the reconstructed placode within the expanded CSF space, we created the cord-sac ratio, defined as the ratio of the diameter of the bulkiest portion of the reconstructed neural placode to the diameter of the dural sac on the post-operative axial MRI. The sacs are graded as loose, with ratios less than 30%; moderately loose, with ratios between 30% and 50%; and tight, with ratios greater than 50% (Fig. 46). In the senior author's series of 315 total resections reported in 2013, 227 (72%) had loose sacs, 73 (23.2%) had moderately loose sacs, and only 15 (4.8%) had comparatively tighter sacs [25].

Redo lipomas are more likely to harbour visible remainder fat and to have higher cord-sac ratios. Very likely, the hard, grasping fibrous scar from prior surgery cements the remainder fat to the dura and makes it extremely difficult to detach. Also, the dull grey colour of the cicatrix, unlike bright yellow virgin fat, can be impossible to distinguish from the white plane . The surgeon thus tends to be over-conservative in the dissection and leaves behind a thick layer of stiff scar-infiltrated fat attached to a bulky placode that is well-nigh impossible to neurulate comfortably. The same unyielding fibrous muddle at the DREZ often leads to "gouging", which may explain the high incidence of post-operative dysesthetic pain in "redo" versus "virgin" patients [1, 2, 19, 52].

Pre-Op   **Post-Op**

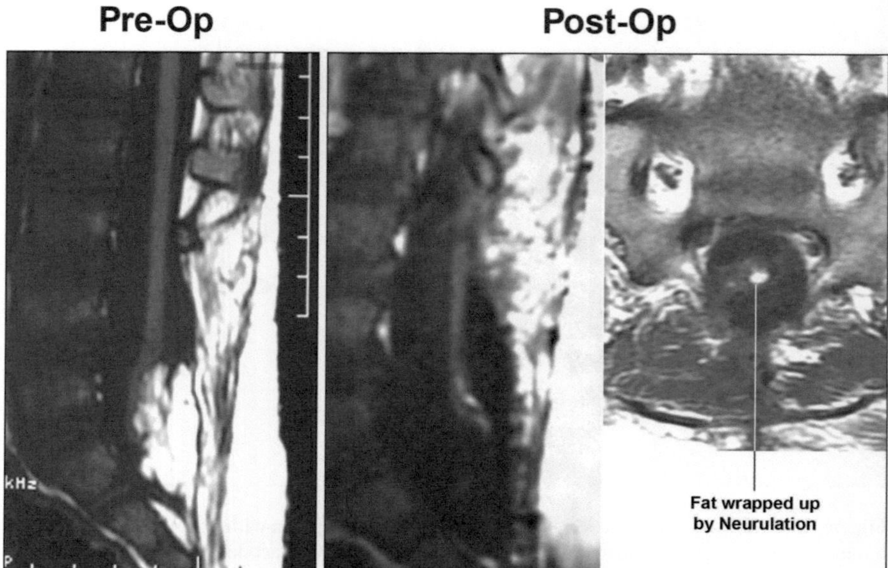

Fig. 45 Pre- and post-operative MRI of a case of complex transitional lipoma with a very small amount (<20 cu mm) of residual fat after resection. Axial image shows the small round piece of fat is wrapped up within the roundly neurulated neural placode and therefore not exposed on the surface. (Reprinted from Pang D. Total resection of complex spinal cord lipomas: how, why, and when to operate. Neuro Med Chir (Tokyo) 55: 695–721, 2015; with permission from the Japanese Neurosurgical Society. CC-BY-NC-ND (https://creativecommons.org/licenses/by-nc-nd/4.0/deed.ja))

Incomplete terminal untethering of the placode predictably ends in early clinical relapse [14, 16, 61]. We ascribe two explanations why this could happen with very large transitional lipomas. In such cases where the caudal placode is mired in fat, its complete detachment cannot be done safely without substantial removal of fat. Also, healthy looking nerves are sometimes seen enmeshed in fat distal to what was reckoned to be the tip of the placode, making it seem impossible to achieve terminal disconnection without sacrificing functional cord. Electrical stimulation of these nerves will more than likely find them to be non-functional vestigial coccygeal roots, and 2–3 sets of "live" anal sphincter roots would have been found on the conus proper above. A decisive transection of the vestigial placode below will achieve complete terminal untethering without sacrificing function [1, 2, 19, 22, 25, 57].

Our experience unequivocally shows that chaotic lipomas are the most treacherous lesions. Some chaotic lesions are easily recognisable by the presence of obvious ventral fat in between pairs of ventral roots on the MRI, but other less blatant ones have sub-resolution trails of fatty infiltration through the DREZ into the ventral motor horn zone, detectable only at surgery. Compared to other lipoma types, chaotic lipomas are more likely to show conspicuous residual fat and high cord-sac

< 30% (72%)   30–50% (23.2%)   > 50% (4.8%)

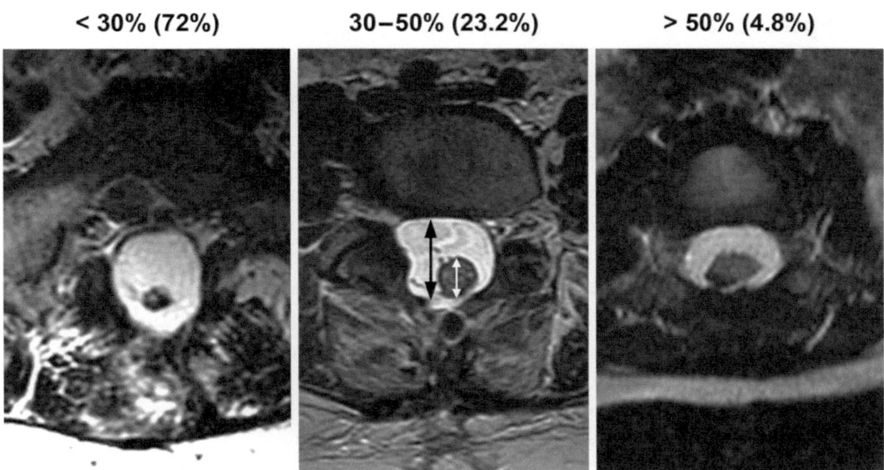

Fig. 46 Cord-sac ratios in the post-operative axial MRI after total/near-total resection of lipoma. This ratio is obtained by dividing the sagittal diameter of the most bulbous portion of the post-neurulated neural placode by the sagittal diameter of the dural sac. 72% in our series have very loose sacs with cord-sac ratios <30%; 23.2% have intermediate ratios 30–50%; and 4.8% have ratios >50% with the least commodious cord-sac relationship. Cord-sac ratio estimates the degree of freedom of motion of the post-neurulated spinal cord within its container sac. (Reprinted from Pang D. Total resection of complex spinal cord lipomas: how, why, and when to operate. Neuro Med Chir (Tokyo) 55: 695–721, 2015; with permission from the Japanese Neurosurgical Society. CC-BY-NC-ND (https://creativecommons.org/licenses/by-nc-nd/4.0/deed.ja))

ratio on the post-operative MRI [1, 2, 19, 22, 25, 52] (Fig. 33d). The strategy for these difficult lipomas, gleaned from more than a few infelicitous encounters, is learning to resist digging too deep once enough dorsal fat has been removed to enable partial neurulation. It is worth stressing that since it is never feasible to totally resect the ventral fat or to achieve even clumsy neurulation, its nascent pial surface that had presumably existed without adhesions since birth should best be kept unabraded so as not to incur iatrogenic tethering (Fig. 33a, c).

Finally, I disagree with Arai et al. [5] and Chapman [61–63] that "lipomyelomeningoceles" have higher surgical risk and worse outcome than regular lipomas. As long as one recognises and gently handles the extruded part of the neural placode beyond the dorsal plane of the spinal canal, the technical steps of fat resection, placode reconstruction, and dural grafting are identical to those used for the more orthodox lipomas, with comparable results. I also think that Kulkarni et al. [3] and Chapman's [63] warnings about lipomas in adults being technically more challenging are unwarranted. Except perhaps for thicker "natural" arachnoid bands in adults and more laborious bone and fascial exposure, most of the microsurgical work is the same as for resecting lipomas on young children and infants.

Complications of Total Lipoma Resection

Our rate of new neurological and urological symptoms following total/near-total resection is 4.1% [25], which compares favourably with the 0.6% to 10% (average of 3–7%) in the literature [5, 7, 9, 11, 15, 16, 18, 21, 26, 64–72], all pertaining to partial resection presumably using less aggressive techniques than ours. Only 1.5% of our patients had new weakness but 4% had neuropathic pain [1, 2, 19, 22, 25, 52], which is likely related to mechanical or thermal perturbation at the DREZ and dorsal root zone from diathermy and gouging. This has taught us to avoid cautery as much as possible and use gentle tamponade and gelfoam, which should handle the majority of bleeding on the cord. If diathermy is absolutely necessary, we use only the ultra-fine tip irrigating bipolar set at the lowest current intensities, always precisely localizing the bleeding spot using the intermittent squirt-irrigation technique from the bubble-squeezer.

Our rates for CSF leak (0.7%) and wound complications (1.1%) with total resection [25] are much lower than almost all of the published series (of partial resection), which report CSF leak rates from 2 to 47% [7, 9, 11, 15, 16, 18, 26, 67, 68] and wound dehiscence and infection rates of 2 to 26% [7–9, 11, 16, 18, 26, 67]. The following time-tested technical points concerning wound closure are worth noting: (1) Adequate caudal laminectomy is necessary to locate a healthy dural edge at least 5–10 mm past the tip of the neural placode to sustain good suture hold for the lower end of the graft anastomosis, which is always the tenuous end. Ideally, this very edge should be sturdy dura and not fat of the distal lipoma stump. A good caudal dural edge is usually available with dorsal lipoma whose fatty stalk ends above the conus as does the dural defect, but in some very large transitional lipomas, the entire conus is involved in the lipoma and the caudal dural edge is partly or wholly infiltrated by fibrous fat. The surgeon will have to improvise on finding the best possible suture hold for the lower end of the graft, occasionally resolving to using "big bites" on fibrous fat or through flakes of the incomplete deep fascial layers. (2) Patience and ingenuity must be used to achieve absolute water-tight closure of the graft with Prolene, followed by Valsalva manoeuvres. (3) We are not as enchanted by synthetic sealants or organic tissue glues for the graft anastomosis as before, for nothing can substitute for solid closure. The use of these agents is optional in cases of tenuous suture line. (4) In large lumbosacral lipomas, gaping muscle and fascial defects may forestall primary approximation of the deep layers at the lower end of the opening. An effective solution is to create generous paramedian relaxing incisions on the flanking lumbodorsal fascia to allow the fascial edges to slide towards the midline and be primarily closed without tension. (5) The large subcutaneous lipoma is never removed during the initial soft tissue dissection to avoid creating a large dead space that could potentially encourage CSF leakage and formation of a tense pseudomeningocele. The latter may compress and flatten the dural sac against the placode or even threaten the viability of the skin flap.

Results of Total Resection

The results of total resection are best analysed by comparing its outcome with that of the traditional technique of partial resection. This has proven to be a convenient enterprise for the senior author, who had performed 116 partial resections prior to 1991, using similar surgical style and rituals and with equal obsession for technical minutiae as for his later total resection series. These comparisons are done in two parts, that of the immediate post-operative results and the long-term outcomes of these two different techniques.

Early Post-Operative Results

The immediate effects of surgery during the first 12 months are very similar between our own total and partial resection groups [1, 2, 19, 22, 25]. For asymptomatic patients, the rates for neurological preservation are 98% for total and 94% for partial resection, respectively. For symptomatic patients, the rates for total resection are 61% for normalisation or improvement and 33% for stabilisation of neurological status, giving a combined rate of 94% for improvement or stabilisation of disease. Similarly, symptomatic patients who had partial resection had a 33% improvement and 62% stabilization rates during the first year, thus also having a 95% rate of short-term protection.

When the early post-operative results are compared between the senior author's total resection group and partial resection series from the literature [5, 7, 9, 15, 16, 18, 71], it is again apparent that both the disease improvement and stabilization rates are very similar, particularly among patients with progressive symptoms. This suggests that the immediate benefits of surgery in the early post-operative period, for both techniques, are owed to the abrupt relief of traction on the cord rather than the extent of lipoma removal or work on the placode. In contrast, surgeons who lamented during partial resection their inability to completely detach the terminal placode from the lipoma stump in some patients, due to massive residual fat and undefinable placode-lipoma interface, also reported their early recurrence of symptoms [16, 26, 61].

When the catalogue of pre-operative symptoms are analysed in regards to their response to total resection, the abatement of pain came out the best and most reliable. Typically, the sharp, dysesthetic pain in the lower limbs and perineum will significantly diminish within 3 months [25]. Relief of low back pain, which may be mechanical in origin, is less reliable [73, 74]. Children do not usually complain of back pain but they do seem to become more active and playful. Active sensory symptoms such as dysesthesia and hyperpathia also respond favourably with surgery. Although only 20% of patients have actual normalisation of motor deficits, the majority with pre-operative weakness will substantially improve [1, 2, 19, 22, 25]. Like tethered cord syndrome in general, recent and milder deficits and symptoms have better chance for good recovery than severe chronic ones. Unlike pain and sensorimotor deficits, bladder dysfunction rarely improves significantly, and if so, the recovery is seldom complete, and partial recovery occurs in no more than 20–30% of patients [19, 22, 25]. Amongst the several subtypes of neuropathic bladder, the spastic, small capacity bladder with uninhibited detrusor contractions tends to respond best to surgery. The atonic bladder virtually never improves to a point of not needing permanent intermittent catheterization, and the response of detrusor-sphincter dyssynergia is at best partial and unpredictable. It is strongly advisable to obtain formal cystometry and voiding cystourethrogram 3–6 months after surgery and yearly thereafter if indicated to assess whether more radical urologic procedures such as bladder augmentation or ureteral conduits might be needed to eliminate reflux and upper urinary tract infections.

Long-Term Outcome

Whilst the *immediate* benefits of both total and partial resection are due to the equivalent relief of traction on the conus in both procedures and are therefore comparable [1, 2, 19, 22, 25], the long-term benefits of total over partial surgery probably come from the sustainment of the untethered state when aggressive fat removal enables the protective reconfiguring of the neural structure, an undertaking obviously unobtainable with partial resection. This is made very plain when the progression-free survivals (PFSs) of the senior author's series of total and partial resection are plotted out for a period of 20 and 11 years, respectively. The PFS after total resection for all lipoma types and clinical subgroups is 88.1%, versus 34.6% for partial resection [25] (Fig. 47). The differences in outcome between the two techniques are even more marked if the subgroup PFSs are individually compared, when the patients in each treatment group are segregated by the presence or absence of pre-operative symptoms, age, and whether previous surgery had been done [1, 2, 19, 22, 25]. Overall, the risk of symptomatic recurrence is 5.94 times higher with partial resection compared with total/near-total resection over 18 years by the Cox Proportional Hazard Regression Model, with a p value of <0.00001. This striking difference in outcomes between total and partial resection is equally obvious when the results of our total resection group are held up against the published results of partial resection [5, 11, 13, 16, 18, 21, 26, 63, 71, 75, 76], especially if the comparisons are done with matched patient profiles (most published series include only virgin cases whereas ours has both virgins and redos) and lesion types (many published series include terminal and filar lipomas which are technically far less complicated and have better prognosis). Barring these and other minor criticisms (e.g. our data are prospective whereas most published series are retrospective), these elaborate comparisons all show far better long-term prognosis with total/near-total resection, which constitutes the best reason for its endorsement over all other treatment options for complex spinal cord lipomas.

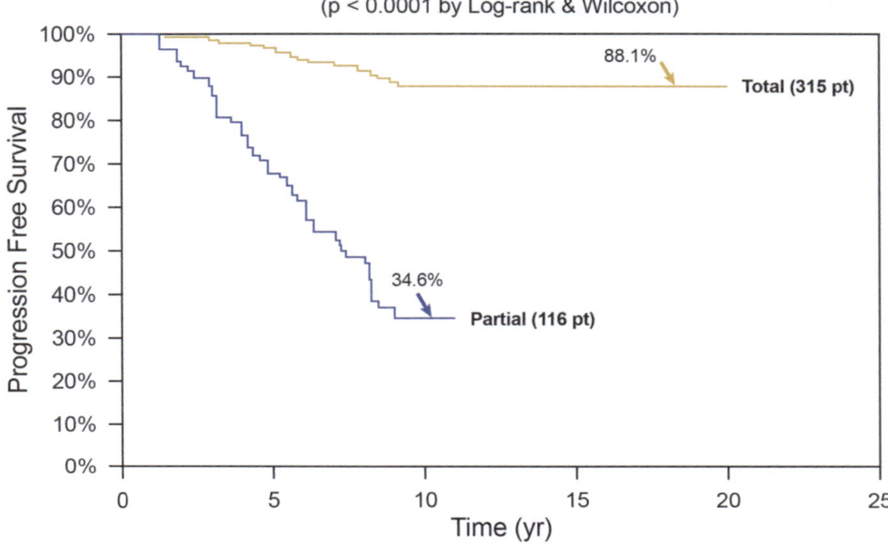

Fig. 47 Outcomes of total versus partial resection. Kaplan-Meier (KM) analysis for progression-free survival probability in total and partial resection of lipoma. The progression-free probability for total resection is 88.1% at 20 years, and 34.6% for partial resection at 10.5 years. The difference is highly significant ($p < 0.0001$ by Log-rank & Wilcoxon). Note stabilization of disease after 8 years with total resection, but inexorable deterioration without disease arrest with partial resection. *Pt* Patients, *Total* Total resection, *Partial* Partial resection. (Reprinted from Pang D. Total resection of complex spinal cord lipomas: how, why, and when to operate. Neuro Med Chir (Tokyo) 55: 695–721, 2015; with permission from the Japanese Neurosurgical Society. CC-BY-NC-ND (https://creativecommons.org/licenses/by-nc-nd/4.0/deed.ja))

Predictor Variables Influencing Outcome

In 2010, we attempted to find the actual reason(s) why total resection gave such a stunning advantage over partial surgery, by investigating the influence of 6 predictor variables on PFS in the series [19]. These variables are gender, age, lipoma type (dorsal, transitional and chaotic), presence or absence of preoperative symptoms, history of previous resection, and cord-sac ratio. Simple Cox univariate analyses show that gender and lipoma type (see later for lipoma type) have no influence on outcome, but that young age, absence of symptoms, no prior surgery, and a low cord sac ratio are all associated with statistically longer PFSs. However, when age, symptoms, and prior surgery (not cord-sac ratio because it is a post-operative entity) are tested with the Cox multivariate model with all 6 variables inserted in the analysis, the significant P-values associated with their univariate PFS curves all disappeared, suggesting these 3 are in fact "non-independent" predictors of outcome [19]. The same statistical exercise was performed in the senior author's 2013 series of 315 patients, with similar results [25]. The inevitable conclusion is that these 3 predictor variables must exert their influence on outcome through some sort of *final common pathway* [1, 2, 19, 22, 25].

Unlike the three non-independent predictor variables of age, symptoms, and prior surgery, cord-sac ratio emerges as the solitary independent predictor of outcome shown clearly by its highly significant influence on progression-free probabilities displayed by the Cox multivariate model [25] (Fig. 48). It is therefore tempting to suggest that cord-sac ratio may in fact be the *final common pathway* for the three non-independent predictors. To test this hypothesis on the influence of prior surgery on outcome, we examine whether redo lipomas' negative effects on PFS can be explained solely by their having high cord-sac ratios. The first positive clue is that redo lipomas tend to end up with much higher post-operative cord-sac ratios than virgin lipomas [19, 22, 25]. Secondly, analysis of covariance (ANCOVA) clearly portrays the same strong correlation between prior surgery and high cord-sac ratios (R^2 correlative coefficient = 0.76; $p < 0.001$) [25]. Last and most revealing, when the Cox multivariate regression analysis is performed on cord-sac ratio for just the redo lipomas, a PFS of 88.4% is still manageable in redo lesions as long as a less than 30% cord-sac ratio can be rendered [25] (Fig. 49). This strongly suggests that redo

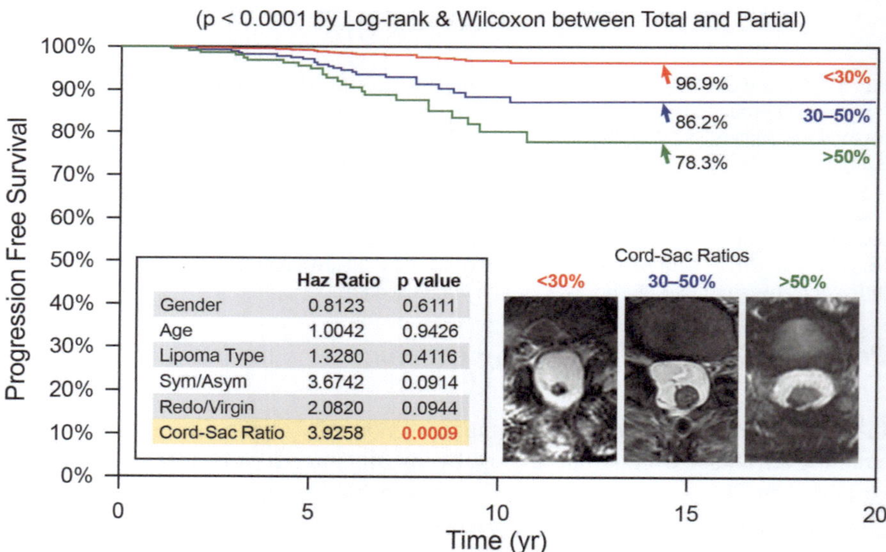

	Haz Ratio	p value
Gender	0.8123	0.6111
Age	1.0042	0.9426
Lipoma Type	1.3280	0.4116
Sym/Asym	3.6742	0.0914
Redo/Virgin	2.0820	0.0944
Cord-Sac Ratio	3.9258	0.0009

Fig. 48 Cox Multivariate Proportional Hazard Regression model analyzing the combined influence of 6 predictor variables (gender; age; lipoma type; symptoms; redo versus virgin; and cord-sac ratio) on PFS after total resection, featuring the resultant effect of the three cord-sac ratios of <30%, 30–50%, and >50%. The hazard ratios and *p* values for all 6 predictor variables are listed in the miniaturized table, showing that cord-sac ratio exerts the *only* significant *independent* influence on outcome. The respective progression-free probabilities, as indicated by the arrows, are 96.9% for low ratio, 86.2% for intermediate ratio, and 78.3% for high ratio. The differences in hazard prediction for the 3 ratios are highly significant ($p = 0.0009$, in bold). <30%; 30–50%, and >50% indicate the 3 cord-sac ratios as shown in MRI insets. *Sym/Asym* Symptomatic versus asymptomatic lipomas. (Reprinted from Pang D. Total resection of complex spinal cord lipomas: how, why, and when to operate. Neuro Med Chir (Tokyo) 55: 695–721, 2015; with permission from the Japanese Neurosurgical Society. CC-BY-NC-ND (https://creativecommons.org/licenses/by-nc-nd/4.0/deed.ja))

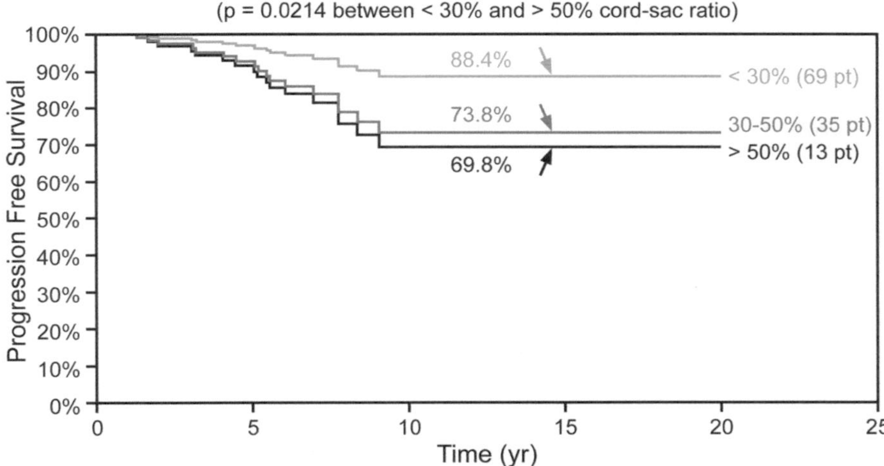

Fig. 49 Cox Multivariate analysis for the influence of cord-sac ratios on outcome in 117 redo lipomas that underwent total resection. Progression-free probabilities are indicated by arrows. A high PFS of 88.4% can still be managed even in redo lipomas if a cord-sac ratio <30% can be achieved, indicating the dominant role of cord-sac ratio, and conversely the subordinate role of other unidentified attributes of previous surgery, on long-term outcome (*p* value = 0.0214 between <30% and >50% cord-sac ratios). *Pt* Patients. (Reprinted from: Pang D, Zovickian J, Wong ST, Hou YJ, and Moes GS. Surgical treatment of complex spinal cord lipomas. Childs Nerv Syst (2013) 29:1485–1513; with Permission from Springer Nature)

lesions can still enjoy good outcome as long as a low cord-sac ratio can be achieved and clearly shows the subordinate role of other unidentified attributes of prior surgery. This same train of analyses, including the respective covariance analysis, can be applied to the other two "non-independent" predictors, age, and symptoms, with similar conclusions.

Cord-Sac Ratio and the Importance of Neurulation

Our own records show a far higher likelihood for total resection to achieve low cord-sac ratios than partial resection, being 72% in the total group versus only 3% in the partial group (Fig. 50), suggesting that cord-sac ratio is probably what determines the difference in outcome between the two techniques [25]. For the total resection group, Cox Multivariate analysis of the combined influence of the 6 predictor covariates shows that cord-sac ratio's highly significant, *independent* influence on outcome is unchanged by howsoever the other effects of age, symptoms, lipoma types, and prior surgery interact (Fig. 48). Regardless of all else, a cord-sac ratio greater than 50% predicts a 5.3 times higher risk for disease progression than a low cord-sac ratio of less than 30%, with a high statistical significance (Figs. 48 and 51). The PFS rises to a reassuring 96.9% for low ratios less than 30% and drops

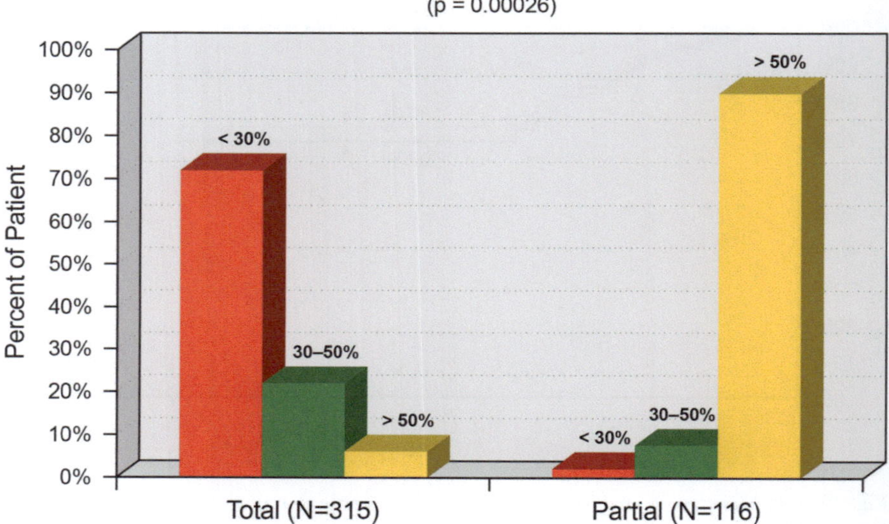

Fig. 50 Distribution of cord-sac ratios between the total resection and partial resection groups. Note 72% of patients who had total resection had cord-sac ratio <30%, versus less than 3% of patients who had partial resection. Conversely, only 6% of patients who had total resection had high ratio of >50%, versus over 90% of patients who had partial resection. The difference is significant ($p = 0.00026$). <30%; 30–50%; and >50% indicate the cord-sac ratios. (Reprinted from Pang D. Total resection of complex spinal cord lipomas: how, why, and when to operate. Neuro Med Chir (Tokyo) 55: 695–721, 2015; with permission from the Japanese Neurosurgical Society. CC-BY-NC-ND (https://creativecommons.org/licenses/by-nc-nd/4.0/deed.ja))

gradually to 86.2% for intermediate ratios between 30% and 50% and 78.3% for ratios higher than 50% [25].

In an operational sense, cord-sac ratio may in fact be the summated product of the other group variables. For example, previous surgery imparts new scar tissue on the remainder fat, whose altered hue and texture undoubtedly makes it near impossible to distinguish lipoma from the white plane and therefore to attain a clean, slender placode and a small cord-sac ratio. Since many symptomatic patients in our total resection group have had prior partial resection, their poorer outcome may be largely due to the negative influence of the "redo factor", which may also account for the disadvantage of old age since most elderly patients had both symptoms and prior surgery before their total resection.

Though a loose fitting sac ensures a greater degree of free movements of the placode within CSF, a condition known to discourage retethering, adhesions can still form if what is facing the dura is a broad, sticky, raw resection surface on a sheet-like placode. Meticulous pia-to-pia neurulation of the neural placode conceals this sticky surface within a smooth pia-covered tube and further lessens the chances of adhesion. Reexploration of both neurulated and unneurulated placodes shows unequivocally that the raw unneurulated slab is much more of a conspicuous nidus for new adhesions than a smooth tube with a discrete seam. Though not an easily

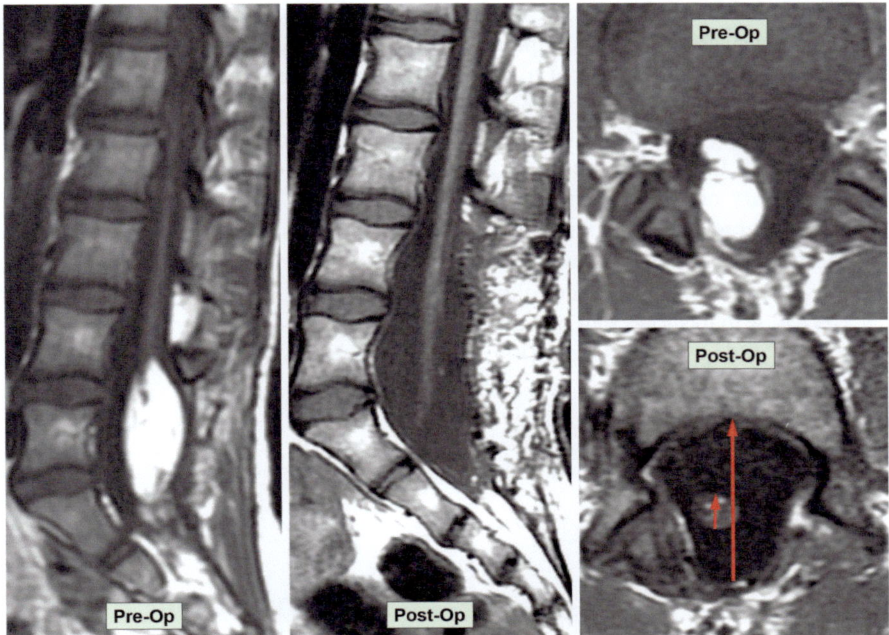

Fig. 51 The pre- and post-operative sagittal and axial MRI of a 10 year old girl who has had 2 previous partial resections of a large transitional lipoma, and who developed new leg weakness. The achieved post-operative cord-sac ratio is 20% (lower right); and she enjoyed long-term progression-free status. (Reprinted from Pang D. Total resection of complex spinal cord lipomas: how, why, and when to operate. Neuro Med Chir (Tokyo) 55: 695–721, 2015; with permission from the Japanese Neurosurgical Society. CC-BY-NC-ND (https://creativecommons.org/licenses/by-nc-nd/4.0/deed.ja))

quantifiable act, concealment of this adhesive surface through minutely careful neurulation must be at least as essential and indispensable as a low cord-sac ratio in guarding against retethering.

Pre-Operative Profiling for Good and Poor Risk Patients

In clinical practice, it is important to inform patients and families of their chances of success before the recommended treatment, and for that, the post-operative index of cord-sac ratio, though by far the most potent outcome predictor, will not be available. To create a pre-surgery *composite* patient profile to differentiate potentially favourable from unfavourable surgical candidates, the strengths of influence on outcome of all pre-operative traits derived from the predictor variables are ranked on a graded map from another multivariate data analysis model, Multiple Correspondence Analyses (MCA). In an MCA 3-dimensional map, the individual strength of influence on outcome of each of the 5 *pre-operative* predictor variables of age, gender, lipoma type, symptoms, and prior surgery is graded so that its magnitude is inversely proportional to its distance from a pertinent outcome category, displayed on a "principal component axis" on the map. A short distance from the outcome category indicates strong influence, and conversely, a long distance indicates minimal influence. Thus, at a glance, the traits clustering closest to the outcome category on the MCA map would have dominant influence and, vice versa, those traits far afield would have little or no influence. Outcome is considered "bad" for those who had post-operative recurrence of symptoms and "good" if no recurrence is documented during the follow-up period [19, 22, 25].

The MCA map shows that bad outcome is strongly associated with lipomas with symptoms and prior resection (Fig. 52). Good outcome is, not unexpectedly,

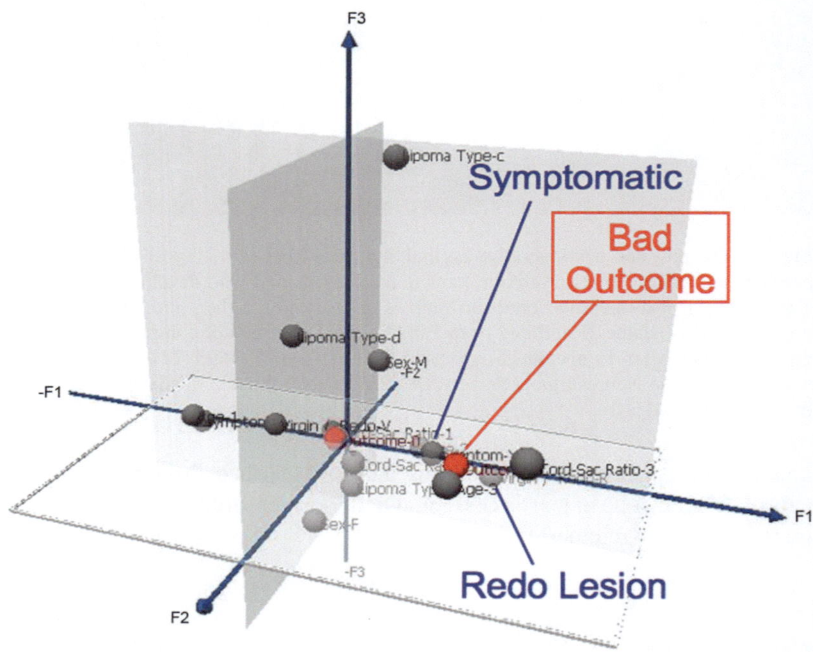

Fig. 52 Pre-operative profiling of good versus poor risk patients for total resection using three dimensional Multiple Correspondence Analysis plot, which displays the respective strength of influence of the 6 predictor variables (gender, age, lipoma type, symptoms, redo versus virgin lipomas, and cord-sac ratio) on outcome after total resection. The grey balls represent predictor variables and red balls represent outcomes. Only the statistically significant predictors are flagged. Bad outcome implies recurrence and good outcome the absence of recurrence during the follow-up period. Close clustering of variables (with flags) around an Outcome signifies strong influence; remote scattering of variables (without flags) from an Outcome signifies weak influence. Bad outcome is associated with pre-operative symptoms and redo lesions. (Reprinted from: Pang D, Zovickian J, Wong ST, Hou YJ, and Moes GS. Surgical treatment of complex spinal cord lipomas. Childs Nerv Syst (2013) 29:1485–1513; with Permission from Springer Nature)

correlated with young age especially less than 2 years, absence of symptoms, and no prior surgery (Fig. 53). Capitalising on the MCA results, we performed Cox regression on various patient groups that had total resection and found that the PFS probability of the 84 patients that fit this ideal profile, i.e. asymptomatic children less than 2 with no previous resection, maintains at a stunning 99.2% at 20 years (Fig. 54). The ideal scenario with the highest probability of obtaining long-term disease control is therefore to perform total resection on very young children before symptoms arise and most definitely before partial resection has been inflicted. Indeed, our subgroup of 139 patients who had their virgin lipomas resected when young all had post-operative cord-sac ratios <30%, and none had recurrence during the 20 years follow-up period.

In stark contrast, older patients with pre-operative neurological dysfunctions and prior surgery will have a much less sanguine future.

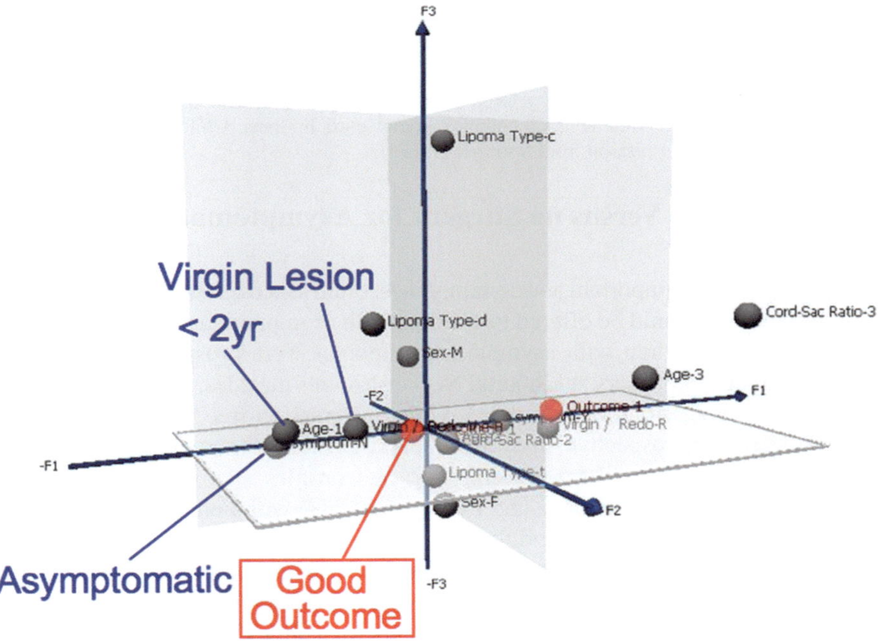

Fig. 53 Same pre-operative profiling as in Fig. 52 for good outcome, using the same Multiple Correspondence Analysis plot. Good outcome is associated with children less than 2 years, asymptomatic lesions, and virgin lipomas. (Reprinted from: Pang D, Zovickian J, Wong ST, Hou YJ, and Moes GS. Surgical treatment of complex spinal cord lipomas. Childs Nerv Syst (2013) 29:1485–1513; with Permission from Springer Nature)

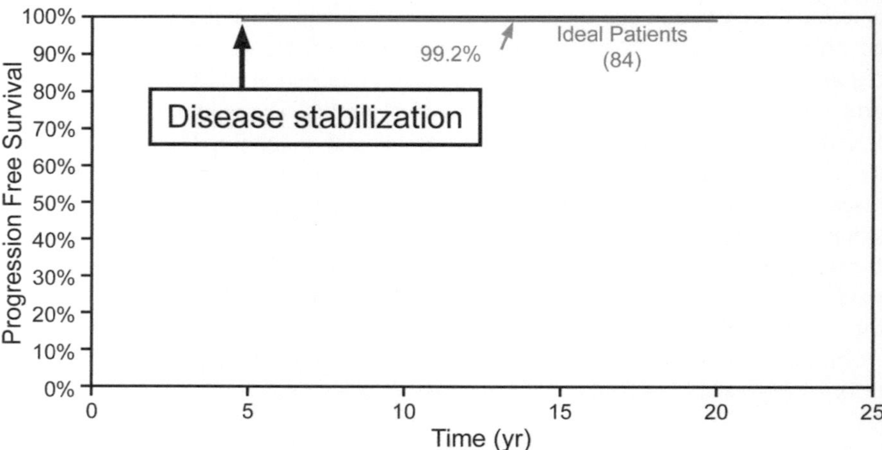

Fig. 54 Kaplan-Meier analysis for progression-free survival showing the predicted outcome of the 84 "ideal patients" who had had total resection; i.e. asymptomatic children younger than 2 years with virgin lipomas. The progression-free probability at 20 years is 99.2%, with disease stabilization after 5 years from surgery. (Reprinted from: Pang D, Zovickian J, Wong ST, Hou YJ, and Moes GS. Surgical treatment of complex spinal cord lipomas. Childs Nerv Syst (2013) 29:1485–1513; with Permission from Springer Nature)

Total Resection Versus no Surgery for Asymptomatic Lipomas

Above all, the most important and certainly most often asked question is undoubtedly whether surgery should be offered to children with asymptomatic lipomas. In 2004, a cohort of 50 children with asymptomatic lipomas were prospectively followed without surgery for 9 years at L'hôpital Necker-Enfants malades, Paris [3], and were found to have a deterioration risk of 33% with a progression-free survival probability of 67% [62]. A retrospective study from Great Ormond Street Hospital, London, with similar patient numbers (56 children) and profiles also reported a 10-year disease progression rate of 40% and PFS of only 60% with non-surgical treatment [4]. The London study also found that the female gender, transitional lipomas, and conus syringes are all associated with a higher rate of deterioration which also occurs earlier than patients not having these traits. Since transitional lesions and females are usually more numerous in most lipoma cohorts, as are conus syringes, one could surmise that there is a large subclass of children with these traits who will have a worse than 40% prospect of disease progression [77] (Fig. 55). Given that children within the lipoma age range have an actuarial life span of 65–70 years and that established neurogenic bladder and motor weakness seldom fully recover following *post factum* salvage surgery [6, 9, 11, 16, 18, 64], the push for pre-emptive total resection for asymptomatic lipomas would seem logical if it can be shown to offer clear-cut outcome advantage over non-surgical management. In our 2019 study [1], the subgroup of young asymptomatic children with virgin lipoma treated with total resection was compared to the results of the Paris and London series of

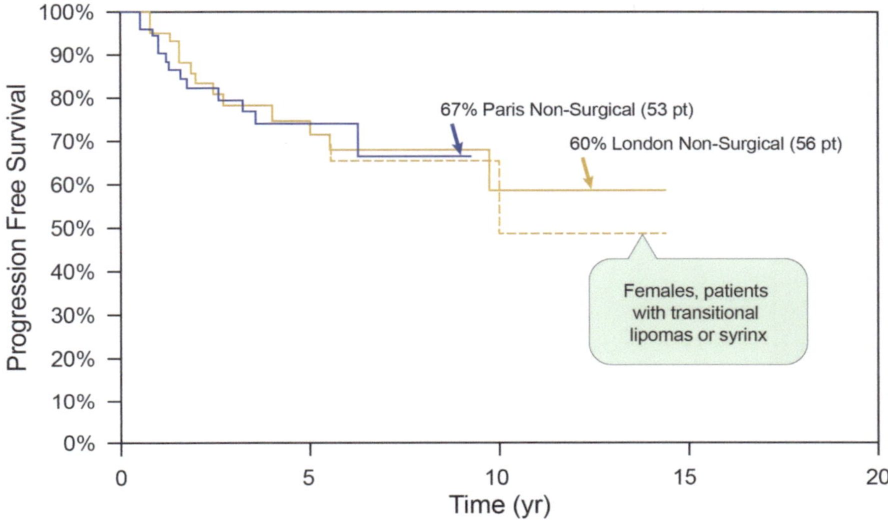

Fig. 55 Non-surgical treatment of asymptomatic lipomas. The blue line denotes the Paris series of 53 patients followed prospectively for 9 years [3], with a PFS of 67%. The yellow line denotes the retrospective London series of 56 patients followed for 10 years [4], with a PFS of 60%. In the London series, females, those with transitional lipomas and conus syrinx did worse, thus with an even worse PFS (dotted yellow line). (Reprinted from Pang D. Total resection of complex spinal cord lipomas: how, why, and when to operate. Neuro Med Chir (Tokyo) 55: 695–721, 2015; with permission from the Japanese Neurosurgical Society. CC-BY-NC-ND (https://creativecommons. org/licenses/by-nc-nd/4.0/deed.ja))

non-surgical management, and the superiority of total resection seemed obvious, with a 20 years PFS of 98.8% [25] compared to the 10 years rates of 67% and 60% for conservative management in Paris and London, respectively [3, 4] (Fig. 56). This prompted our initial endorsement of total resection as prophylactic treatment for asymptomatic children with dorsal and transitional lipomas.

The caveat of that blanket endorsement is that none of the three series in question, our total resection group of asymptomatic virgin lesions, or the London and Paris series were segregated according to the actual morphology of the lipoma-cord relationship either on pre-operative radiographic imaging or at surgery, and thus the PFS data for all three cohorts were those representing mixed lipoma types. Recently, Thompson et al. [72] followed a subgroup of 21 asymptomatic children with lipomas whose MRI showed a reasonably clear-cut profile of the conus relatively unmolested by fat and found that their PFS after a follow-up period of 20 years was 77.2%, far better than the PFS of 60% of the mixed group reported by the same centre in 2012 [4]. This raises the question whether this subgroup of children whose conus displays clean outline on pre-operative MRI have better prognosis for preservation of bladder

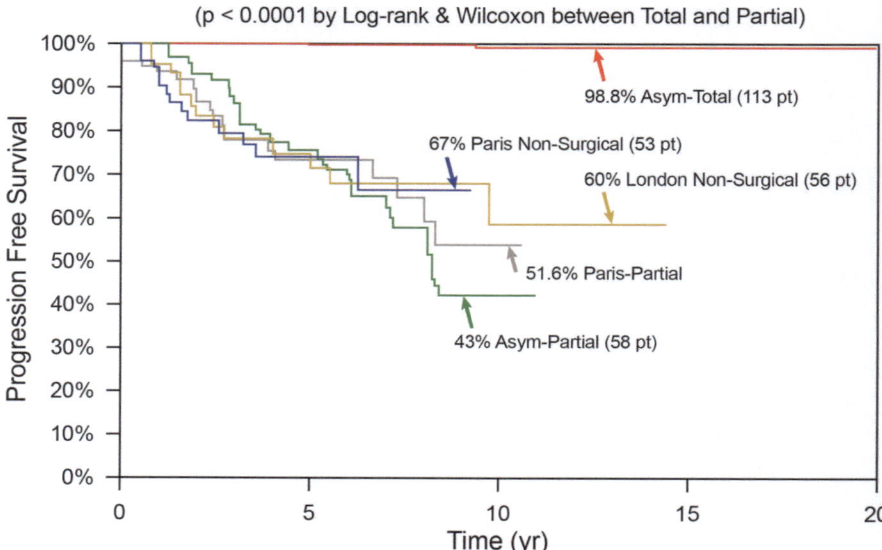

Fig. 56 Outcome differences between total resection, partial resection, and non-surgical management of asymptomatic virgin lipomas by Kaplan-Meier analysis. The non-surgical progressive-free survival graphs ("Paris Non-Surgical Asym") from the Parisian study [3] and from the London study [4] ("London Non-Surgical Asym")are inserted for visual comparison only and not meant to imply a true "head-to-head" comparison. Progression-free probability at 20 years for the 113 asymptomatic virgin lipomas that had undergone total resection is 98.8%, much better than 67% of the Parisian series or the 60% of the London series, and far superior to the 43.3% of our own partial resection series and the 51.6% of the Parisians' own partial resection series. The difference between total and partial resection for asymptomatic virgin lipomas is highly significant ($P < 0.0001$). *Pt* Patients, Asym − Total = asymptomatic virgin lipomas treated by total resection; Asym − Partial = asymptomatic virgin lipomas treated by partial resection; Paris Non-surgical Asym = asymptomatic virgin lipomas managed non-surgically in Paris [3]; London non-surgical Asym = asymptomatic virgin lipomas from London [4]. The Paris partial resection and our own partial resection series are as labelled. (Reprinted from Pang D. Total resection of complex spinal cord lipomas: how, why, and when to operate. Neuro Med Chir (Tokyo) 55: 695–721, 2015; with permission from the Japanese Neurosurgical Society. CC-BY-NC-ND (https://creativecommons. org/licenses/by-nc-nd/4.0/deed.ja))

function without surgery, i.e. have a tamer natural history, and perhaps be spared prophylactic surgery and its attendant risks of iatrogenic complications.

The slight shortfall of this revised endorsement is that the cohort size in the study of Thompson et al. is small [72] and that the impression of the "clean-cut conus" on MRI is rather subjective, more dependent on the experience of the observer than any measurable "standard parameters". All things considered, the final decision whether to offer prophylactic total resection for lipomas must rest on the seasoned surgeon's overall assessment, including whether the conus possesses distinct outlines on the pre-operative MRI.

There are currently no data on the rate or probability of disease progression for adults with asymptomatic lipomas, and their actuarial life span is obviously shorter than that of children, so the cumulative risk for adults should be far smaller. A forceful argument therefore cannot be made for prophylactic surgery in asymptomatic adults, but when a lipoma becomes symptomatic, further deterioration is usually inevitable, and aggressive resection can then be justified for both children and adults.

Is Partial Resection Worse Than No Resection?

We would very much like to register our definitive answer to this question and hopefully put the issue of partial resection to rest. To start, the 11 years PFS probability of 34.6% from the senior author's own partial resection series of 116 lipomas [19, 22, 25] is clearly inferior to the Paris (PFS of 67%) and London (PFS of 60%) series [3, 4] of observation alone. If we now calculate outcome only on our asymptomatic virgin cases who had partial resection to match the profiles of the other two series, in essence eliminating the fastidious redo lipomas, their 11-year PFS after partial surgery is only 43% [19], still far short of the Paris and London numbers [3, 4, 25]. Moreover, the Parisian series of partial resection [3] managed only a slightly higher PFS of 51% (Fig. 56), and other similar series report equally dismal or worse PFSs, far worse than no surgery. Minus the good-risk terminal lipomas, Colak et al.'s series [13] would have a less than 50% PFS, as would Pierre-Kahn's partial resection series a less than 40% PFS [26]. Cochrane et al.'s [15] partial resection of transitional lipomas had a 10-year PFS of only 20%, and Cornette et al. [75] conceded unaltered progression of disease after partial resection.

The explanation for the above statistics is quite plain if one had the unpleasant experience of exploring these redo lipomas, as the senior author did more than 150 times, and witnessed how the abraded but unneurulated placode could be solidly welded to the dura by rigid scar much more than in an unoperated lipoma with its nascent surface. If the frequency and speed of symptomatic recurrence are proportional to the extent and firmness of fixity of the placode, one would certainly expect partial resection to incur sooner and more severe functional impairment than if no surgery had been done, which is clearly shown in the senior author's 2013 analysis [25]. The time course of in situ scar formation also explains why partial resection typically gives immediate clinical improvement owing to the *initial* relief of tethering but is unable to sustain these short-lived benefits against the slow but inexorable course of chronic scar formation, ending in an unrelenting downhill path that is clearly worse than the natural history of the disease.

Our extensive literature search suggests that the current global practice of lipoma surgery comprises a continuum of techniques ranging from perfunctory whittling of fat with no chance of placode refurbishment, to aggressive total resection of lipoma, elaborate microsurgical reconstruction of the placode, and capacious dural grafting, as is endorsed here. In between these two extremes, there is at least one historical series that describes the half-measured protocol of "subtotal fat removal" and "partial neurulation" and reports somewhat better results than non-surgical treatment [9]. It is thus tempting to hypothesise that the thoroughness of "clean" placode reconstruction, which is estimable by MRI, is commensurate with the clinical benefits, and that the projected outcome of non-surgical treatment lies somewhere between the two extremes of skimpy and complete fat removal. This would also imply that partial resection will in the long run prove more harmful than no surgery for the patient. In this context, we rather strongly think that partial resection should be discouraged.

New Doubts, New Insights, and Some New Recommendations

Since our 2019 report [1], the ever enlarging data pool on total resection has induced us to consolidate a few recommendations regarding treatment that were, at best, tentatively entertained before.

Lipoma Types and Surgical Outcome and the Dubious Rank of Chaotic Lipomas

According to the senior author's total resection data, the type of lipoma should not affect outcome projection [19, 25], but in reality it probably does, as previously alluded to. One of the limitations of biostatistics is its inherent fallacy of rigidly assigning finite variables to represent the almost infinite vicissitudes of biological forms. For example, under the same umbrella of transitional lipomas, there are lesions with relatively orderly alignment of DREZ and nerve roots, a predictable lipoma-cord interface, and manageable quantities of fat, and there are also lipomas with plume-like billows of smothering fat that defy designation. The success and complication rates for these two extremes cannot be the same, and indiscriminately blending their divergent statistical weights is accordingly misleading. Thus, the blanket statement of "no statistical difference" in outcome between lipoma types should not be taken too literally, nor should it supplant an experienced surgeon's impression, despite comforting statistics, that some sprawling, intractable transitional lipomas demand much more exacting skill and portend a graver prognosis than a tamer, friendlier dorsal lipoma.

By far the most difficult and treacherous lipomas we have ever resected are of the chaotic type. The demarcation between fat and neural tissue is sometimes indiscernible even within the dorsal portion of these lesions, and the resection should be more conservative and aim only to remove just enough dorsal fat to enable a comfortable neurulation of the dorsal part. We have repeatedly emphasised restraint and avoid doing damage to the pia covering the ventral fat since its complete resection and ventral neurulation are never possible. Consequently, it is not uncommon for chaotic lipomas to have higher cord-sac ratios and display more residual fat than the other two lipoma types on the post-operative MRI (Fig. 33d).

When in 2010 we compared the total resection outcomes of the three lipoma types in a cohort of 238 patients, we found no actual statistical differences between them [19]. However, even with the caveat of small sample size of only 10 chaotic lesions, the PFS curve for chaotic lipomas ran considerably lower than the curves for dorsal and transitional lesions, and the *P* values between chaotic and the other two lesions were only very slightly higher than 0.05, giving us the preliminary suspicion that chaotic lipomas had worse prognosis than the others. In our more recent series of 315 total resections published in 2013 [25], the number of chaotic lipomas has risen to 28. The PFSs for dorsal and transitional lipomas of 92.2% and 86%, respectively, remained very similar to the 2010 figures, and again they had clearly no statistical difference, with a *P* value of 0.458. However, the PFS for chaotic lesions has dropped slightly to 54%, and its regression curve separates even further away from the other two curves than in 2010 (Fig. 57). Within this chaotic group, there were no patients with cord-sac ratios lower than 50%, and their postoperative MRI often showed a hefty placode with a loathsome amount of remainder ventral fat and a tight container fit [25]. By strict standard, the outcome differences

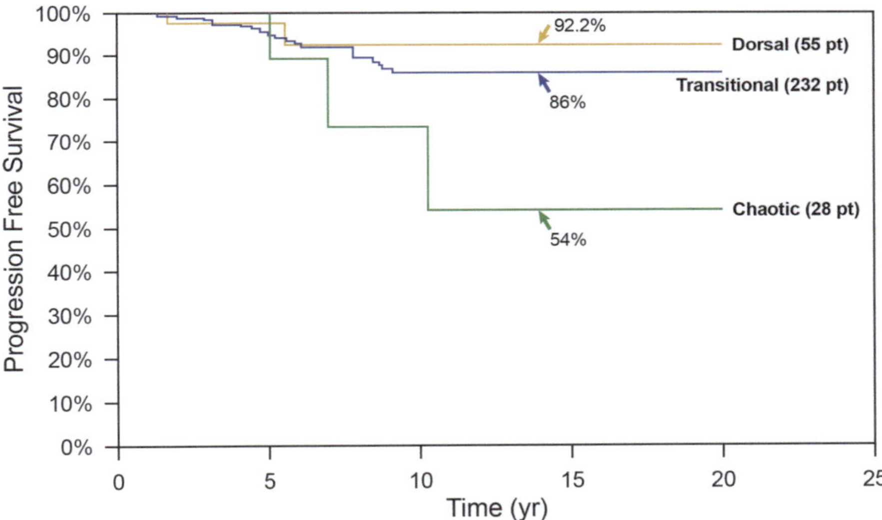

Fig. 57 The influence of lipoma type on outcome after total resection by KM analysis. The progression-free probabilities for the 3 lipoma types are indicated by arrows. There is no significant difference in outcome between dorsal and transitional lipomas ($p = 0.458$ by Log-rank and 0.904 by Wilcoxon) even after adjusting for sample size. There are "tentative" differences between chaotic and the other lipoma types when compared individually ($p = 0.0472$ with dorsal lipomas and 0.0422 with transitional lipomas). *Pt* Patients. (Reprinted from Pang D. Total resection of complex spinal cord lipomas: how, why, and when to operate. Neuro Med Chir (Tokyo) 55: 695–721, 2015; with permission from the Japanese Neurosurgical Society. CC-BY-NC-ND (https://creativecommons.org/licenses/by-nc-nd/4.0/deed.ja))

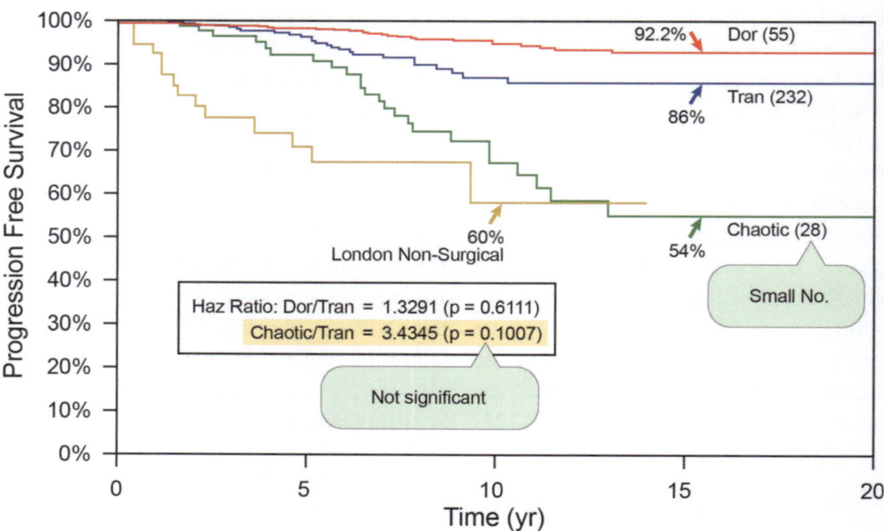

Fig. 58 The London non-surgical treatment progression-free survival curve [4] is inserted on to the 3 PFS curves of the different lipoma types obtained with the Cox proportional hazards analysis. The hazard ratio between chaotic and transitional lipomas is not statistically significant but that may be due to the small number in the chaotic group. The 10-year PFS from the London series is very similar to the PFS of the chaotic lipomas, which raises the question whether there is merit in resecting asymptomatic chaotic lipomas. (Reprinted from Pang D. Total resection of complex spinal cord lipomas: how, why, and when to operate. Neuro Med Chir (Tokyo) 55: 695–721, 2015; with permission from the Japanese Neurosurgical Society. CC-BY-NC-ND (https:// creativecommons.org/licenses/by-nc-nd/4.0/deed.ja))

between chaotic and the other 2 lipoma types only barely reach statistical significance (*P*-value of 0.0492 with dorsal lipoma and 0.0481 with transitional lipoma), but given larger numbers in the future, the rank of chaotic lesions might very well be definitively downgraded to the most sinister of the three lipoma types.

In Fig. 58, we inserted the London outcome curve of non-surgical treatment on to the PFSs of the 3 lipoma types. The 54% PFS of chaotic lipomas, after aggressive resection, is actually worse than both the London and Paris series of non-surgical treatment, which begs the question whether asymptomatic chaotic lipomas should be treated with any prophylactic surgery, regardless of technique. This sobering observation has stricken another lipoma type out of our prophylactic surgery category, and we now recommend that asymptomatic chaotic lesions, if unmistakably diagnosed on MRI, should be closely observed without surgery until symptoms develop.

Pre-Operative Symptoms and Surgical Outcome

For all the lofty statistics and extravagant analyses, there remains the unanswered question whether symptomatic lipomas do worse than asymptomatic ones after total resection. In the senior author's 2013 series of 315 patients [25], multivariate analysis finds no statistical difference in outcome between symptomatic and asymptomatic lesions, but univariate analysis, in contrast, shows that asymptomatic lesions had significantly better outcome than symptomatic lesions, as we have found in his earlier series of 238 patients [19] (Fig. 59). Even when the analysis is run just on the virgin lesions to eliminate the "redo factor" among symptomatic patients, asymptomatic patients still came out much better [25] (Fig. 60).

Besides our own results, several large series in the literature [9, 12, 26] also report considerably better outcome for asymptomatic than symptomatic patients. It was once argued that children with symptoms tend to be older and are thus more likely to undergo growth spurts and take up rigorous sports, both situations subject the spinal cord to pernicious tugging known to trigger symptoms in other tethered cord conditions, whereas asymptomatic children are much younger. The post-resection profiles of the two groups are thus not comparable as the symptomatic older child is being followed at a more vulnerable age [9]. Whilst this may explain some cases of early recurrence in the symptomatic group, Byrne et al.'s series of 100 infants, which eliminated the age difference in the two groups, still shows a markedly better outcome for asymptomatic infants [6]. Current consensus seems to support the notion that there are indeed prognostic differences between symptomatic and asymptomatic lipomas following total resection.

To date, no consistent dissimilarity in size, architecture, or histology has been found between symptomatic and asymptomatic lipomas, but there may be invisible differences in susceptibility inherent within their respective spinal cords. Perhaps the already injured cord that is showing symptoms has become more "fragile" and possesses a lower threshold for new symptoms with even "slight" retethering. Perhaps those spinal cords which develop early symptoms are also intrinsically predisposed to sustain new injuries to even minor future insults and are thus destined to have earlier disease recurrence.

Interestingly, this observation of a better post-resection outcome for asymptomatic over symptomatic lipomas somewhat argues against the earlier recommendation of awaiting surgery until the onset of symptoms for classic dorsal lipomas and those associated with distinct conus outlines on MRI. This, unfortunately, shall remain one of the several untidy issues regarding these treacherous lesions, at least till a much larger follow-up study reveals the actual long-term fate of those lipomas with clean conus outlines. It needs reiterating here that lipomas that clearly involve part or most of the conus, or those in which the conus is barely recognisable except as non-fat streaky crescents within the fatty mass on T_1 axial MRI images, must still be operated on before symptoms arise.

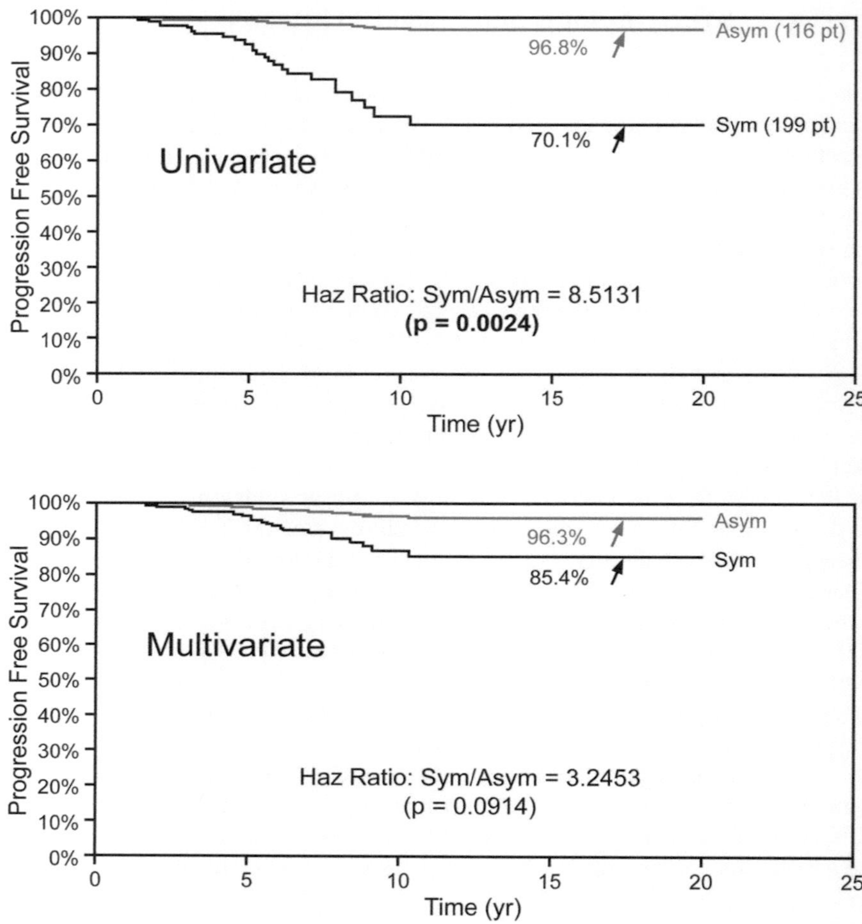

Fig. 59 Paired Cox Univariate (upper) and Multivariate (lower) analyses of the influence of pre-operative symptoms on PFS. The respective progression-free probabilities for asymptomatic and symptomatic lipomas are indicated by arrows, and their hazard ratios and relevant *p* values are listed for each Cox analysis. This shows the individual influence (expressed in univariate analysis) of pre-operative symptoms on outcome disappears when the influences of the other predictor variables are jointly considered (by multivariate analysis). *Pt* Patients, *Asym* Asymptomatic lipomas, *Sym* Symptomatic lipomas. (Significant *p* values are in bold) (Reprinted from: Pang D, Zovickian J, Wong ST, Hou YJ, and Moes GS. Surgical treatment of complex spinal cord lipomas. Childs Nerv Syst (2013) 29:1485–1513; with Permission from Springer Nature)

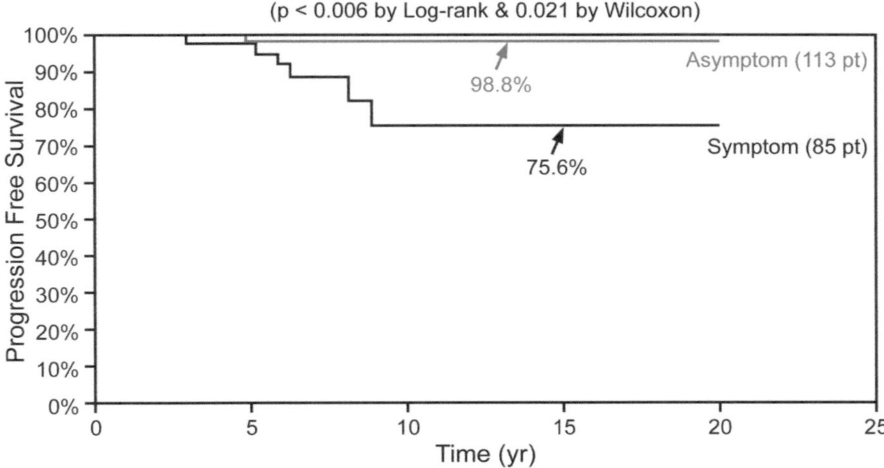

Fig. 60 The influence of pre-operative symptoms on outcome for virgin lipomas after total resection. Kaplan-Meier analysis for asymptomatic virgin and symptomatic virgin lipomas after total resection. Progression-free probability at 20 years for asymptomatic virgin lipomas is 98.8%, versus 75.6% for symptomatic virgin lipomas. The difference is significant ($p = 0.006$ by Log-rank and 0.021 by Wilcoxon). *Pt* Patients, *Asymptom* Asymptomatic virgin lipomas, *Symptom* Symptomatic virgin lipomas. (Reprinted from: Pang D, Zovickian J, Wong ST, Hou YJ, and Moes GS. Surgical treatment of complex spinal cord lipomas. Childs Nerv Syst (2013) 29:1485–1513; with Permission from Springer Nature)

The True Value of BCR in Intraoperative Electrophysiology Monitoring

Notwithstanding our tireless endorsement of intraoperative electrophysiology monitoring in total lipoma resection, the true value of BCR is, at best, undetermined at present. It has already been mentioned above that the electrical circuit for the BCR involves somatic sensory and motor neurons and is distinct from the visceral bladder wall stretch receptor-detrusor connections responsible for reflexive micturition. Because the two circuits are "anatomical neighbours" both residing within the same compact sacral cord segments, the hope is that clinical injury to the bladder circuit, which is technically not easily measurable, is reflected in disturbance in the somatic BCR circuit which is eminently measurable. However, it is not at all certain whether the conduction efficiencies of the two circuits are comparable, or more importantly, whether their injury thresholds to mechanical and ischaemic insults are similar enough to warrant reliance on monitoring just the BCR as a fair index to the integrity of both. We have seen cases where the BCR either is severely blunted or altogether disappears at the end of surgery, yet the patient has retained normal or near-normal bladder function; or vice versa, patients have partial loss of continence in face of a robust BCR. Also, surgically induced bladder dysfunction often improves with time, but there is obviously no possibility of tracking changes in the BCR *pari passu* with the corresponding improvement in voiding efficiency. At Great Ormond Hospital in London, we are currently collecting prospective data in our total resection group on the baseline and end-of-surgery BCR and the corresponding pre-and postoperative bladder function and hope to elicit a more cohesive correlation between the two.

Conclusion

Total/near-total resection of complex spinal cord lipomas and complete reconstruction of the neural placode produce a much better long-term symptom-free survival than partial resection. There is, in fact, incontrovertible evidence that partial resection causes new and exuberant scarring between the cut surface of the remainder fat and dura, resulting in earlier and firmer retethering and consequently a worse prognosis compared to no surgery. Our post-operative neuro-urological and wound complications for total resection are either comparable to, or lower than, most series of partial resection.

In matching our results of total resection to published results of non-surgical management of lipomas, we find that total resection confers much greater long-term benefits than no surgery in children with asymptomatic virgin lipomas. The ideal patient profile for total resection predictive of early disease stabilisation and the longest recurrence-free survival has been identified to be a child less than 2 years old who is without symptoms or prior surgery. We therefore still recommend prophylactic total resection for most asymptomatic dorsal and all transitional lipomas in children. Whether those dorsal lesions with clearly defined conus outline on MRI should be put in a wait-and-see category will have to await longer follow-up of a larger cohort of these patients without surgery. Multivariate analysis also shows that a low post-operative cord-sac ratio is highly predictive of good long-term outcome. Our firm impression is that a well-executed neurulation is just as important in preventing re-tethering.

Our experience so far shows that chaotic lipomas are the most treacherous, and the majority are simply not amenable to thorough resection or optimal placode reconstruction, let alone attaining the goal of a low cord-sac ratio. Their poor statistics are unlikely to improve even with larger numbers, and consequently we do not recommend prophylactic surgery for asymptomatic chaotic lipomas.

A lengthy analysis like this one is futile unless it can provide at least a few serviceable "truths", perhaps as succinct answers to the often asked questions of how, why, and when to perform total resection on spinal cord lipomas. The "how" of total resection, i.e. its technical aspects, can be learned by any willing neurosurgeon with a modicum of patience, tenacity, and open-mindedness. Those who have observed the surgery will attest that other than a few unaccustomed manoeuvres and tricks, which can be learned, the rest is strictly standard microsurgery. The intraoperative electrophysiology work can be managed by any trained neurophysiologist, and the equipment should be purchasable at reasonable cost.

As to the "why" and "when" questions, our massive outcome data collected over 30 years should have given eloquent reasons to endorse total resection for most asymptomatic dorsal and transitional lipomas in children and for all symptomatic lipomas in all ages. The surgery should be done soon after diagnosis, except in very young infants with stable neurology, for whom surgery is delayed till 6–12 months of age to minimise surgical and anaesthetic morbidity. Surgery for asymptomatic chaotic lipomas is withheld until symptoms develop.

Lastly, to conclude the conclusion, we should put in mind that "seeing is believing", and anyone wishing to witness first hand our technique, appended with personal tutelage, is welcomed to contact us to make arrangements.

Conflict of Interest Statement The author states that he has no conflicts of interests associated with the making of this manuscript.

References

1. Pang D. Surgical management of complex spinal cord lipomas: how, why, and when to operate. A review. J Neurosurg Pediatr. 2019;23:537–56. Journal of Neurosurgery Pediatrics 75th Anniversary Invited Review Article.
2. Pang D. Surgical management of complex spinal cord lipomas: a new perspective. J Korean Neurosurg Soc. 2020;63(3):279–313.
3. Kulkarni HV, Pierre-Kahn A, Zerah M. Conservative management of asymptomatic spinal lipomas of the conus. Neurosurgery. 2004;54:868–75.
4. Wykes V, Desai D, Thompson DNP. Asymptomatic lumbosacral lipomas—a natural history study. Childs Nerv Syst. 2012;28:1731–9.
5. Arai H, Sato K, Wachi A. Surgical management in 81 patients with congenital intraspinal lipoma. Childs Nerv Syst. 1992;8:171.
6. Byrne RW, Hayes EA, Georg TM, McLone DG. Operative resection of 100 spinal lipomas in infants less than 1 year of age. Pediatr Neurosurg. 1995;23:182–7.
7. Hoffman HJ, Taecholarn C, Hendrick EB, Humphreys RP. Management of lipomyelomeningoceles. J Neurosurg. 1985;62:1–8.
8. James CCM, Williams J, Brock W, Kaplan GW. U HS: radical removal of lipomas of the conus and cauda equina with laser microsurgery. Neurosurgery. 1984;13:340–5.
9. La Marca F, Grant JA, Tomita T, McLone DG. Spinal lipomas in children: outcome of 270 procedures. Pediatr Neurosurg. 1997;26:8–16.
10. McLone DG, Mutluer S, Naidich TP. Lipomeningoceles of the conus medullaris. In: Karger S, editor. Concepts in pediatric neurosurgery. Basel, Switzerland: Karger; 1982. p. 171–7.
11. Sutton LN. Lipomyelomeningocele. Neurosurg Clin N Am. 1995;6:325–38.
12. Dorward NL, Scatliff JH, Hayward RD. Congenital lumbosacral lipomas: pitfalls in analyzing the results of prophylactic surgery. Childs Nerv Syst. 2002;18:326–32.
13. Colak A, Pollack IF, Albright AL. Recurrent tethering: a common long-term problem after lipomyelomeningocele repair. Pediatr Neurosurg. 1998;29:184–90.
14. Pierre-Kahn A, Lacombe J, Pichon J, et al. Intraspinal lipomas with spina bifida: prognosis and treatment in 73 cases. J Neurosurg. 1986;65:756–61.
15. Cochrane DD, Finley C, Kestle J, Steinbok P. The patterns of late deterioration in patients with transitional lipomyelomeningocele. Eur J Pediatr Surg. 2000;10(suppl 1):13–7.
16. Xenos C, Sgouros S, Walsh R, Hockley A. Spinal lipomas in children. Pediatr Neurosurg. 2000;32:295–307.

17. Bruce DA. Schut L: spinal lipomas in infancy and childhood. Childs Brain. 1979;5:192–203.
18. McLone DG, Naidich TP. Laser resection of fifty spinal lipomas. Neurosurgery. 1986;18:611–5.
19. Pang D, Zovickian JG, Oviedo A. Long term outcome of total and near total resection of spinal cord lipomas and radical reconstruction of the neural placode part II: outcome analysis and preoperative profiling. Neurosurgery. 2010;66:253–73.
20. Schoenwolf GC. Histological and ultrastructural observations of tail bud formation in the chick embryo. Anat Rec. 1979;193:131–48.
21. Stolke D, Zumkeller M, Seifert V. Intraspinal lipomas in infancey and childhood causing a tethered cord syndrome. Neurosurg Rev. 1988;11:59–65.
22. Pang D, Zovickian JG, Ovieda A. Long term outcome of total and near Total resection of spinal cord lipomas and radical reconstruction of the neural placode part I: surgical technique. Neurosurgery. 2009;65:511–29.
23. Brunelle F, Sebag G, Baraton J, Carteret M, Martinat P, Pierre-Kahn A. Lumbar spinal cord motion measurement with phase-contrast MR imaging in normal children and in children with spinal lipomas. Pediatr Radiol. 1996;26:265–70.
24. Dick EA, deBruhn R. Ultrasound of the spinal cord in children: its role. Eur Radiol. 2003;13:552–62.
25. Pang D, Zovickian JG, Wong ST, Hou YJ, Moes GS. Surgical treatment of complex spinal cord lipomas. Childs Nerv Syst. 2013;29(Special Annual Issue):1485.
26. Pierre-Kahn A, Zerah M, Renier D, Canalli G, Sainte-Rose C, Lellough-Tubiana A, Brunelle F, Le Merrer M, Giudicelli Y, Pichon J, Kleinknecht B, Nataf F. Congenital lumbosacral lipomas. Childs Nerv Syst. 1997;13:298–334.
27. Dias M, Pang D. Human neural embryogenesis: a description of neural morphogenesis and a review of embryonic mechanisms. In: Pang D, editor. Disorders of the pediatric spine. New York: Raven Press; 1994.
28. Hamilton HL, Boyd JD, Mossman HM. Human embryology. 4th ed. Baltimore: Williams & Wilkins; 1972.
29. Kunitomo K. The development and reduction of the tail and of the caudal end of the spinal cord. Contributions to Embryology, Carnegie Institute. 1918;8:163–98.
30. Streeter GL. Factors involved in the formation of the filum terminalis. Am J Anat. 1919;25:1–12.
31. Barson AJ. The vertebral level of termination of the spinal cord during normal and abnormal development. J Anat. 1970;106:489–97.
32. Jones PH, Love JG. Tight filum terminale. Arch Surg. 1956;73:556–66.
33. Caldarelli M, McLone DG, Colins JA, Suwa J, Knepper PA. Vitamin a induced neural tube defects in a mouse. Concepts Pediatr Neurosurg. 1985;6:161–71.
34. McLone DG, Suwa J, Collins JA, Poznaski S, Knepper PA. Neurulation: biochemical and morphological studies on primary and secondary neural tube defects. Concepts Pediatr Neurosurg. 1983;4:15–29.
35. Marin-Padilla M. Clinical and experimental rachischisis. In: Vinken PS, Bruyn GW, editors. Handbook of clinical neurology, vol. 32. Amsterdam: North-Holland; 1978. p. 159–91.
36. Marin-Padilla M. Mesodermal altercations induced by hypervitaminosis A. J Embryol Exp Morpholog. 1966;15:261–9.
37. Marin-Padilla M. Morphogenesis of anencephaly and related malformations. Curr Top Pathol. 1970;51:145–74.
38. Marin-Padilla M. Morphogenesis of experimentally induced Arnold-Chiari malformation. J Neurol Sci. 1981;50:29–55.
39. Marin-Padilla M. Morphogenesis of experimentally induced encephalocele (cranioschisis occulta). J Neurol Sci. 1980;46:83–99.
40. Marin-Padilla M. Notochordal-basochondrocranium relationships: abnormalities in experimentally induced axial skeletal (dysraphic) disorders. J Embryol Exp Morpholog. 1979;53:15–38.
41. Marin-Padilla M. The tethered cord syndrome: developmental considerations. In: Holtzmann RNN, Stein BM, editors. The tethered spinal cord. New York: Thieme; 1985. p. 3–13.

42. McLone DG, Knepper PA. Role of complex carbohydrates and neurulation. Pediatr Neurosci. 1986;1:2–9.
43. Morris-Kay GM, Crutch B. Culture of rat embryos with B-D-xyloside: evidence of a role for proteoglycans in neurulation. J Anat. 1982;134:491–506.
44. O'Shea KS, Kaufmann MH. Phospholipace C-induced neural tube defects in the mouse embryo. Experientia. 1980;36:1217–9.
45. Toole BP. Glycosaminoglycans in morphogenesis. In: Hay E, editor. Cell biology of extracellular matrix. New York: Plenum Press; 1981. p. 229–94.
46. Detwiler SR, Hotzer H. The inductive and formative influence of the spinal cord upon the vertebral column. Bull Hosp Jt Dis Orthop Inst. 1954;15:114–23.
47. Kallen B. Early embryogenesis of central nervous system with special reference to closure defects. Dev Med Child Neurol. 1968;19(suppl):44–53.
48. McLone DG, Naidich TP. Spinal dysraphism: experimental and clinical. In: Holtzman RN, Stein BM, editors. The tethered spinal cord. New York: Thieme-Stratton; 1985.
49. Pang D. Spinal cord lipoma. In: Batjer H, Loftus C, editors. textbook of neurological surgery. Lippincott, Williams and Wilkins; 2002.
50. Pang D. Spinal cord lipomas. In: Pang D, editor. Disorders of the pediatric spine. New York: Raven Press; 1995. p. 175–201.
51. Pang D: Tethered cord syndrome, in Hoffman HJ (ed): Advances in pediatric neurosurgery. Philadelphia: Hanley and Belfus, Inc,1986: pp. 45–79.
52. Pang D. Total resection of complex spinal cord lipomas: how, why, and when to operate. Neurol Med Chir. 2015;55:695–721.
53. Schoenwolf GC, Nichols DH. Histological and ultrastructural studies of secondary neurulation in mouse embryos. Am J Anat. 1984;169:361–76.
54. Muller F, O'Rahilly R. The development of the human brain, the closure of the caudal neuropore, and the beginning of secondary neurulation at stage 12. Anat Embryol. 1974;176:413–30.
55. O'Rahilly R, Meyer DB. The timing and sequence of events in the development of the human vertebral column during the embryonic period proper. Anat Embryol. 1973;157:167–76.
56. Talwalker VC, Datsur DK. Ectopic spinal cord myelomeningocele with tethering: a clinicopathological entity. Dev Med Child Neurol. 1974;16(s32):159–60.
57. Pang D. Retained medullary cord in humans—late arrest of secondary neurulation. Neurosurgery. 2011;68:1500–19.
58. Pang D. Electrophysiological monitoring for tethered cord surgery. In: Yamada S, editor. Tethered cord syndrome. 2nd ed. New York, Stuttgart: Thieme Medical Publishers; 2010. p. 199–209.
59. Pang D. Intraoperative neurophysiology of the conus medullaris and cauda equina. Childs Nerv Syst. 2010;26:411–2.
60. Pang D. Use of an anal sphincter pressure monitor during operations on the sacral spinal cord and nerve roots. Neurosurgery. 1983;13:562–8.
61. Chapman PH, Davis KR. Surgical treatment of spinal lipomas in childhood. Pediatr Neursurg. 1993;19:267–75.
62. Chapman PH. Comments in: Kulkarni HV, Pierre-Kahn A, Zerah M: Conservative Management of asymptomatic spinal lipomas of the conus. Neurosurgery. 2004;54:868–75.
63. Chapman PH. Congenital intraspinal lipomas. Anatomic considerations and surgical treatment. Child's Brain. 1982;9:37–47.
64. Atala H, Sato K, Wachi A. Bladder functional changes resulting from lipomyelomeningocele repair. J Urol. 1992;148:592–5.
65. James CCM, Lassman LP. Diastematomyelia and the tight filum terminale. J Neurol Sci. 1970;10:193–6.
66. James HE, Canty TG. Human tails and associated spinal anomalies. Clin Pediatr. 1995;34:286–8.
67. Kanev PM, Lemire RJ, Loeser JB, Berger MS. Management and long-term follow-up review of children with lipomyelomeningocele, 1952-1987. J Neurosurg. 1990;74:48–52.

68. Koyanagi I, Iwasaki Y, Hida K, Abe H, Isu T, Akino M. Surgical treatment supposed natural history of the tethered cord with occult spinal dysraphism. Childs Nerv Syst. 1997;13:268–74.
69. McGuire EJ. The innervation and function of the lower urinary tract. J Neurosurg. 1986;65:278–85.
70. McGuire EJ, Woodside JR, Borden TA, Weiss RM. Prognostic value of urodynamic testing in myelodysplastic patients. J Urol. 1981;126:205–9.
71. Sathi S, Madsen JR, Bauer S, Scott RM. Effect of surgical repair on neurologic function in infants with lipomeningocele. Pediatr Neurosurg. 1993;19:256–9.
72. Thompson DNP, Spoor J, Schotman M, Maestic S, Craven CL, Desai D. Does conus morphology have implications for outcome in lumbosacral lipomas? Childs Nerv Syst. 2021;37:2025–31.
73. Hoffman HJ, Hendrick EB, Humphreys RP. The tethered spinal cord: its protean manifestations, diagnosis and surgical correction. Childs Brain. 1976;2:145–55.
74. Pang D, Wilberger JE. Tethered cord syndrome in adults. J Neurosurg. 1982;57:32–47.
75. Cornette L, Verpoorten C, Lagae L, Plets C, Van Calenbergh F, Casaer P. Closed spinal dysraphism: a review on diagnosis and treatment in infancy. Eur J Paediatr Neurol. 1998;2:179–85.
76. Schut L, Bruce DA, Sutton LN. The management of the child with lipomyelomeningocele. Child Neurosurg. 1983;30:440–76.
77. Pang D. Commentary to the article: asymptomatic lumbosacral lipomas—a natural history study; by Wykes V, Desai D, Thompson D.N.P. Childs Nerv Syst. 2012;28:1741–2.

Secondary Neurulation Defects: Retained Medullary Cord

Kyung Hyun Kim, Ji Yeoun Lee, and Kyu-Chang Wang

Introduction

Secondary neural tube formation has long been understood to take place over a series of steps. It begins first with a medullary cord formation phase (condensation, vacuolization, canalization), followed by a regression phase involving partial dissolution of the medullary cord. Related anomalies can therefore occur either from a failure of formation or that of regression. Malformations caused by a failure of regression include thickened filum terminale, which is the incomplete regression of the medullary cord (complete regression reduces it to a normal thin filum); filar cyst, which is a delayed luminal collapse of the caudal medullary cord; retained medullary cord (RMC), which results from total failure of regression of the

K. H. Kim
Division of Pediatric Neurosurgery, Seoul National University Children's Hospital,
Seoul, Republic of Korea

Department of Neurosurgery, Seoul National University College of Medicine,
Seoul, Republic of Korea
e-mail: nskhkim@snu.ac.kr

J. Y. Lee
Division of Pediatric Neurosurgery, Seoul National University Children's Hospital,
Seoul, Republic of Korea

Department of Anatomy and Cell Biology, Seoul National University College of Medicine,
Seoul, Republic of Korea

K.-C. Wang (✉)
Department of Neurosurgery, Seoul National University College of Medicine,
Seoul, Republic of Korea

Neuro-oncology Clinic, National Cancer Center, Goyang, Republic of Korea
e-mail: kcwang@snu.ac.kr

D. Pang, K.-C. Wang (eds.), *Spinal Dysraphic Malformations*, Advances and Technical Standards in Neurosurgery 47,
https://doi.org/10.1007/978-3-031-34981-2_7

215

medullary cord when it is still attached to the cul-de-sac of the vertebral axis; and finally, terminal myelocystocele and terminal myelocele when failed regression occurs at the stage when the medullary cord detaches from the skin before or after collapse of the terminal balloon, respectively [1–5]. These anomalies are all due to problems with the regression process, which chiefly involves programmed apoptosis, and each lesion varies depending on the exact timing when the developmental error occurs. For example, terminal myelocystocele results when the apoptosis arrest happens during a relatively early phase of medullary cord regression, while thickened filum terminale is caused by a much later apoptosis arrest.

Definition of RMC

The term retained medullary cord has now been widely accepted since Pang et al. coined it in 2011 [6]. A recent search for 'retained medullary cord' in PubMed showed 17 articles, and this number has been trending upward in recent years. While active research is presently being conducted, most of the recent publications are based on case reports. Piece by piece, this research has added much information pertaining to the understanding of RMC. Current literature shows cases of RMC associated with caudal lipoma, filar cyst, limited dorsal myeloschisis, congenital dermal sinus, subcutaneous meningocele (which is actually terminal myelocele or terminal myelocystocele), caudal agenesis, and split cord malformation [1, 6–10]. Despite many case reports, further studies are still needed to show the clinical ramifications of RMC. Also, we question whether it is appropriate that any non-functional cord-like structure caudal to the true conus should be classified as retained medullary cord. For example, caudal or transitional lumbosacral lipoma, and terminal myelocele or terminal myelocystocele may all have a non-functioning cord-like segment between the attached fat tissue and functioning conus, and the surgically removed parts may well contain non-functioning neural components but they are not RMCs and should not be termed such to avoid confusion.

Embryologically, RMC can be considered a rudimentary and redundant medullary cord that has persisted as a robust structure in smooth continuity with the 'true' conus, and which extends to the dural cul-de-sac. Superficially, it resembles the mature spinal cord, and it is thicker than the filum terminale, showing a slight caudal tapering. Its colour, pial covering, and outgoing rootlets are indistinguishable from those of the true conus, but it does not function as a neural structure. Its magnetic resonance imaging (MRI) signal intensity is the same as that of the conus, so the exact junction between the conus and RMC cannot be demarcated on MRI or by cursory inspection at surgery but only by direct electrical stimulations. Only through intraoperative neurophysiological monitoring (IONM) that shows a non-functioning cord-like structure can RMC be unerringly diagnosed [6].

The original description by Pang et al. [6] describes the retained medullary cord extending down to the dural cul-de-sac. Kim et al. [11] instead reported cases in which the caudal non-functioning cord-like structures were low-lying but did not reach the dural cul-de-sac. In this context, any non-functioning part of the neural structure that is caudal to the electrophysiologically proven true conus can be called an RMC even if it is not stretching the full length of the dural tube.

Thus, RMC is probably a result of regression failure at a certain stage of secondary neural tube development, but the exact genetic mechanism of this failure is currently unknown [6].

Cystic RMC

A typical filar cyst is a spindle-shaped cyst located at the junction between the tip of the conus and the upper end of the filum. It is regarded as a benign lesion without necessity of follow-up imaging unless a second tethering lesion is present [12]. This cystic dilatation sometimes extends almost the whole length of the filum, but the patient typically does not present with neurological deficits at birth [13, 14]. Previously, the terms 'terminal syrinx with low-lying conus' and 'giant filar cyst' were used for these cases [11, 15, 16]. Based on pathological findings, it is more reasonable to include them in the RMC category because they usually contain glioependymal tissues similar to those of RMC. A cystic RMC may therefore be seen as an intermediate form between a typical (non-cystic) RMC and a terminal myelocystocele. Kim et al. [1] described a patient with an intraspinal extradural-looking cyst that was actually an upwardly curved continuation of the caudal portion of a cystic RMC (Figs. 1, 2, 3). The thin wall of the cyst was fused with the wall of the dorsally expanded dura. On electrical stimulation, no response was obtained from the cystic structure. Histopathological examination of the resected cystic segment confirmed the presence of spotty, disorganized glioependymal tissue. Shim et al. [4] reported a case of RMC with cystic dilatation of its caudal end extending to the S4-5 level resembling a persistent terminal balloon of the chick embryo, complete with trumpet-like flaring of the terminal cyst filled with cerebrospinal fluid (CSF) resembling the trumpet of a terminal myelocystocele but without extra-spinal extrusion of its caudal part. These reports suggest that filar cyst, cystic RMC and terminal myelocystocele are a continuum of malformations resulting from successive regression failure of the medullary cord, with terminal myelocystocele being the earliest and filar cyst the latest in the time scale (Figs. 4, 5, 6).

'Possible RMC'

We define 'possible RMC' as a lesion in which the radiologic features suggest those of RMC by its distal cord-like structure, but the presence of a non-functioning caudal portion (the 'true RMC') has not been confirmed electrophysiologically. This confusion is due either to a reliance on pure MRI appearance without surgical confirmation, or, at surgery, the exposure is so limited that only the distal part of the

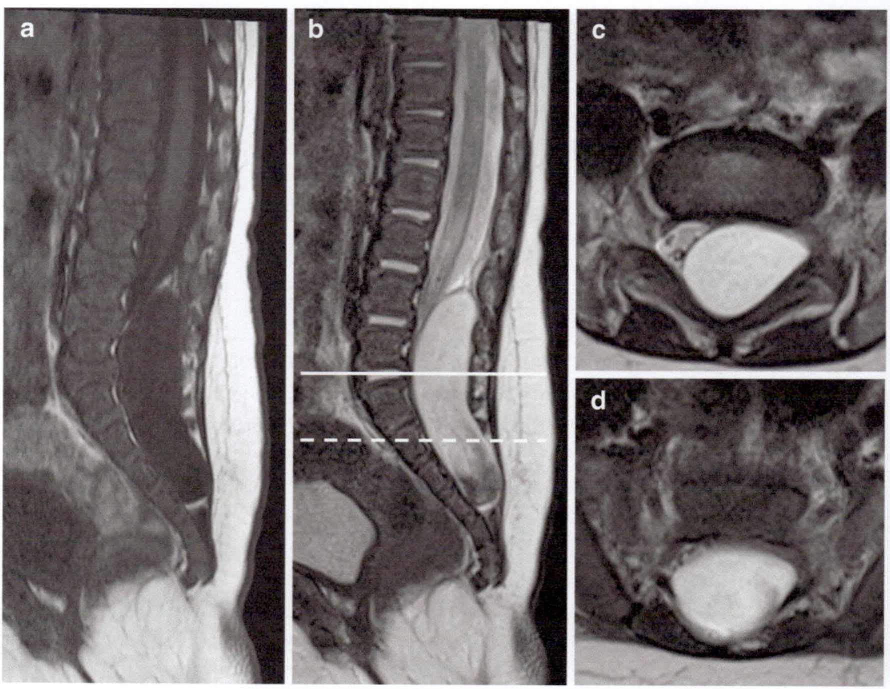

Fig. 1 A 7.2-cm-sized extradural-looking dorsal cystic lesion in the spinal canal, from L4 to S4 level, and the low-lying conus medullaris. (**a**) T1-weighted sagittal image, (**b**) T2-weighted sagittal image, (**c**) T2-weighted axial image at the L5-S1 level (white solid line in **b**), (**d**) T2-weighted axial image at the S1–2 level (white dashed line in **b**) (**d**). (Reprint permission from Springer Nature [1])

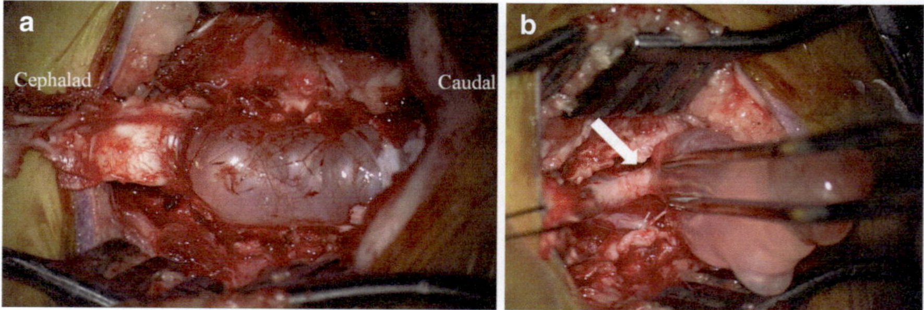

Fig. 2 Intraoperative photographs of the patient shown in Fig. 1. (**a**) A cerebrospinal fluid-filled cyst popped out after pulling up the laminotomy flap, before dural opening. The cyst turns out to be intradural, being folded up on itself and enclosed within an extremely thin overlying dura. (**b**) The rostral portion of the cyst, together with its thin overlying dura, was pulled down gently towards the caudal end of the spine to show its rostral end (still within the thin dura), where it appears to be continuous with the dural layer (white arrow). (Reprint permission from Springer Nature [1])

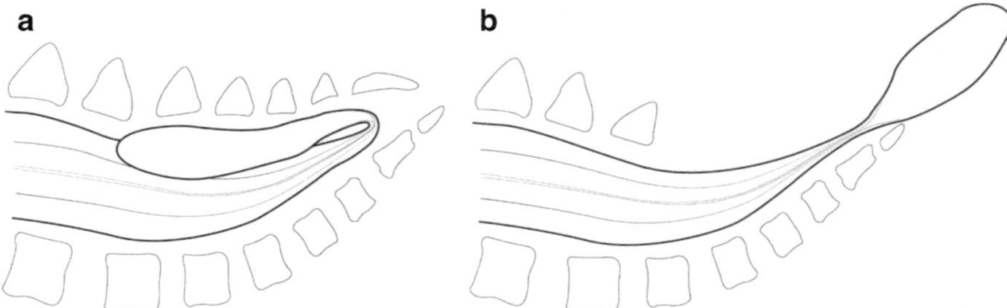

Fig. 3 A schematic illustration of the atypical cystic retained medullary cord seen in Figs. 1 and 2: (**a**) as it was within the intraspinal space, and (**b**) when it was stretched straight after the dura was opened. (Reprint permission from Springer Nature [1])

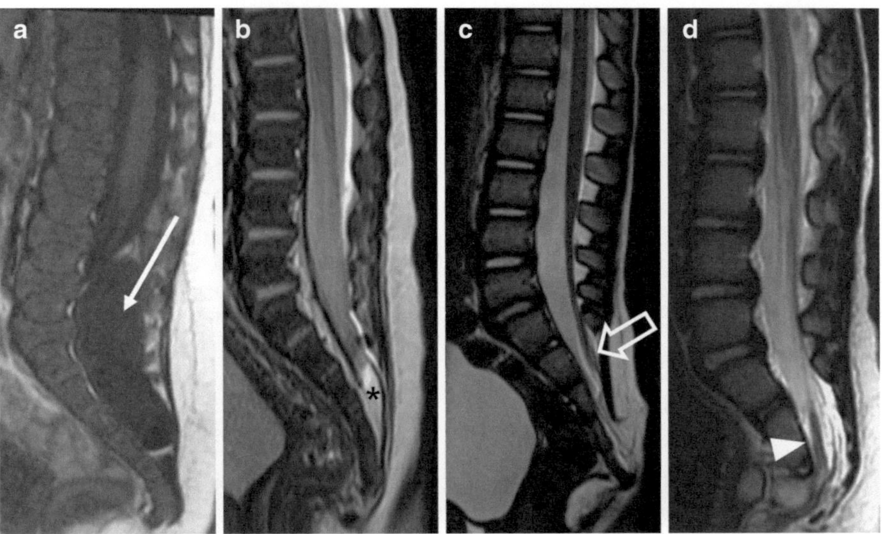

Fig. 4 MR images showing various forms of retained medullary cord (RMC). (**a**) A dorsally reflected intraspinal distal cystic RMC (arrow), (**b**) a small cystic RMC (asterisk) attached to the distal end of the thin filum, (**c**) a typical non-cystic RMC (outlined arrow) extending to the dural cul-de-sac, and (**d**) a non-cystic RMC (arrowhead) attached to the distal end of the thin filum. (Reprint permission from Springer Nature [1, 4] for (**a**) and (**b**), from Korean Neurosurgical Society [11] for (**c**), and from Oxford University Press [6] for (**d**))

filum is identified. These two scenarios happen in a conservative practice in which patients with a low-lying conus (not reaching the cul-de-sac) are observed without surgery, or if surgery is performed, only the distal end of the filum is exposed through minimal exposure. Without wide exposure and benefit of intraoperative electrophysiology, a simple low-lying conus cannot be distinguished from an RMC that does not extend to the dural cul-de-sac.

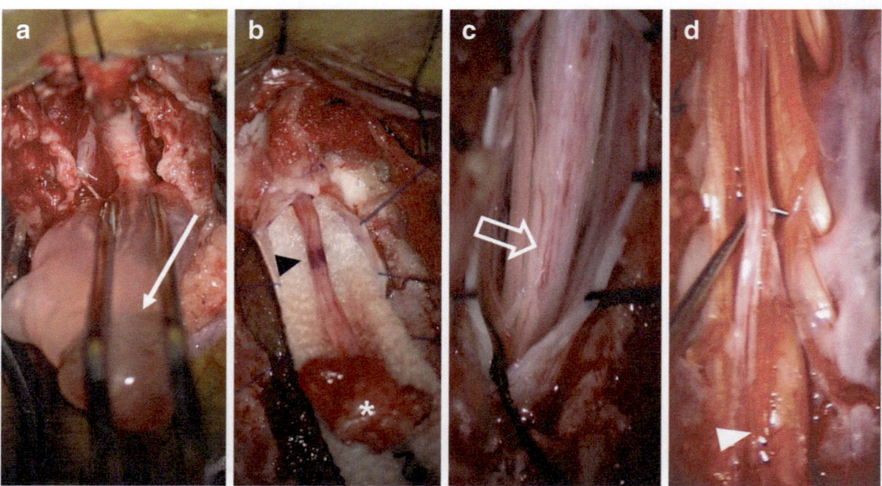

Fig. 5 Intraoperative photographs showing various forms of retained medullary cord (RMC). The figures with the same alphabetic character in Fig. 4 and this figure are from the same patient. (**a**) A dorsally reflected intraspinal distal cystic RMC with an overlying ultrathin, translucent dural layer, the whole structure now stretched straight (arrow) by the bayonet forceps, (**b**) a small cystic RMC (asterisk) attached to the distal end of the thin filum. The purple mark on the filum (black arrowhead) is the site of untethering cut. (**c**) A typical non-cystic RMC (outlined arrow) extending to the dural cul-de-sac, and (**d**) a non-cystic RMC (white arrowhead) attached to the distal end of the thin filum which was lifted by a hook. (Reprint permission from Springer Nature [1, 4] for (**a**) and (**b**), from Korean Neurosurgical Society [11] for (**c**), and from Oxford University Press [6] for (**d**).)

Surgical Treatment of RMC

The clinical symptoms of RMC are due to the cord tethering effects. If the patient has motor deficits, foot deformities, frequent urinary tract infections and other signs of neurogenic bladder and bowel, dysesthesia, leg pain, or coccydynia, surgery is recommended to untether the RMC. Even if there are no symptoms, surgery should be contemplated to prevent the emergence of neurological symptoms.

In choosing surgical strategy, it is important to note that an RMC typically is a cord-like structure that is seamlessly continuous with the conus medullaris, and it may not be easy to identify the boundary between functional conus and defunct neural tissue with the naked eye [6]. A few superficial features may help in characterizing typical RMCs. The first one concerns the appearance of surface blood vessels. Blood vessels on the conus medullaris tend to be serpentine, whereas the vasculature on the RMC is relatively straight. However, the unmistakable boundary between the true conus and the non-functioning retained medullary cord can only be made with intraoperative neurophysiological mapping. To identify the extent of the functioning conus, a concentric bipolar coaxial stimulator probe should be used. Selected rootlets should be isolated and surrounding CSF adequately

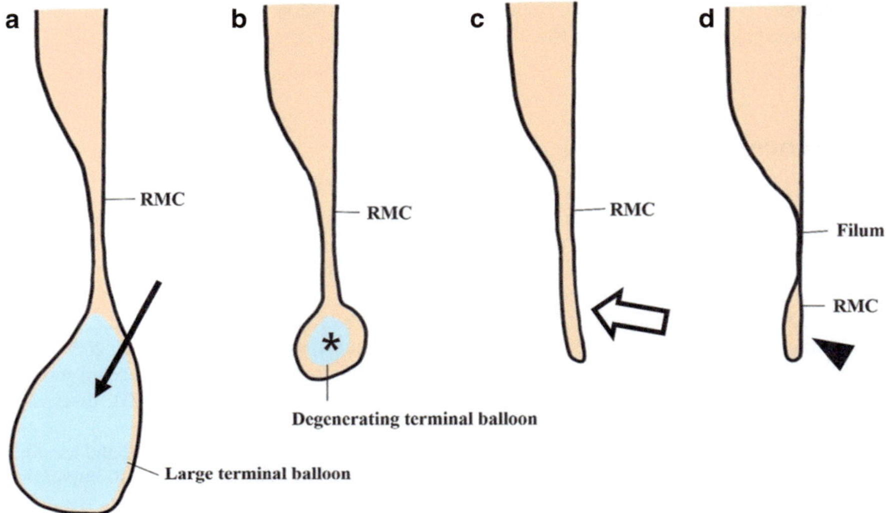

Fig. 6 Schematic drawings for various forms of retained medullary cord (RMC) shown in Figs. 4 and 5. The figures with the same alphabetic character in Figs. 4, 5 and this figure are from the same patient. (**a**) A dorsally reflected intraspinal distal cystic RMC (arrow) which has been stretched straight, (**b**) a small cystic RMC (asterisk) attached to the distal end of the thin filum, (**c**) a typical non-cystic RMC (outlined arrow) extending to the dural cul-de-sac, and (**d**) a non-cystic RMC (arrowhead) attached to the distal end of the thin filum. (Reprint permission from Springer Nature [4])

suctioned away to minimize the spread of electrical current to nearby rootlets [17]. Direct stimulation on the cord-like structure itself is also done with current intensities as high as 6–7 milliamperes. Locations on the cord which show responses must be clearly distinguished from those showing no response through repetitive stimulation, and only then could safe transection of the distal non-functioning part be made at this boundary line. We do not recommend extensive laminotomy to expose the entire length of the RMC distal to this boundary line. In the event that the bony exposure is below this boundary line, we will execute the untethering sectioning directly on the non-functioning part if only this part of the defunct cord is exposed. We recommend not cutting any rootlet even if it shows no function on stimulation unless it appears to impart the impression of tethering.

If surgery is deemed necessary for a 'possible RMC', limited unilateral partial hemilaminectomy is usually adequate as used in simple filum sectioning, again to avoid excessive bony exposure. If the non-cystic conus tip is a fair distance above the cul-de-sac, and there is an obvious caudal filum not resembling an RMC, the filum can be cut without IONM through a small laminectomy [18]. In general, the result of RMC surgery is excellent, barring unexpected misadventures.

Acknowledgements We are indebted to Professor Dachling Pang for his meticulous review of our manuscript.

This work was supported by the National Research Foundation of Korea (NRF) grant funded by the Korea government (MSIT) (No. 2021R1F1A1058932).

References

1. Kim KH, Lee JY, Yang J, Park SH, Kim SK, Wang KC. Cystic retained medullary cord in an intraspinal J-shaped cul-de-sac: a lesion in the spectrum of regression failure during secondary neurulation. Childs Nerv Syst. 2021;37(6):2051–6. https://doi.org/10.1007/s00381-020-04943-6.
2. Lee JY, Kim KH, Wang KC. Terminal myelocystocele: pathoembryogenesis and clinical features. J Korean Neurosurg Soc. 2020;63(3):321–6. https://doi.org/10.3340/jkns.2020.0063.
3. Pang D, Zovickian J, Lee JY, Moes GS, Wang KC. Terminal myelocystocele: surgical observations and theory of embryogenesis. Neurosurgery. 2012;70(6):1383–404; discussion 404-5. https://doi.org/10.1227/NEU.0b013e31824c02c0.
4. Shim Y, Park HJ, Kim KH, Park SH, Wang KC, Lee JY. Retained medullary cord and terminal myelocystocele as a spectrum: case report. Childs Nerv Syst. 2022;38(6):1223–8. https://doi.org/10.1007/s00381-021-05351-0.
5. Yang J, Lee JY, Kim KH, Wang KC. Disorders of secondary neurulation: mainly focused on pathoembryogenesis. J Korean Neurosurg Soc. 2021;64(3):386–405. https://doi.org/10.3340/jkns.2021.0023.
6. Pang D, Zovickian J, Moes GS. Retained medullary cord in humans: late arrest of secondary neurulation. Neurosurgery. 2011;68(6):1500–19; discussion 19. https://doi.org/10.1227/NEU.0b013e31820ee282.
7. Kurogi A, Murakami N, Morioka T, Mukae N, Shimogawa T, Kudo K, et al. Two cases of retained medullary cord running parallel to a terminal lipoma. Surg Neurol Int. 2021;12:112. https://doi.org/10.25259/sni_626_2020.
8. Morioka T, Murakami N, Kanata A, Tsukamoto H, Suzuki SO. Retained medullary cord with sacral subcutaneous meningocele and congenital dermal sinus. Childs Nerv Syst. 2020;36(2):423–7. https://doi.org/10.1007/s00381-019-04301-1.
9. Murakami N, Morioka T, Shimogawa T, Hashiguchi K, Mukae N, Uchihashi K, et al. Retained medullary cord extending to a sacral subcutaneous meningocele. Childs Nerv Syst. 2018;34(3):527–33. https://doi.org/10.1007/s00381-017-3644-2.
10. Shirozu N, Morioka T, Inoha S, Imamoto N, Sasaguri T. Enlargement of sacral subcutaneous meningocele associated with retained medullary cord. Childs Nerv Syst. 2018;34(9):1785–90. https://doi.org/10.1007/s00381-018-3812-z.
11. Kim KH, Lee JY, Wang KC. Secondary neurulation defects-1: retained medullary cord. J Korean Neurosurg Soc. 2020;63(3):314–20. https://doi.org/10.3340/jkns.2020.0052.
12. Seo K, Oguma H, Furukawa R, Gomi A. Filar cysts in rare cases may progress in size, particularly when associated with filar lipoma. Childs Nerv Syst. 2019;35(7):1207–11. https://doi.org/10.1007/s00381-019-04148-6.
13. Irani N, Goud AR, Lowe LH. Isolated filar cyst on lumbar spine sonography in infants: a case-control study. Pediatr Radiol. 2006;36(12):1283–8. https://doi.org/10.1007/s00247-006-0317-9.
14. Zeinali M, Safari H, Rasras S, Bahrami R, Arjipour M, Ostadrahimi N. Cystic dilation of a ventriculus terminalis. Case report and review of the literature. Br J Neurosurg. 2019;33(3):294–8. https://doi.org/10.1080/02688697.2017.1340585.
15. Pencovich N, Ben-Sira L, Constantini S. Massive cystic dilatation within a tethered filum terminale causing cauda equina compression and mimicking syringomyelia in a young adult patient. Childs Nerv Syst. 2013;29(1):141–4. https://doi.org/10.1007/s00381-012-1911-9.

16. Sade B, Beni-Adani L, Ben-Sira L, Constantini S. Progression of terminal syrinx in occult spina bifida after untethering. Childs Nerv Syst. 2003;19(2):106–8. https://doi.org/10.1007/s00381-002-0672-2.
17. Sala F, Barone G, Tramontano V, Gallo P, Ghimenton C. Retained medullary cord confirmed by intraoperative neurophysiological mapping. Childs Nerv Syst. 2014;30(7):1287–91. https://doi.org/10.1007/s00381-014-2372-0.
18. Wang KC. Spinal dysraphism in the last two decades: what I have seen during the era of dynamic advancement. J Korean Neurosurg Soc. 2020;63(3):272–8. https://doi.org/10.3340/jkns.2020.0068.

Secondary Neurulation Defect: Terminal Myelocystocele, a Biological Leviathan

Ji Yeoun Lee, Kyu-Chang Wang, and Dachling Pang

Introduction

Terminal myelocystocele (TMC) is an anomaly in the sacrococcygeal region usually forming a subcutaneous hump of various sizes. Due to its ponderous appearance, there had been confusion regarding its embryogenesis and classification in the broad subject of spinal dysraphism [1–4]. We have demystified the TMC by defining the essential and nonessential features to explain the diverse morphology [5]. Essential features seen in every TMC constituting the core malformation are as follows (Fig. 1): First, the caudal spinal cord is elongated and protrudes dorsally into the extraspinal space attached to the subcutaneous fat. Second, the extruded distal part of the spinal cord is a trumpet-shaped, CSF-filled cyst lined with some form of neuroepithelium. Most important, on a surgical standpoint, the terminal part of the extruded spinal cord is nonfunctional and can be removed without loss of function;

J. Y. Lee
Department of Anatomy and Cell Biology, Seoul National University College of Medicine,
Seoul, Republic of Korea

Division of Pediatric Neurosurgery, Seoul National University Children's Hospital,
Seoul, Republic of Korea

K.-C. Wang
Division of Pediatric Neurosurgery, Seoul National University Children's Hospital,
Seoul, Republic of Korea

Neuro-oncology Clinic, Center for Rare Cancers, National Cancer Center,
Goyang, Republic of Korea
e-mail: kcwang@snu.ac.kr

D. Pang (✉)
Department of Paediatric Neurosurgery, University of California, Davis, Davis, CA, USA

Great Ormond Street Hospital for Children, NHS Trust, London, UK

© The Author(s), under exclusive license to Springer Nature
Switzerland AG 2023
D. Pang, K.-C. Wang (eds.), *Spinal Dysraphic Malformations*, Advances and
Technical Standards in Neurosurgery 47,
https://doi.org/10.1007/978-3-031-34981-2_8

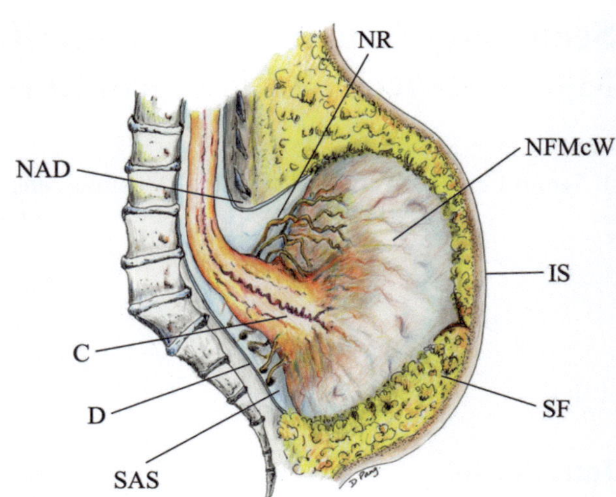

Fig. 1 Schematic drawing of the essential features of a terminal myelocystocele. The elongated spinal cord is extruded to the extraspinal space, attached to the subcutaneous fat in the shape of the opening of a trumpet. *C* Conus, *NR* Nerve roots, *NFMcW* Nonfunctional myelocystocele wall, *SAS* Subarachnoid space, *D* Dura, *IS* Intact skin, *SF* Subcutaneous fat

and finally, the overlying skin is always full thickness, although may be endowed with stigmata including hemangioma or fleshy appendages. The nonessential features include various degrees of hydromyelia within the spinal cord rostral to the extraspinal extrusion, variable sizes of protruded subarachnoid spaces, thickness of the subcutaneous fat overlying the mouth of the trumpet, and sacral bone anomalies. The nonessential features tend to determine the size and morphology of the malformation's visible presence.

Although the incidence of TMC is low, there was never flagging interest in treading the arduous path to construct theories of its embryogenesis, in understanding its seemingly bewildering structural and functional compartmentalisations, and, from thence, to achieve its safe repair, the whole enterprise inducing us in a previous publication [5] to anoint TMC as a 'biological leviathan', after Thomas Hobb's legendary sea monster [6]. In this chapter, the theory of TMC's embryogenesis will be described, followed by the surgical strategy in accordance with the embryology. The clinical features and prognosis will also be presented in detail.

Pathoembryogenesis

A tentative theory on the embryogenesis of TMC suggested by McLone and Naidich postulated that the bulging terminal trumpet might be the result of the entrapped CSF which failed to exit from the early neural tube before the canalization phase [7]. However, the mechanism of the dorsal distension of the CSF-filled terminal ventricle was not explained in the context of the events of normal embryogenesis of the secondary neural tube normal embryogenesis. The fact that most of the TMC cases reported do not harbour holocord syringes or have large defects of the vertebral column makes this theory less likely.

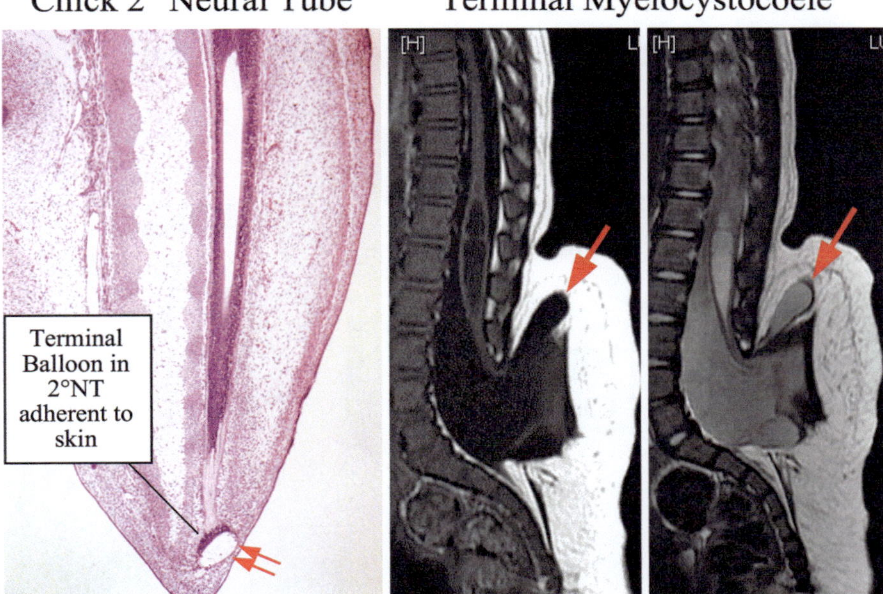

Fig. 2 Comparison between the longitudinal section of a chick embryo of late secondary neurulation (left) showing the terminal balloon (small arrows) and the sagittal MRIs of a terminal myelocystocele patient (middle and right). The mouth of the myelocystocele (arrows on the middle and right) resembles the terminal balloon of the chick embryo

The real breakthrough came when the resemblance of the TMC with the terminal balloon (see below) was noted, a structure previously noted during secondary neurulation of the chick embryo [5] (Fig. 2). Secondary neurulation is divided into three stages (or phases): condensation, cavitation, and regression of the medullary cord [8, 9] (Fig. 3). During the condensation phase, the tail bud, which is a multipotential cell mass of undifferentiated mesenchyme at the caudal end of the embryonic axis becomes segregated into central and peripheral cells [10–12]. The peripheral cells tend to show an apicobasal orientation, and later constitute most of the neuroepithelium of the secondary neural tube, called the medullary cord at this stage. The cavitation phase starts with the formation of small cavities within the cephalad end of the medullary cord due to gradual dissolution of the central cells, and the cavities then coalesce into a central lumen. This process is soon extended to the most caudal end of the medullary cord, while the proximal single lumen merges with the central canal of the more cephalad primary neural tube. Gradual progression of this process ultimately results in the completion of the secondary neural tube, and the primary and secondary neural tubes are connected as a single luminal structure (Fig. 4a). After the conjoining of the two neural tubes, the regression phase of the medullary cord begins. During the regression phase, a focal dorsal bulging of the

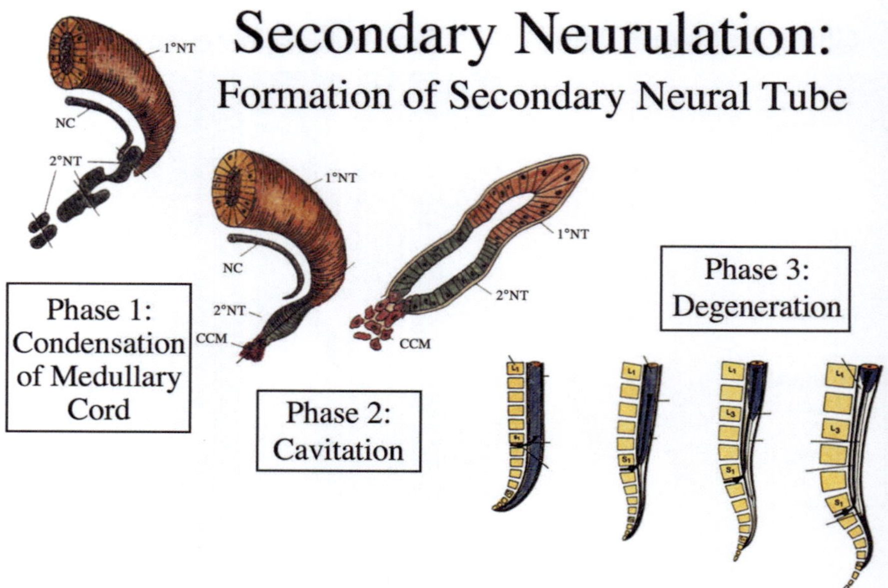

Fig. 3 Schematic drawing of secondary neurulation showing the three phases: condensation, cavitation, and degeneration

central canal at the very tip of the medullary cord is consistently noted and has been coined the 'terminal balloon' [12, 13] (Fig. 4b). At the peak of distention of the central neural canal, the dorsal wall of this terminal balloon becomes so close to the surface ectoderm of the embryo that the two layers appear almost fused as one. As regression of the medullary cord continues, the caudal neural tube shortens and the terminal balloon eventually disappears [14–16] (Fig. 4c, d).

The main essential feature of TMC, its cerebral spinal fluid (CSF)-filled trumpet of distended neural tissue abutting against the subcutaneous fat, is vividly reminiscent of the terminal balloon of the caudal neural tube in chicks just before its final dissolution, as the CSF-filled dorsal bulging of the mouth of the trumpet of TMCC is attached to the subcutaneous ectoderm [5] (Fig. 2). Hence, we postulate that TMC may be caused by an abrupt cessation of the final degenerative process of secondary neurulation, resulting in a time-frozen arrest of secondary neurulation at the stage of the terminal balloon [13]. This hypothesis also provides plausible explanations for some of the nonessential features of TMC: for example, the variable thickness of the subcutaneous fat, and the different degrees of hydromyelia within the spinal cord rostral to the trumpet. As the thickness of the subcutaneous layer will increase during degeneration of the caudal end of the medullary cord, the subcutaneous fat at the site of the attachment of the trumpet may be thicker if the apoptosis arrest occurs in the later phase of the degeneration. The variable size of the hydromyelia may also be explained by the observation that the relative

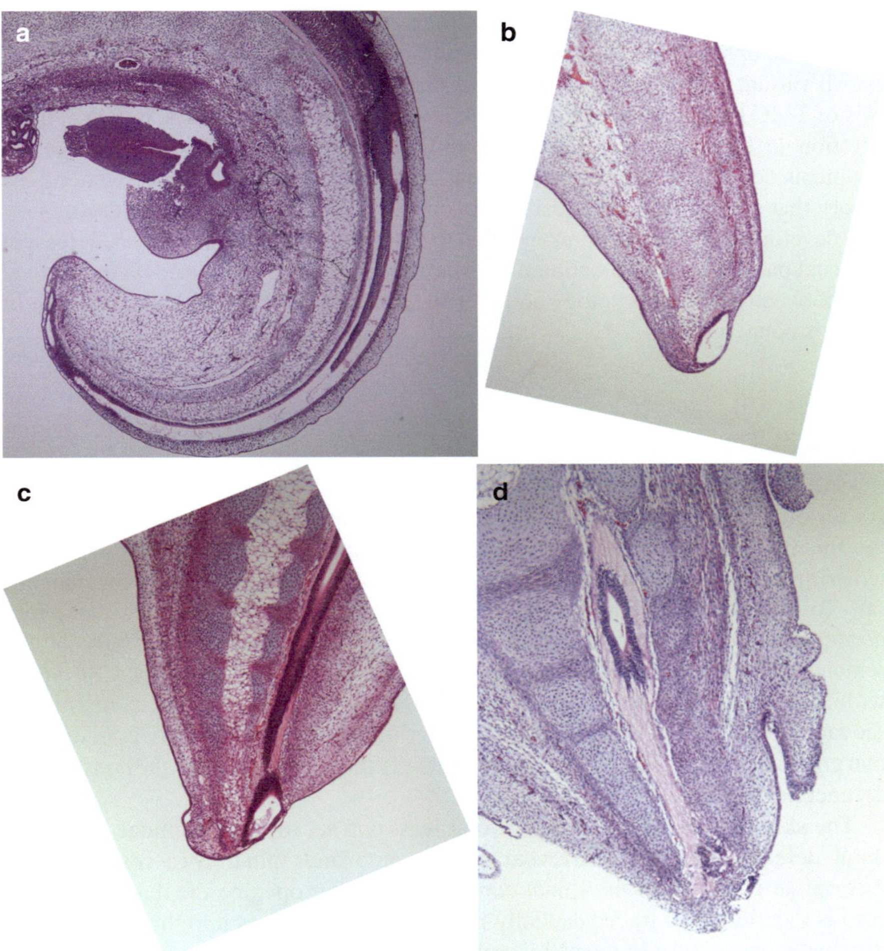

Fig. 4 Histological sections of chick embryos showing the formation and degeneration of the terminal balloon during secondary neurulation. (**a**) Coalescence of the lumen of primary and secondary neural tubes (×40). (**b**) Terminal balloon with very thin dorsal wall attached to the skin (×100). (**c**) Degeneration of the medullary cord and shrinkage of the terminal balloon (×40). (**d**) Degeneration of the terminal balloon and detachment of the medullary cord from the skin ectoderm (×40)

spatiotemporal order of medullary cord degeneration and dissolution of the terminal balloon varies greatly between chick embryos in our laboratory cohort. Thus, in some cases, the terminal balloon disappeared before the degeneration and collapse of the central canal of the medullary cord, and the arrest of dissolution of the terminal balloon in such cases will result in a large and extensive hydromyelic cavity. In contrast, some of the chick embryos were found to have almost completely degenerated medullary cord canal when the terminal balloon was still in full bloom. Arrested apoptosis in such cases will result in a TMC with minimal hydromyelia.

All variant features aside, the core of our present hypothesis of the embryogenesis of TMC lies in the presumption that its characteristic trumpet is, in fact, a preservation in human of the equivalent terminal balloon in chicks due to arrested apoptosis during the late stages of secondary neurulation. One may also extend the theory that since the terminal balloon in chicks is slated to be absorbed during normal development, one may presume that the analogous trumpet in human, at least in its distal part, is also nonfunctional and may be disposable. It is based on this crucial link between avian embryology and human malformation that our surgical repair of TMC is conceived.

Surgical Technique

As for other spinal dysraphic entities, complete untethering and reconstruction of the functional portion of the neural tube are the main goals of surgery. The worst tethering is at the attachment site of the mouth of the trumpet to the subcutaneous fat. To accomplish complete untethering, it is necessary to resect the entire nonfunctional portion of the distal trumpet so as to minimize the bulk of the remaining functional tissue. Also, it is important to obtain abundant CSF space within the reconstructed thecal sac to achieve the lowest (spinal) cord-to-(thecal) sac ratio, thus to reduce the chance of retethering. The critical issue for both of these two goals is therefore to separate intraoperatively the functional from the nonfunction defunct neural tissues.

The skin incision is performed and at least one set of intact laminae above the dural defect is exposed, to reveal normal dura and spinal cord rostral to the extraspinal extrusion of the spinal cord trumpet. After opening the dura, the spinal cord is identified and traced caudally to where the cord flares into the trumpet. The trumpet is then carefully opened longitudinally at its thinnest part. The inner lining of the trumpet is then stimulated with a concentric bipolar stimulation probe using currents from 4–6 mA with checking for responses from the anus and the lower legs. This crucial manoeuvre with the stimulation probe ultimately identifies a linear junctional demarcation, or boundary, between nonfunctional and functional neural tissues, the latter always endowed with 'live' nerve roots issuing from its corresponding pial surface opposite to the inner velvety lining of the trumpet. Only after such a solid boundary line is drawn with certainty (using intraoperative electrophysiology) that bold resection of the distal nonfunctional part can be done with impunity. Usually, the extraspinal portion of the trumpet is nonfunctional, but not always. The residual stump of the remaining functional trumpet is then carefully neurulated with 8-0 nylon microsutures. The dural defect is closed primarily if there is adequate material to achieve a capacious sac for the neural placode, or a redundant graft is sewn in to achieve the same end, that is, a low cord-sac ratio. The whole assembly is then returned back into the spinal canal (Fig. 5).

Although the syringomyelia may be quite extensive in some cases, direct syringotomy is virtually never necessary since resecting the distal trumpet is equivalent to terminal drainage of the syrinx.

The timing of surgery is usually within the first 6 months of life or shortly upon radiographic diagnosis. However, one bitter lesson we have learned from our combined experience is that rapid distention of the subcutaneous bulk due to massive accumulation of CSF can cause precipitous and irreversible neurological worsening caused by internal stretching of the distal cavitated spinal cord. Emergency operation should be instituted at once on such a contingency [5, 17].

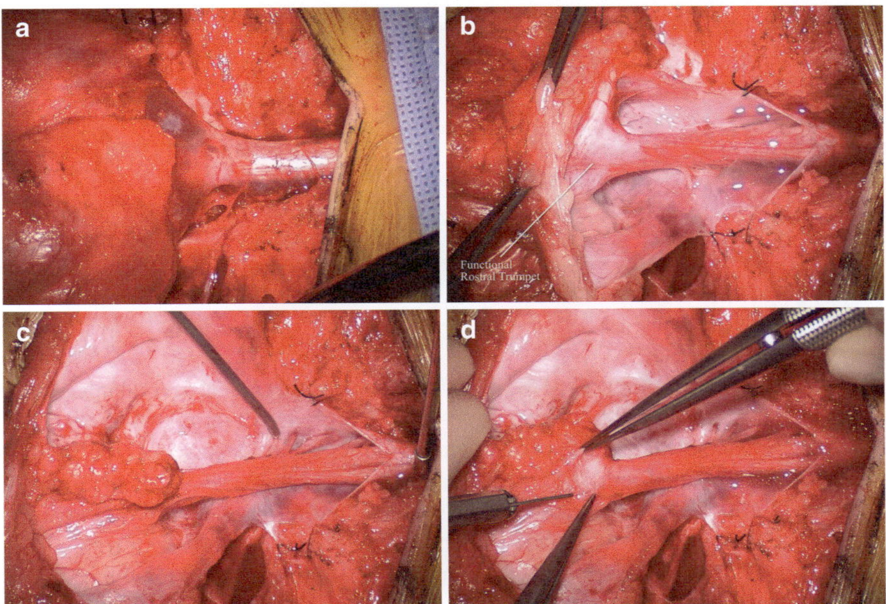

Fig. 5 The sequence of the operation for a typical TMC. (**a**) Exposure of the extradural space and the attachment of the subarachnoid space to the subcutaneous fat. (**b**) Intradural exposure of the extended spinal cord and the rostral trumpet of the myelocystocele. (**c**) Stimulation of the nerve roots to identify the last functional level. (**d**) Opening of the rostral trumpet as a vertically directed slit to expose the inner surface of the myelocystocele. (**e**) Stimulation of the inner surface of the trumpet to identify the junction between the functional and nonfunctional trumpet. (**f**) Visualization of the opening of the hydromyelic cavity after untethering by resecting the nonfunctional portion of the trumpet. (**g**) Neurulated stump of the rostral trumpet. (**h**) Duroplasty with bovine pericardial dural graft

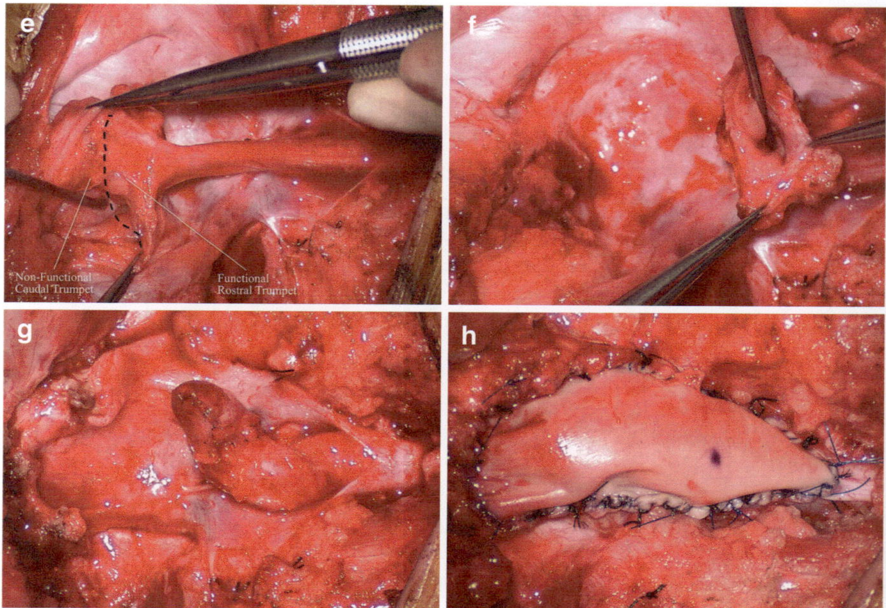

Fig. 5 (continued)

Histopathology

The histopathological features of the resected distal trumpet reveal several interesting features [5]. First, although the name implies the presence of an ependymal lining, most of the samples are devoid of ependyma. Second, instead of the typical neuroepithelial tissue found in a normal neural tube, the lining of a TMC commonly consists of glial tissue with dense fibrous stroma and thick-walled blood vessels. Only a small number of abnormal-looking neurons are scattered within this glial core without any organizational pattern. Third, although both myelinated and unmyelinated nerves are found, they are arranged in a haphazard fashion without any resemblance to the classic nerve root entry and exit zones in a functional spinal cord. These abnormal features support the electrophysiological conclusion that most of the extraspinal protruded neural tissue is nonfunctional.

Associated Anomaly

Patients with TMC may have various forms of sacral anomaly such as sacral agenesis, supernumerary sacrum, and sacrum with abnormal curvature or morphology [5, 18, 19]. The association with hydrocephalus or Chiari malformation is rare. Reports with severe cloacal anomalies can also be found, but in general, the tendency for co-occurrence of other congenital anomalies does not seem significantly high compared to other spinal dysraphic malformations.

Conclusion

TMC is a rare but important entity of spinal dysraphism as it is a good example of how a thorough knowledge in embryology can demystify a seemingly unknowable conundrum of a complex malformation, and at the same time provide insight into its clinical management. Complete resection of the extraspinally extended, nonfunctional, and distended retained medullary cord should be done. With meticulous electrophysiological monitoring, maximal removal of the redundant malformed neural tissue can be performed to reduce the chance of retethering.

References

1. Byrd SE, Harvey C, Darling CF. MR of terminal myelocystoceles. Eur J Radiol. 1995;20(3):215–20.
2. Gupta DK, Mahapatra AK. Terminal myelocystoceles: a series of 17 cases. J Neurosurg. 2005;103(4 Suppl):344–52.
3. Sim KB, Wang KC, Cho BK. Terminal myelocystocele—a case report. J Korean Med Sci. 1996;11(2):197–202.
4. James HE, Lubinsky G. Terminal myelocystocele. J Neurosurg. 2005;103(5 Suppl):443–5.
5. Pang D, Zovickian J, Lee JY, Moes GS, Wang KC. Terminal myelocystocele: surgical observations and theory of embryogenesis. Neurosurgery. 2012;70(6):1383–404; discussion 404–5.
6. Hobbes T. Leviathan, or, The matter, forme, & power of a common-wealth ecclesiasticall and civill:/by Thomas Hobbes. London: Printed for Andrew Ckooke [sic] ... 1651.
7. McLone DG, Naidich TP. Terminal myelocystocele. Neurosurgery. 1985;16(1):36–43.
8. Costanzo R, Watterson RL, Schoenwolf GC. Evidence that secondary neurulation occurs autonomously in the chick embryo. J Exp Zool. 1982;219(2):233–40.
9. Saitsu H, Yamada S, Uwabe C, Ishibashi M, Shiota K. Development of the posterior neural tube in human embryos. Anat Embryol (Berl). 2004;209(2):107–17.
10. Griffith CM, Wiley MJ, Sanders EJ. The vertebrate tail bud: three germ layers from one tissue. Anat Embryol (Berl). 1992;185(2):101–13.
11. Schoenwolf GC, Delongo J. Ultrastructure of secondary neurulation in the chick embryo. Am J Anat. 1980;158(1):43–63.
12. Yang HJ, Wang KC, Chi JG, Lee MS, Lee YJ, Kim SK, et al. Neural differentiation of caudal cell mass (secondary neurulation) in chick embryos: hamburger and Hamilton stages 16-45. Brain Res Dev Brain Res. 2003;142(1):31–6.
13. Lee JY, Kim SP, Kim SW, Park SH, Choi JW, Phi JH, et al. Pathoembryogenesis of terminal myelocystocele: terminal balloon in secondary neurulation of the chick embryo. Childs Nerv Syst. 2013;29(9):1683–8.
14. Chung YN, Lee DH, Yang HJ, Kim SK, Lee YJ, Lee MS, et al. Expression of neuronal markers in the secondary neurulation of chick embryos. Childs Nerv Syst. 2008;24(1):105–10.

15. Miller SA, Briglin A. Apoptosis removes chick embryo tail gut and remnant of the primitive streak. Dev Dyn. 1996;206(2):212–8.
16. Mills CL, Bellairs R. Mitosis and cell death in the tail of the chick embryo. Anat Embryol (Berl). 1989;180(3):301–8.
17. Lee JY, Phi JH, Kim SK, Cho BK, Wang KC. Urgent surgery is needed when cyst enlarges in terminal myelocystoceles. Childs Nerv Syst. 2011;27(12):2149–53.
18. Pang D. Sacral agenesis and caudal spinal cord malformations. Neurosurgery. 1993;32(5):755–78; discussion 78–9.
19. Kuo MF, Tsai Y, Hsu WM, Chen RS, Tu YK, Wang HS. Tethered spinal cord and VACTERL association. J Neurosurg. 2007;106(3 Suppl):201–4.

Updates on Intraoperative Neurophysiology During Surgery for Spinal Dysraphism

Claudia Pasquali, Federica Basaldella, and Francesco Sala

Introduction

Tethered cord syndrome (TCS) is the term first coined in 1976 by Hoffman and colleagues, which indicates a functional disorder characterized by motor and sensory changes in the legs, sphincter incontinence, low back pain, and skeletal deformities, usually caused by an embryologic failure of spinal cord development. This ultimately results in a radiculo-medullary mechanical stretch which generates vascular changes and consequently ischemic damage to the nervous structures of the conus-cauda region [1–6].

Clinical presentation is heterogenous, and is related to the patient's age. Moreover, it is difficult to predict which patients will remain asymptomatic for their entire lives, or those who will clinically deteriorate. For this reason, the treatment of patients with asymptomatic tethered cord remains controversial [7]. On the other hand, the finding of symptomatic lumbosacral lipomas (LSLs) in adult patients suggests that the risk of neurologic deterioration exists at any age and it increases with time [8, 9]. For this reason, prophylactic surgery has been offered in asymptomatic patients, but this should warrant high treatment standards in order to avoid iatrogenic neurological deficits. In this regard, the use of intraoperative neurophysiology (ION) contributes to the safety of tethered cord surgery [7, 10]. ION has established itself as a discipline aimed to not merely predict but possibly prevent or minimize neurological deficits by providing the surgeon with immediate feedback on the functional status of neural structures during the manipulation of the spinal cord and nerve roots (via monitoring techniques), as well as by identifying

C. Pasquali · F. Basaldella · F. Sala (✉)
Section of Neurosurgery, Department of Neurosciences, Biomedicine and Movement Sciences, University Hospital, Verona, Italy
e-mail: francesco.sala@univr.it

© The Author(s), under exclusive license to Springer Nature Switzerland AG 2023
D. Pang, K.-C. Wang (eds.), *Spinal Dysraphic Malformations*, Advances and Technical Standards in Neurosurgery 47,
https://doi.org/10.1007/978-3-031-34981-2_9

ambiguous anatomical structures (via mapping techniques). Some studies suggest that the use of ION will ultimately reduce the risk of inadvertent nervous injuries, and improve long-term outcomes [11, 12] both in children and adults [13, 14], although providing strong evidence for the benefit of ION remains problematic.

Tethered Cord Aetiopathogenesis and Classification

Spinal dysraphism develops early during pregnancy. The development of the neural system begins during the second and the third week of gestational age with the formation of the mesoderm between the endoderm and ectoderm (gastrulation). The primary neural tube originates from the ectoderm, together with the skin, eye and inner ear. From mesodermal mesenchymal cells arises the notochord, which stimulates the thickening of overlying ectoderm and the growth of the neural plate [15]. The primary neural plate folds up, and separates itself from the adjoining cutaneous ectoderm, becoming the primary neural tube. Its extremities, called neuropores, close at day 25 (the cranial one) and at day 28 (the caudal one), determining the ends of primary neurulation and the beginning of secondary neurulation at the caudal end of the spinal cord [16, 17].

Following a process of mesenchyme-epithelium transformation, condensation and intra-chordal cavitation during secondary neurulation, the caudal conus and the non-neural terminal filum is formed [18]. Meninx and vertebral column grow faster than the neural tube; therefore the conus ascends progressively, reaching its final position between birth and the second month of postnatal life, on average between the lower third of the T12 and the middle third of the L2 vertebrae [18–22]. Spinal dysraphism originates from abnormalities occurring during either primary or secondary neurulation, and are divided into "open" defects characterized by the neural placode being open to the outside, and "occult" defect, when the neural placode is covered under the skin. In the latter, the overlying skin often displays typical cutaneous anomalies such as hypertrichosis, sacral dimple, subcutaneous lipomas, haemangiomas, port-wine stain, Mongolian spot, and deviation of the gluteal fold, which suggests an underlying defect [23, 24].

Spinal dysraphism can be classified both according to clinical and radiological aspects, and to the timing of the neurulation defect (Table 1) [25–29].

Tethered cord syndrome has an incidence of 0.004–0.008% in the general population, which increases up to 0.1% when we consider only primary school children [30, 31]. Lumbosacral lipomas (LSLs) represent 70% of the lesions associated with tethering [32, 33] and are the most challenging type of spina bifida occulta (SBO).

As originally suggested by Pierre-Kahn, we should distinguish lipomas into conus lipomas and filum lipomas [34, 35]. A lipomatous or thickened filum often becomes stretched and inelastic, therefore affecting the mobility of the conus. Filum lipomas rarely involve nerve roots, which are usually free and with a normal course. In addition, they are rarely associated with increased subcutaneous fat [34].

Table 1 Classification of spinal dysraphism

Clinical and radiological classification	Embryological classification

Open spinal dysraphisms
– Myelomeningocele
– Myelocele
– Hemimyelomeningocele
– Hemimyelocele
Closed spinal dysraphisms:
  With subcutaneous mass
  – Lipomas with dural defect
  – Lipomyelomeningocele
  – Lipomyelocele
  – Terminal myelocystocele
  – Meningocele
  – Nonterminal myelocystocele
  Without subcutaneous mass
  – Dorsal enteric fistula
  – Neurenteric cysts
  – Diastematomyelia
  – Dermal sinus
  – Intradural lipoma
  – Filar lipoma
  – Tight filum terminale
  – Abnormally elongated spinal cord
  – Persistent terminal ventricle
  – Caudal agenesis (caudal regression syndrome)
  – Segmental spinal dysgenesis
	Anomalies of gastrulation:
	– Disorders of midline notochordal integration
	– Dorsal enteric fistula
	– Neurenteric cysts
	– Diastematomyelia
	– Dermal sinus
	– Disorders of notochordal formation
	– Caudal agenesis (caudal regression syndrome)
	– Segmental spinal dysgenesis
	Anomalies of primary neurulation:
	– Myelomeningocele
	– Myelocele
	– Lipomas with dural defect
	– Lipomyelomeningocele
	– Lipomyelocele
	– Intradural lipoma
	– Nonterminal myelocystocele
	Anomalies of secondary neurulation:
	– Filar lipoma
	– Tight filum terminale
	– Abnormally elongated spinal cord
	– Persistent terminal ventricle
	– Terminal myelocystocele
	– Anomalies of unknown origin
	– Meningocele

Adapted from: Rossi A, Biancheri R, Cama A, Piatelli G, Ravegnani M, Tortori-Donati P. Imaging in spine and spinal cord malformations. Eur J Radiol. 2004;50(2):177–200, and Reghunath A, Ghasi RG, Aggarwal A. Unveiling the tale of the tail: an illustration of spinal dysraphisms. Neurosurg Rev. 2021;44(1):97–114

The classification of conus lipomas is much more complex. In agreement with Chapman [25] and Pang [26, 27], we could distinguish four entities according to the interaction of the lipoma with the spinal cord: dorsal, caudal (terminal), transitional and chaotic lipomas.

Dorsal lipomas adhere to the dorsal surface of the lumbar spinal cord, separate from the conus. The lipoma could extend in subcutaneous tissue through a dorsal dural defect.

Caudal lipomas adhere to the distal part of the conus medullaris and to the cauda equina. They do not involve sacral roots nor the dural sac, but they usually involve the filum, which appears thickened.

Transitional lipomas represent a combination of the caudal and the dorsal types. Asymmetry is often present. The lesion involves nerve roots, which in some cases become indistinguishable from fibrous bands.

Finally, chaotic lipomas, like other variants, have a dorsal origin but they extend ventrally and engulf neural tissue and nerve roots. These represent the most challenging conus lipomas, surgically wise, due to a complex engulfment of both dorsal roots, ventral roots and the conus itself.

Lipomyelomeningocele is another variant described in the literature. It is a complex form of transitional lipomas, characterized by an extraspinal extension of the lesion, combined with a cystic subcutaneous component [27, 36].

In 1981, Yamada demonstrated that the presence of any abnormality tethering the caudal spinal cord causes chronic hypoxic-ischemic damage to the lumbosacral cord. This presents clinically as the so-called TCS, described by Hoffman. Yamada demonstrated further that untethering the cord could improve mitochondrial oxidative metabolism, reducing the hypoxic stress [3, 37].

The timing of the onset of clinical symptoms is dependent on the degree of stretch on the conus medullaris and cauda equina, and it is not predictable. In the paediatric age group, symptoms may occur as early as the first months of life, although in most cases there is a progressive appearance of neurological deficits over the years. An important observation, though, is the fact that adult patients with a tethered cord are rarely asymptomatic, and the risk of neurologic deterioration increases over time [7, 8].

Functional Neuroanatomy of the Conus-Cauda Region

In normal anatomy, the lower end of the spinal cord, the conus medullaris, is located at the L1-L2 vertebral level. This consists of the S2 to S5 segments. Together with the upper lumbar segments, the motor-sensory neurons in the caudal end of the spinal cord contribute to the origin of the lumbosacral plexus (D12-L5) for the lower extremities, and to the external urethral and anal sphincters .

The majority of muscles of the anterior hip and thigh, in particular the iliacus, sartorius, and the four quadriceps femoris, are innervated by the femoral and sciatic nerves. The femoral nerve originates from the lumbar plexus (L2-L4) and its branches, the saphenous and femoral-cutaneous nerves, innervate the skin of the front and medial sides of the leg. The sciatic nerve innervates the skin of the posterior and lateral surfaces of the thigh, the posterior surface of the leg, as well as the skin of the perineum. It originates from the sacral plexus (L4-S3) and innervates the posterior thigh muscles, and the muscles of the leg and foot. Its most important branches are the common fibular nerve for the innervation of the tibialis anterior and the extensor hallucis longus muscles, and the tibial nerve for the innervation of the posterior muscular compartment of the leg: gastrocnemius, popliteus, soleus, plantaris, tibialis posterior, flexor digitorum longus, and flexor hallucis longus. Articular branches of the tibial and deep fibular nerves innervate the ankle region.

The obturator nerve (L2-L4) innervates the adductor muscles as well as the skin on the medial aspect of the thigh. The gluteal nerves (L1-S3) innervate the three gluteus muscles and the skin of the gluteal region.

The conus medullaris also supplies fibres for the lumbar sympathetic, sacral somatic, and sacral parasympathetic nerves.

The course of the somatic and autonomic nervous systems is separate in the pelvic cavity, while, with the exception of the sympathetic fibers, they run together at the level of the cauda equina and conus level, except for the sympathetic fibres. This explains why monitoring of the external anal sphincter, innervated by the pudendal nerve, a somatic nerve, gives information to the status of the activity of the autonomic nervous system, which controls detrusor activity through a reflex pathway.

The functional anatomy of the genitourinary and anogenital systems is quite complex. The pudendal nerves carry somatic afferent fibres from the mucosa and skin of the genitoperineal region. Sensory fibres are from the dorsal nerves of the penis (or clitoris) which run to the spinal cord through the dorsal spinal roots of S2-S5. The afferent information then ascends via the spinothalamic tracts of the dorsal column, and then to the thalamo-cortical tracts to the somatosensory cortex.

The motor cortex controls the sphincteric lower motor neurons located in the midventral spinal grey matter of the S2 to S4 spinal cord segments (the "Onuf's nucleus") from which the somatic motor roots arise for the innervation of the levator ani muscle and the external anal sphincter.

The innervation of the lower urinary tract is represented by three sets of peripheral nerves: the pelvic parasympathetic nerves, the sympathetic nerves, as well as the somatic efferent and afferent nerves from the S2-S4 sacral roots. Anatomically, the urethral sphincter consists of the internal and the external sphincters. The internal urethral sphincter is under involuntary control and is innervated by the autonomic nervous system; the external urethral sphincter is under voluntary control and receives innervation from the somatic pudendal nerve from the S2 to S4 nerve roots.

The pelvic parasympathetic nerves originate at the sacral level of the spinal cord: their function is to excite the bladder and relax the urethra. The sympathetic nerves originate from the upper lumbar segments: their function is to inhibit the bladder musculature, modulate transmission in bladder parasympathetic ganglia, and excite the bladder base and urethra. The somatic fibres from the S2-S4 sacral roots supply the innervation of the pelvic floor muscles both through direct branches and the pudendal nerve. The latter also innervates the external anal and urethral sphincters and through its inferior hemorrhoidal branches also carry afferent signal from the anal canal.

Pelvic visceral nerves transport sensory fibres from the rectum and the bladder to the sacral cord.

Functionally, the internal anal sphincter is responsible for about 85% of the resting pressure in the lumen of the canal. It receives motor innervation from the sacral parasympathetic fibres originating from the mediolateral columns of the sacral cord segments S2-S4 and likely provides autonomic control of its function.

The external anal sphincter is innervated mainly by the pudendal nerve and in a minor part by a perineal branch of S4.

From the above summary, it clearly depicts the complex involvement of sphincter innervation and control. This complexity accounts for the lack of ION techniques capable of reliably assessing all these neural pathways. Yet, some techniques are available to lessen the risk of urinary incontinence or retention as well as the loss of sensation to the pudendal region.

Why and When to Operate

The general aim of tethered cord surgery is to eliminate the mechanical traction and release the filum and the conus in order to avoid or arrest the progression of symptoms, and, to a lesser degree, to revert the existing neurological deficits. After surgery, low back pain improves between 86% and 95% of cases [27, 38–41], motor impairments improve up to 71% of cases [38, 40–43]. Sensory deficits rarely improve but they tend to stabilize [41].

Bladder and bowel dysfunctions are the most socially disabling conditions, their prevalence is found in more than 70% in adult patients, while it ranges from 22% to 60% in children [44]. These conditions tend to be refractory to surgery and improve in only 16–60% of the cases; this is one reason not to delay untethering once the diagnosis of TCS is made [39, 41, 45–49].

Adult patients are rarely asymptomatic at the time of surgical treatment, whilst in children with asymptomatic dysraphic malformations, the timing of surgery is still a matter of debate [7, 10].

The Necker group in Paris has advocated a conservative management for lumbosacral lipomas, based on a close clinical-radiological-urological follow-up. This is based on their study in which the authors compared the incidence of neurological decay in patients treated with prophylactic surgery to those who have not been treated: after a nine-year follow-up, they observed that 33% of conservatively treated patients and 46% of surgical treated patients presented neurological symptoms. Whilst this difference was not statistically significant, they suggested that surgical treatment was not better than the natural history [9]. An important aspect of this study, however, was that the surgical technique used by this group was partial resection of the lipomas, and that no neuromonitoring was used.

Further studies have demonstrated that not all asymptomatic paediatric patients will develop symptoms throughout their lives [27, 50]. In some cases, symptoms will appear only during adulthood, with a more favourable progress but it is almost exceptional to find a truly asymptomatic adult patient, and this argument is relevant when considering prophylactic surgery.

Later on, Pang published a considerably large series of patients with spinal cord lipomas presenting the long-term outcome following total and near-total resection together with a reconstruction of the neural placode. This seminal paper pointed out that total resection of lipomas achieves better long-term outcome than partial resection and, following total resection, asymptomatic patients do better than symptomatic patients. It also highlighted that the non-surgical French series compared their outcome results between non-surgical and partial resection groups, not total resection. Therefore, in a asymptomatic child, if one advocates for surgery it should aim for a total or near-total resection; otherwise conservative management is preferable [50].

Although rarely emphasised in the never-ending debate on the surgical indication for asymptomatic children with conus lipomas, ION was not used in the French study, whereas Pang systematically used, and strongly advocated, ION to achieve total resection of the lipomas.

Untethering techniques are variable and mainly depend on the underlying type of dysraphism: they go from simple cutting of the filum terminale, to more complex resections of lipomas, which often firmly adhere to and encase neural structures. Depending on the type of dysraphism, various degrees of manipulation of the neural roots and conus are required, and this ultimately increases the risk of neural injury due to traction, coagulation or inadvertent section of functional rootlets [13, 24, 30, 34, 37].

The incidence of transient complications following tethered cord surgery has been reported between 10.9% and 13%, but it drops to 0–4.5% when only permanent neurological injuries are considered [26, 43, 50–52]. Yet, these rates of complications are significant, especially for asymptomatic patients, as both sensorimotor deficits and sphincterial disturbances may negatively and permanently impact on the quality of life.

Anaesthesia

Anaesthetic agents interfere with synaptic function and alter the conduction of signals during ION. Therefore, the correct choice of the anaesthesiologic regimen and a thorough communication between the anaesthesiologists and the neuromonitoring team is critical for the success of ION.

Halogenated gases such as isoflurane, sevoflurane and, recently, desflurane are not recommended as they negatively affect the reproducibility of neuromonitoring, in particular with SEP and MEP monitoring. Halogenated gases, compared to total intravenous anaesthesia (TIVA), cause a significantly greater reduction of the amplitude of SEPs and at times can completely suppress the amplitude of the evoked potential, and, to a lesser degree, delay the latency [53].

Short to intermediate-acting myorelaxant is used only for intubation, and then, in adults, the maintenance of anaesthesia is reached with a constant infusion of propofol (100–150 µg kg min^{-1}) and opioid (e.g. fentanyl 1 µg kg h^{-1}). In patients with opioid tolerance, some anaesthesiologists supplement TIVA with low dose of halogenated gases suggesting that the depression of the responses associated with low dose of halogenated agents (e.g. 3% desflurane) is offset by the effect of the lower propofol dosage [54].

In the paediatric population, especially within the first 2 years of life, the prolonged infusion or high dosage of propofol is linked to PRIS (Propofol infusion syndrome), characterized by reversible lactic acidosis associated with acute refractory bradycardia, potentially leading to asystole. For this reason, within the paediatric population the use of TIVA is controversial and the use of halogenated agents is preferred in this age group [55].

On the other hand, it should be noted that halogenated gases do not affect mapping techniques, which represent the real pillar of ION in tethered cord surgery:

in particular, direct motor mapping of the cauda equina is less affected by anaesthetics as it does not involve polysynaptic pathways.

ION Techniques During Tethered Cord Surgery

The ION techniques utilized in tethered cord surgery includes a combination of monitoring and mapping techniques. Mapping techniques aim at functionally identifying ambiguous anatomical structures, for example, in differentiating whether or not a rootlet-looking structure is truly functional or is a nonfunctional fibrous band or vestigial root. Similarly, mapping is essential to determine the functional level between the true conus medullaris and a retained medullary cord [18, 56]. Mapping techniques therefore provide specific information at a given point in time during surgery, but do not assess the functional integrity of a neural pathway. This is achieved through monitoring techniques such as Somatosensory Evoked Potentials (SSEPs), free-running EMG, motor evoked potentials (MEPs) and the bulbocavernosus reflex (BCR).

Historically, Somatosensory Evoked Potential (SEPs) and Free-Running EMG were the first techniques introduced to monitor the functional integrity of the neural structures [12]. This was further implemented, at the end of the 1990 s, by the introduction of MEPs and BCR [57–60].

In general, the major role in tethered cord surgery is played by mapping techniques in which nonfunctional vestigial roots or fibrous bands could be cut to achieve cord untethering. Monitoring techniques are certainly valuable, especially with regard to mMEPs and the BCR, while SSEPs might be more difficult to monitor, especially in very young children, and are generally less relevant in guiding the surgical strategy [57, 58, 61–63].

The sensitivity of SSEPs ranges between 28.6 and 50% and specificity between 94.7 and 100% [11, 64, 65]. MEPs have been reported to have a sensitivity range between 75% and 100%, with a specificity from 25% to 100%. Muscle MEPs are characterized by a positive predictive value (PPV) ranging from 63% to 100%, and a negative predictive value (NPV) ranging from 75% to 97% [11, 12, 57, 64]. Free-running EMG sensitivity is reported as high as 87.5% and specificity as high as 83.3%, with a PPV of 87.5% and NPV of 83.3%, respectively [64].

A summary of mapping and monitoring techniques in the lumbosacral region is presented in Fig. 1.

The variety in the rates of specificity and sensitivity rates reported for the different ION techniques likely reflects not only the different patient population in these studies but also different warning criteria and different experiences within the neuromonitoring team. In general, the lower the experience, the higher the chance of falsely positive alarms. So, it is important to rule out technical and anaesthesiological caveats before providing feedback to the surgeon.

Tethered cord surgery is mainly performed in the paediatric population. As such, the developing nervous system may still be immature from a neurophysiological

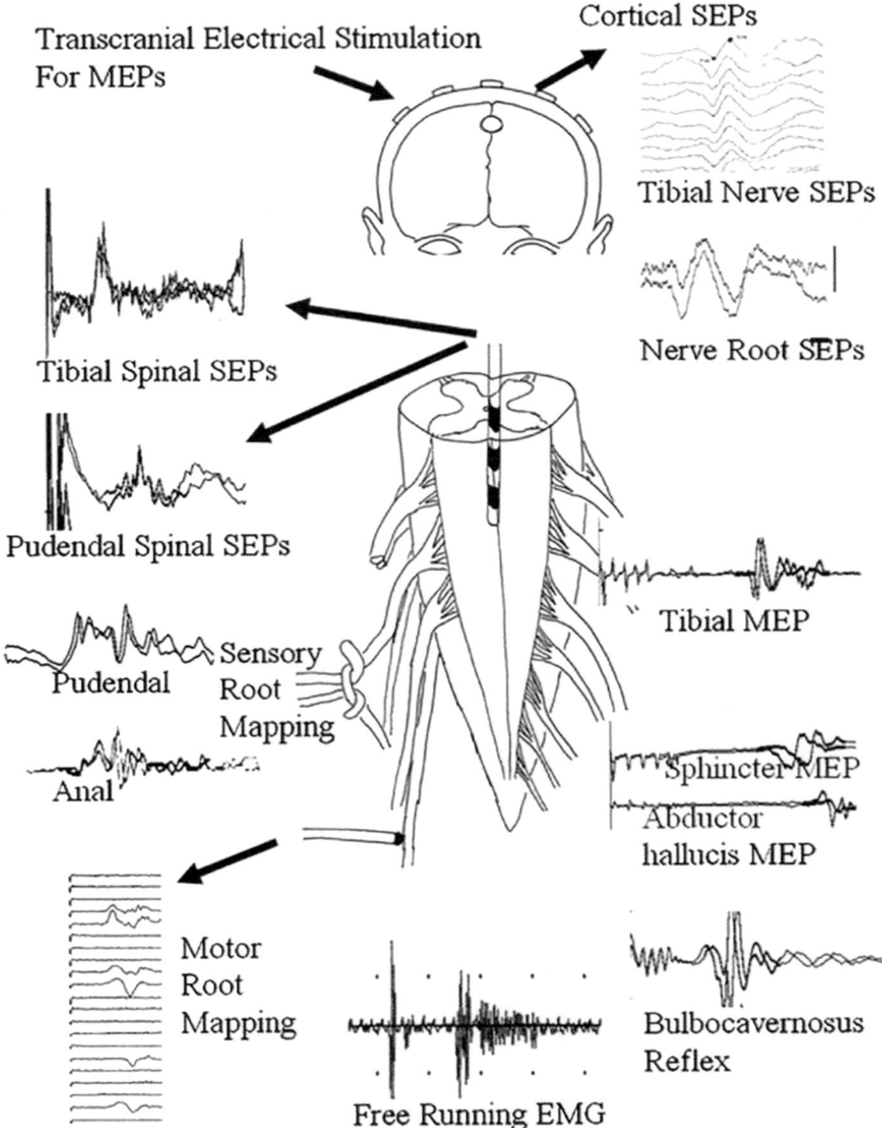

Fig. 1 Schematic illustration of neurophysiological techniques for conus and cauda equina monitoring and mapping. From Kothbauer KF, Deletis V. Intraoperative neurophysiology of the conus medullaris and cauda equina. Child's Nerv Syst 2010;26(2):247–53. https://doi.org/10.1007/s00381-009-1020-6

standpoint and this can affect ION techniques, especially in children below the age of 4–5 years. Therefore, tailoring ION techniques to the child's age is critical [51, 56, 66, 67].

It is known that the myelination of corticospinal motor pathways completes around the age of 11–13 years, and therefore ION in young children (especially below age 6) is more challenging. The low monitorability of transcranial MEPs in younger children can be overcome by techniques aimed to improve temporal and spatial facilitation [57, 68]. Some protocols consider the reduction or elimination of propofol with the addition of ketamine. This approach seems to increase the success in acquiring responses from 78% to 96% in children over the age of 6 and up to 86% in children under the age of 6 [55, 69–73]. Another factor that, to some extent, likely counterbalances the higher threshold for cortical activation of the corticospinal tract in younger children is the fact that their skull is much thinner and therefore the impedance for transcranial electrical stimulation (TES) is lower. Yet, in the first years of life, eliciting transcranial muscle MEPs may require higher stimulation intensities than in older children.

Monitoring Techniques

Somatosensory Evoked Potentials

Somatosensory Evoked Potentials (SSEPs) allow a continuous monitoring of the dorsal column pathways, recording the nervous response from the scalp (Cz′–Fz) or directly from the spinal cord with an epidural electrode, following stimulation of peripheral nerves.

SSEPs are elicited by stimulation of the posterior tibial nerve at the knee or at the ankle with an intensity of 20–40 mA, a pulse duration of 0.20–0.25 ms and a frequency of 4.3–4.7 Hz. Such stimulation also allows monitoring of the L5-S1 sensory roots.

Baseline responses are recorded after patient positioning and before skin incision. A reduction in amplitude of the cortical P40/N50 waves of more than 50% and/or a 10% prolongation in latency is considered significant for an increased risk of injuries to the posterior roots or to the dorsal column pathway.

A drawback of SSEP monitoring during tethered cord surgery is the inability of SSEPs to monitor for any single root because the overlap by an adjacent root could mask a single root injury [37, 58, 74].

Also, unlike MEPs, SSEPs require signal averaging to eliminate the background electrical noise. Since 1–200 signals are averaged, this requires time and results in delayed feedback to the surgeon, as compared to the immediate response achievable with both MEPs and the BCR.

Occasionally in babies, both the wrist and the ankle can be very puffy and the stimulation of the peripheral nerve at these sites is not efficacious. In the presence of poor baseline SSEPs, it is always advisable to check that actual stimulation is being delivered and ensure that a real twitch of the wrist or the ankle is visible.

In our experience, although routinely used, SSEPs are of less value than other monitoring techniques in tethered cord surgery. There is also the difficulty in recording robust and consistent responses in young children. Overall, it is very uncommon to modify the surgical strategy only on the basis of SSEPs changes.

Motor Evoked Potentials

Functional integrity of the upper and lower motoneurons is monitored by activating the motor cortex by TES, using a short train of stimuli and recording MEPs from needle electrodes placed into the limb muscles.

The preferred scalp electrodes utilized during this procedure are corkscrew-like: they have low impedances and little risk of being displaced during patient positioning, compared to cup or needle electrodes.

In newborn babies and children, with an open fontanel or in those harbouring ventriculoperitoneal shunts, attention should be taken to avoid injuring the shunt system with corkscrew or needle electrodes; alternatively, cup electrodes could be used.

Stimulation electrodes are placed at C1 and C2 scalp sites (according to the International 10–20 EEG system (Fig. 2)) and, through them, short trains of 5–7 square-wave stimuli of 0.5-ms duration with an inter-stimulus interval of about 4 ms are applied at a repetition rate of 1–2 Hz. Intensity usually does not exceed 200 mA. In neurologically intact children, lower limb mMEPs are occasionally recordable with stimulation intensities as low as 60–70 mA.

In very young children, the presence of immature myelinated corticospinal fibres could desynchronize the movement of action potentials on their way to the lower motor neurons, and this often ends in failure to elicit muscle MEPs. Technical adjustments such as the double-train stimulation technique utilises the relative hyperpolarization of motoneurons to achieve stable MEP responses with higher amplitudes [75, 76].

Prior to surgery, the neurophysiologist registers the baseline MEPs at threshold (namely, the lowest stimulation intensity required to elicit an MEP response).

A C1/C2 montage elicits MEPs on the muscles of the right side, whereas C2/C1 permits recordings from muscles on the left side. By switching the polarity of stimulation from left to right, MEPs are selectively generated. Often, in order to monitor lower extremities muscles, a Cz′ (placed 1 cm behind the typical Cz point)-C6 cm montage is preferred, as this montage has the advantage of inducing less muscle twitching when compared to the C1/C2 and even more so the C3/C4 ones [37, 51, 61, 77, 78].

To assess the integrity of the efferent motor pudendal nerves and of parapyramidal motor fibres (for volitional control of the anal sphincters), a pair of wire or needle electrodes are inserted bilaterally in the external anal sphincter. When needle electrodes are used, it is important to place them just a few millimetres beneath the skin since this muscle is very thin (Fig. 3).

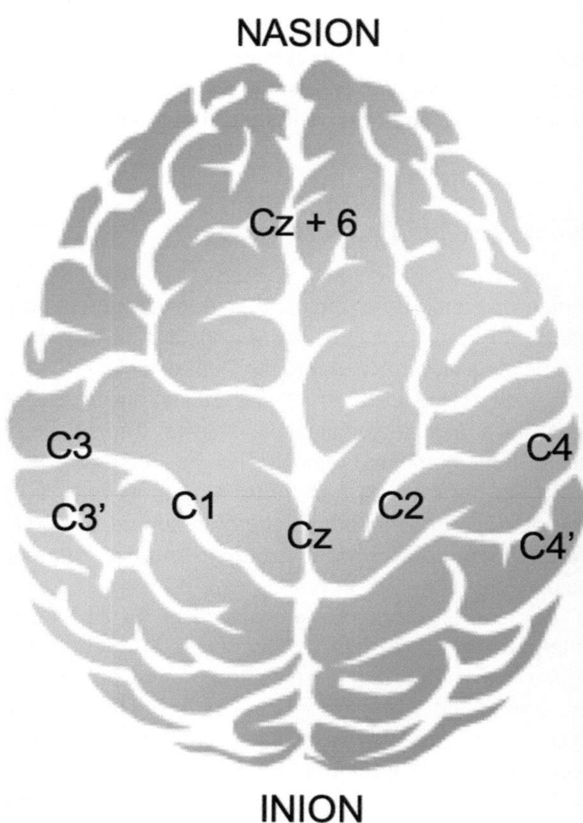

Fig. 2 Schematic illustration of corkscrew electrode position for recording SSEP and eliciting transcranial MEPs

Additional recording needle electrodes are then inserted bilaterally in the rectus abdominis, quadriceps, gastrocnemius, tibialis anterior and abductor hallucis to ensure the other spinal cord levels are also monitored (Table 2, Fig. 4).

During tethered cord surgery, mMEPs and SSEPs from one of the upper extremities is advisable as a control modality to verify anaesthetic interferences and rule out non-surgically related problems.

While it is generally accepted that the presence of mMEPs correlates with preserved motor control in all instances, it should be remembered that muscle innervation is provided by different roots which all contribute to the amplitude of the MEP. Therefore, a single root injury, which could occur during tethered cord surgery, might not be well reflected by MEP monitoring and, although rare, discrepancies between intraoperative MEPs data and postoperative motor outcome are possible.

In addition, transcranial-MEP amplitude is usually smaller than the amplitude of the compound muscle action potentials (CMAPs) evoked by maximal peripheral nerve stimulation, suggesting that only a limited number of spinal motor neurons innervating the target muscle are activated by transcranial stimuli. For this reason, a

STIMULATION

TES for anal MEP monitoring

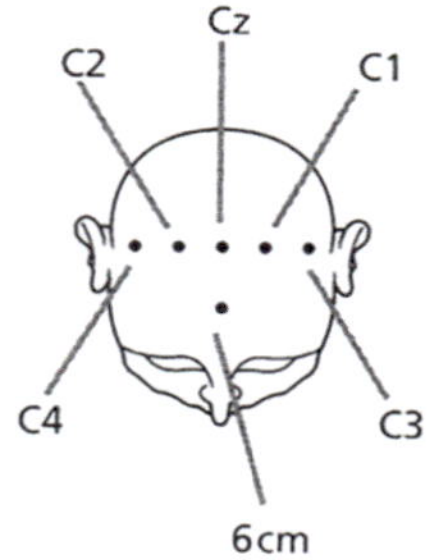

Mapping of pudendal motor roots for the anal sphincter

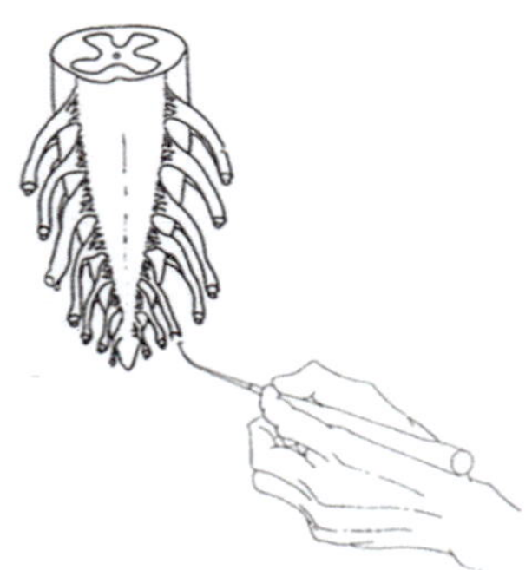

RECORDING

Anal MEP

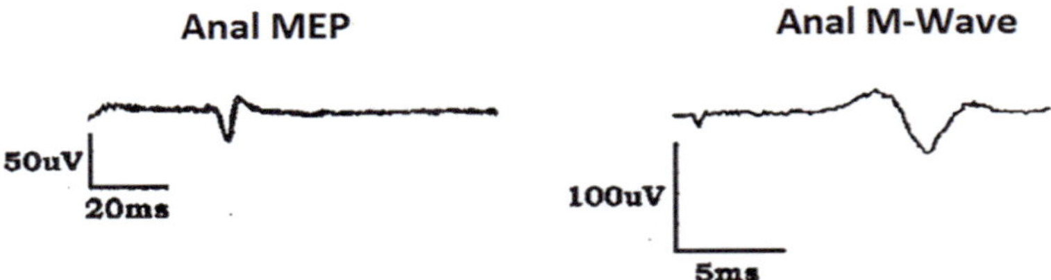

Anal M-Wave

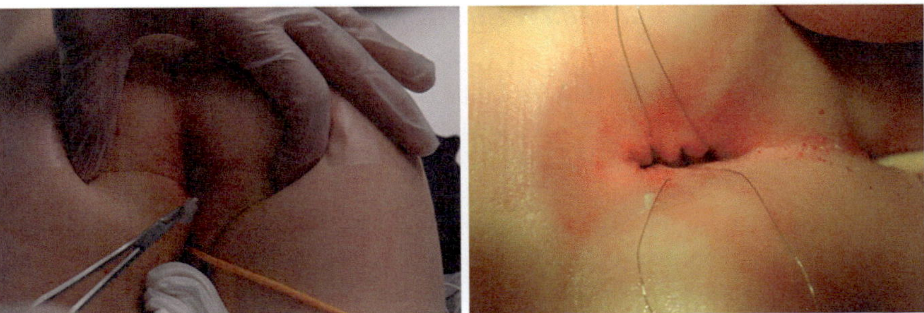

Fig. 3 Monitoring and mapping for the anal sphincter muscleUpper and middle left panels, transcranial electrical stimulation (TES) is delivered through scalp electrodes, and the anal MEP is recorded from pairs of wire electrodes inserted bilaterally in the anal sphincter (lower panels). Upper and middle right panels, direct stimulation of the pudendal nerve for the anal sphincter at the level of the cauda equina. An anal M-wave is recorded from the muscle. Note how the anal MEP has a longer latency and a lower amplitude, as compared to the anal M-Wave. Reprinted from reference [61] (Sala et al., 2013)

Table 2 Target recording muscles and their spinal cord level innervation

Spinal level	Muscle(s)
L1	Iliopsoas, rectus abdominis
L2	Iliopsoas, gracilis, pectineus, quadriceps femoris
L3	Iliopsoas, quadriceps femoris, adductors
L4	Iliopsoas, quadriceps femoris, tibialis anterior
L5	Tibialis anterior, extensor hallucis longus Gastrocnemius, gluteus maximus
S1	Gastrocnemius, biceps femoris, gluteus maximus
S2	Gluteus maximus, soleus, external anal sphincter
S3	Abductor hallucis, external anal sphincter
S4	External anal sphincter

reliable interpretation of the critical changes in TcMEPs remains controversial and as there lacks a well-defined neurophysiological criterion of reversible damage during surgery in the conus-cauda region, it is imperative to preserve MEPs throughout the procedure [79].

On the other hand, when a loss of a segmental lower motor neuron occurs, distal plasticity and the secondary increase in the size of motor units from neighbouring spinal cord segments could compensate for the affected segments, resulting in a long-term tendency to partial motor recovery [74].

A multitrain transcranial electrical stimulation (mtTES), in which a multipulse transcranial electrical stimulus is preceded by a preconditioning pulse train, has been described to achieve sufficient depolarization of motor neurons and enhance TcMEP responses during surgery [76, 80].

Free-Running (Spontaneous) Electromyography

Continuous monitoring of the lower limbs is permitted by the use of free-running electromyography (EMG) which continuously registers neuronal discharges from peripheral nerve roots from L1 to S4. The same recording needle electrodes are used for MEPs.

EMG recording of the external anal sphincter (EAS) is currently recommended during intraoperative neuromonitoring: it provides, by extrapolation, information also on the sacral motor pathways of the external urethral sphincter (EUS), as they have the same somatic innervation through the pudendal nerve and S2, S3, and S4 roots [81]. A time window of 100 millisecond/division (1 s/full screen) frequency filters set at 10 Hz for high-frequency pass filter, and at 2–5 kHz for low-frequency filter, are used [82].

There is no robust criteria for EMG interpretation in tethered cord surgery but different patterns of free-running EMG activity have been described and considered indicative of either reversible or irreversible neural injury. Sustained EMG activity

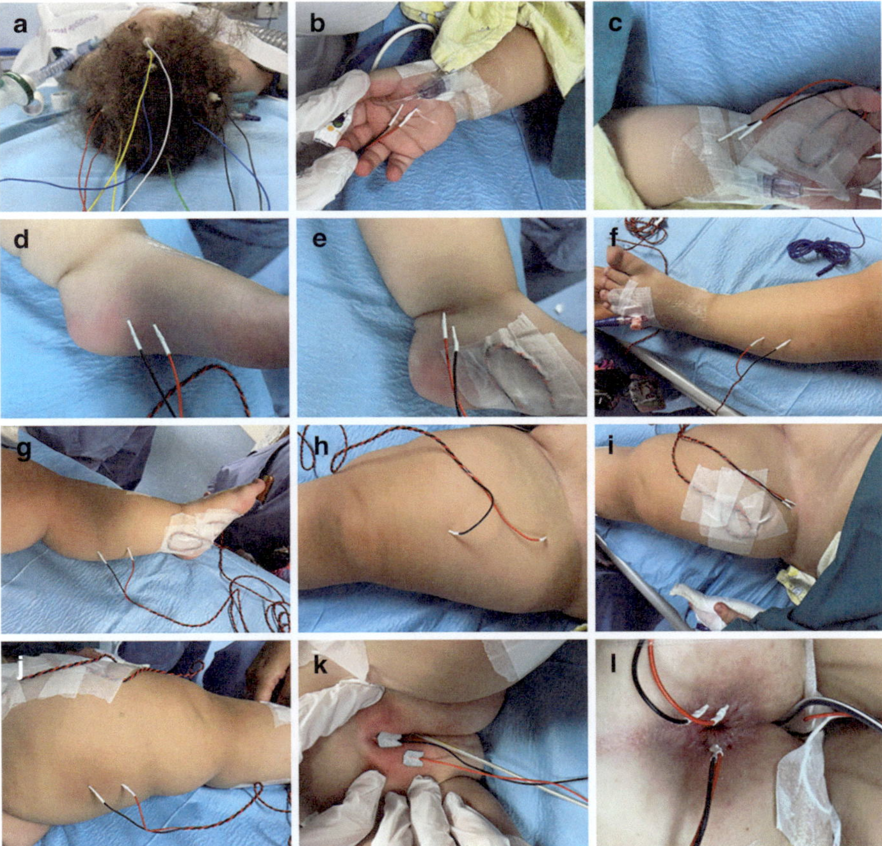

Fig. 4 Placement of needles for SSEPs, MEPs and BCR monitoring as well as for recordings of CMAPs following stimulation of motor roots in the cauda equina. (**a**) Transcranial electrodes positioning (see Fig. 3). (**b**) Needle electrodes inserted in the abductor pollicis brevis to record MEPs from one upper extremity as a control modality to exclude MEP changes due to non-surgical factors such as technical problems, anaesthesia, temperature, …. (**c**) Needle electrodes inserted at the wrist to evoke median nerve SSEPs. (**d**) Needle electrodes inserted in the abductor hallucis to record MEPs from S3 miotome. (**e**) Needle electrodes inserted at the ankle to evoke posterior tibial nerve SSEPs. (**f**) Needle electrodes inserted in the tibialis anterior to record MEPs from L4-L5 miotomes. (**g**) Needle electrodes inserted in the medial gastrocnemius to record MEPs from L5-S1 miotomes. (**h**) Needle electrodes inserted in the quadriceps femoris to record MEPs from L3-L4 miotomes. (**i**) Needle electrodes inserted in the Iliopsoas to record MEPs from L1-L4 miotomes. (**j**) Needle electrodes inserted in the adductor longus to record MEPs from L3 miotomes. (**k**) Surface electrodes applied to the clitoris (anode) and the great labia (cathode) to stimulate pudendal afferents for monitoring of the BCR. (**l**) Pairs of wire electrodes inserted bilaterally in the Anal Sphincter (S2-S4) to record the BCR as well as transcranial MEPs for the Anal Sphincter

may be indicative of mechanical irritation and typically precedes changes in evoked potentials, acting as a warning sign for potential injury [13, 37] with a sensitivity reported up to 100% in some studies, but also a lower specificity of 19% in other studies [83], which also illustrates the risk of false positive alarms. In general, free-running EMG may be difficult to interpret as spontaneous, sustained, activity could be induced not only by dangerous surgical manoeuvres but also merely by cold irrigation or by placing a cottonoid on the nerve. Nevertheless, free-run EMG continues to be of additional value when integrated with other monitoring modalities and high-frequency neuronal discharges, which persist after the surgical manipulation of the root has stopped. These should be seriously considered as a sign of impending injury to the nerve.

When continuous free-running EMG activity occurs, this may compromise the interpretation of mMEPs. Under these circumstances, we prefer to temporarily pause surgery and wait a few minutes until the spontaneous EMG activity has significantly reduced. Alternatively, recording in a cascade mode helps to differentiate random EMG activity from a time-locked, consistent CMAP or mMEP.

Bulbocavernous Reflex

One of the most socially disabling conditions in tethered cord syndrome is bladder incontinence or retention, due either to the progression of the pathology or the surgery. The use of ION reduces the risk of sphincter impairment during detethering procedures. The functional integrity of motor and sensory sacral nerve roots from S2-S4 spinal cord segments is evaluated via the bulbocavernous reflex (BCR).

This reflex pathway is made up of an afferent portion represented by sensory pudendal nerve fibres, and an efferent portion represented by motor fibres to the pelvic floor (bladder and urethral sphincters), levator ani (variable), and the external anal sphincter (via the inferior rectal nerve).

The reflex response of perineal muscles, including the external anal sphincter, after stimulation of the dorsal penile or clitoris nerves, demonstrates the integrity of this reflex arc located within the sacral segments of S2-S4. This reflex can be extremely sensitive and disappear due to manipulation of any of the three structures without a clear clinical correlation [57, 58, 61].

As the BCR is a polysynaptic reflex, it is susceptible to the influence of anaesthesia: muscle relaxants and halogenated agents should be avoided. An important advantage of this technique is that it can be recorded in newborns with the proviso that they have a higher latency than adults.

The intraoperative use of BCR was first described by Deletis and Vodusek in 1997 [59, 84]. Currently, the parameters for BCR monitoring are a train stimulation of 2–5 pulses of 500 ms duration, with 3 ms interpulse interval, and a stimulation current from 5 to 45 mA. To enhance the response, it is possible to use a double train stimulation with an intertrain interval from 150 to 200 ms. When a maximal stimulation (45 mA) is given with no response, BCR is considered unmonitorable

[58, 74]. When monitorable, it is monitored every 10–20 s during the intradural procedure and at 1- to 3-min intervals for the remainder of the surgery, tailoring the timing of monitoring to the surgical steps.

Skinner et al. (2007) proposed a double train strategy to improve the monitorability of the BCR and, though an optimal inter-train interval was not defined, this approach may facilitate BCR recordings when the standard stimulation parameters are unsuccessful.

Two surface electrodes, with an electrode impedance lower than 5 Ohm, are used to stimulate the dorsal penile/clitoral nerve. In males, the electrodes are placed on the dorsum of the penis; in females, the cathode is placed over the clitoris and the anode on the adjacent labium on one side. Recording on the external anal sphincter requires the placement of needles or hook wires in the external anal sphincter muscle [85]. The recordings may display two components: the first (R1) is an oligosynaptic pathway, more resistant to anaesthesia; the second (R2) is polysynaptic and therefore more vulnerable to anaesthesia.

Monitoring the BCR in babies is challenging, due to the difficulties in keeping the impedance of stimulating electrodes low. As reported by Sala et al. they found that they were able to monitor BCRs in children as young as 10 months old [61], but recently Shinjo et al. reported on the successful monitoring of the BCR in children as young as 4 days old. The latter group reported a remarkable success rate (close to 91%) in a group of children aged between 4 days to 10 years (mean 2.7 years) [86]. Of note is that they were able to maintain a total intravenous anaesthesia in 18 out of 22 children using propofol, which may have been the key to success, as halogenated gases or nitrous oxide preferentially used in infants invariably impair the monitorability of the BCR.

The inferior rectal nerve, a branch of the pudendal nerve, which receives contributions from sacral roots S2–S4, innervates the external anal sphincter. Iatrogenic injury of these roots represents a significant morbidity of TCS surgery leading to faecal incontinence. The perineal branch of the pudendal nerve supplies the external urethral sphincter, which is located at the proximal urethra and it is difficult to access for neurophysiological monitoring. Since, like the external anal sphincter, the external urethral sphincter is innervated by the pudendal nerve, some authors (Quinones-Hinojosa in 2004 and then Husain and Ashton in 2008) suggested that monitoring only the external anal sphincter is reliable to prevent pudendal nerve injuries [13, 67, 82]. Others (Gunnarsson and Krassioukov in 2004) maintained that, as different branches of the pudendal nerve supply the two sphincters, these can be damaged separately and therefore individually monitoring of each sphincter is safer [12].

Special ring electrodes on the Foley catheter are necessary for the monitoring of the external urethral sphincter. Parasympathetic fibres activate bladder detrusor contraction and the relaxation of the internal urethral sphincter, permitting bladder voiding. These parasympathetic fibres do not travel with the pudendal nerve, and a separate monitoring of the detrusor muscle can help in detecting damage at this level. Although not routinely used because of its complexity, the integrity of the detrusor muscle can be evaluated by changes in the urinary bladder pressure measured through a manometer connected to a Foley catheter. Before the surgery, the patient has to undergo a cystometrogram to assess bladder capacity. At the time of surgery, the bladder is filled to capacity through a Foley catheter. A manometer is then connected to the Foley catheter, where it measures changes in urinary bladder pressure due to detrusor muscle contraction. A sustained, high-frequency stimulus is required to produce this response [51, 84].

Consistent alarm criteria for altered intraoperative BCR still does not exist in the literature. If anaesthetic conditions are unchanged and perfusion is preserved, the amplitude and waveform complexity of BCR should remain stable. Alteration in waveform complexity, such as decreased duration, as well as amplitude drop, can anticipate signal disappearance or indicate an incomplete degree of conduction.

Morota recently showed that a cutoff value of BCR amplitude reduction of 75% has a PPV of 53.8% and a NPV of 98.5%, whilst a cutoff value of BCR amplitude reduction of 100% has a PPV of 100% and a NPV of 97.9% suggesting that a BCR amplitude reduction of 75% could be considered a safe warning criterion [85].

Loss of BCR recordings during the surgery may indicate low sacral segment damage, and postoperative urinary dysfunctions are highly probable. Nevertheless, frequently these deficits are transient and urinary retention (or, more rarely, incontinence) resolves over time. The interpretation of BCR monitoring remains challenging because micturition is controlled at various levels along the central and peripheral nervous system, so that the preservation of BCR is important but does not, per se, guarantee an intact sphincter control.

Mapping Techniques

Mapping techniques permit the direct identification of functional neural structures by direct electrical stimulation of the structure in the surgical field and recording from the innervated muscles. Often, during untethering procedures, the surgeon has to deal with structures which contribute to tethering of the cord, that have the macroscopic features of normal nerve roots, and/or other nervous structures.

To identify motor nerve roots and differentiate them from fibrous bands, a direct stimulation of nerve roots can be done, by recording the Compound Muscle Action Potential (CMAP) from segmental target muscles [51, 58] (Fig. 5). We prefer to use a bipolar concentric electrode for it has a better spatial resolution, as compared to the classical bipolar forceps, and a lower risk of current spreading when compared to monopolar stimulation.

The electrical stimulation should be slowly increased from 0.01 mA to a maximum stimulation of about 3 mA, with 1 Hz frequency and a stimulus duration of 200 us, until a CMAP response is elicited [61].

Different strategies and thresholds have been suggested by different authors, and there is no established threshold intensity ratio to distinguish functional from nonfunctional rootlets.

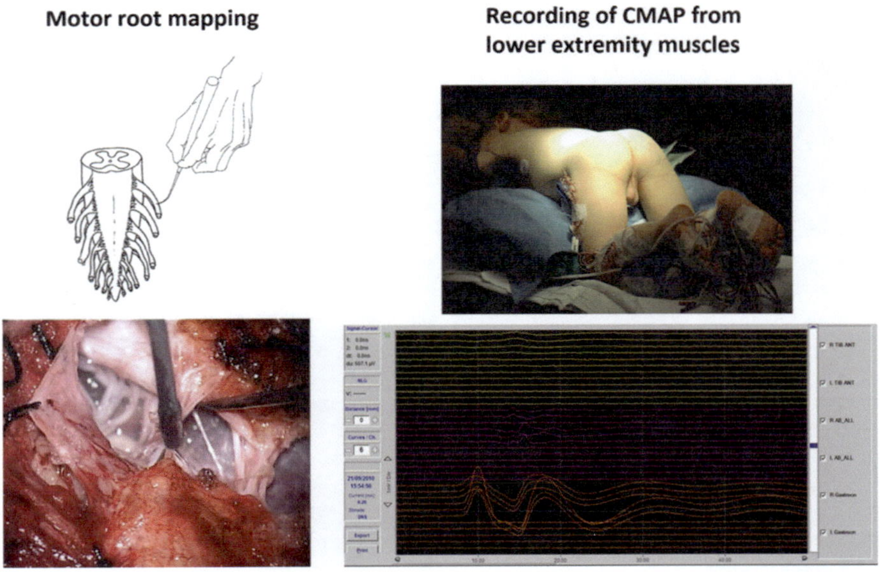

Motor root mapping

Recording of CMAP from lower extremity muscles

Fig. 5 Mapping of the cauda equina. Left upper panel, schematic illustration of direct stimulation of cauda equina roots. Left lower panel, intraoperative view of direct stimulation of the rootlets during surgery for a lumbosacral lipoma. Right upper panel, pairs of needle recording electrodes are inserted bilaterally in lower extremity muscles to record compound muscle action potentials (CMAPs) following stimulation of lumbosacral roots. Right lower panel, screenshot showing a CMAP recorded from the right gastrocnemius muscle using a single stimulus of 0.2-ms duration and 0.2-mA intensity. The stimulus was delivered through a hand-held monopolar electrode, with reference needle electrode in paraspinal muscles. Reprinted from reference 61 (Sala et al., 2013)

Our preferred strategy when determining whether or not a rootlet involved in the pathology is functional is the following. First, we stimulate a motor rootlet not engulfed in the lipoma or any other tethering lesion. This will define the threshold intensity for motor mapping in that specific patient at the given anaesthesiologic regimen. Usually 0.05–0.1 mA suffices to elicit a muscle response. We then stimulate the ambiguous tissue and determine whether or not a CMAP is elicited as well as establishing the specific intensity required to elicit a response. If no response is elicited at intensities up to 2–3 mA, we usually consider this not functional and therefore resectable (Fig. 6).

In order to minimize the risk of spreading of the current and, therefore, of falsely positive mapping, it is important to isolate the structure we want to map from all other neural structures and from the cerebrospinal fluid [37].

We prefer to place a cottonoid under the rootlet, keeping the field dry and then stimulate. It is always advisable to repeat the stimulation a few times to confirm either the positive or negative result.

If motor mapping is straightforward, sensory mapping with peripheral stimulation and recording from the surgical site may be more challenging. A motor response

C. Pasquali et al.

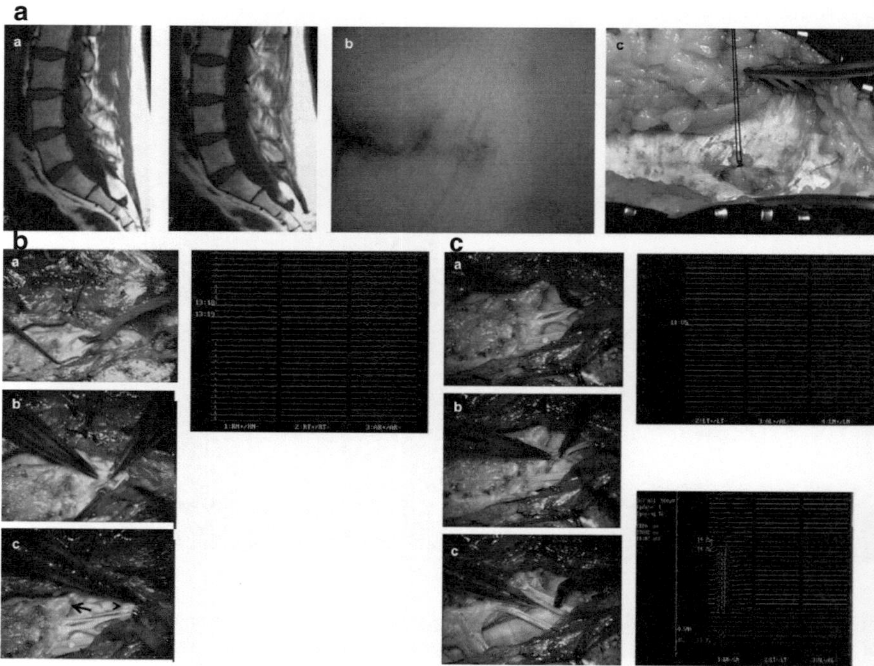

Fig. 6 Mapping functional rootlets and nonfunctional tissue to improve cord untethering during resection of a conus lipoma. (**A**) T1-weighted sagittal MRI of a 34-year-old man with a cord tethered by a sacral conus lipoma (hyperintense) (**a**). The patient presented skin markers of occult spinal dysraphism (**b**), including a dermal sinus that was evident during the surgical approach. The surgical stitch is holding the dermal sinus where it passes through the muscular fascia (**c**). (**B**) Intraoperative picture of the cord tethered by the lipoma. The lipoma has been separated from the dura, along the adhesion line. Neurophysiological mapping is now used to determine which anatomic structures retain function and which can be sacrificed—because not functional—to untether the cord; (**a**) Direct mapping of a thick and fatty filum tethering the cord on the midline is performed using a monopolar hand-held stimulating probe, with reference needle in nearby paraspinal muscles (not shown) and stimulation intensity up to 2 mA. On the right, cascade mode showing no compound muscle action potentials (CMAPs) from the right tibialis anterior (RT), abductor hallucis (AR) and sphincter muscles (RN). Similarly, no CMAPs were recorded from the left side muscles (not shown). Based on negative mapping results, the filum is coagulated and cut (**b**). Partial untethering of the cord is obtained. The proximal (black arrow) and distal (arrowhead) stumps of the fatty filum are indicated (**c**). (**C**) Fibrous bands tethering the cord are directly stimulated. Some of these may still retain the macroscopic features of nerve rootlets, but no response is elicited from the left side (left panel) and right side muscles (not shown) (**a**). The fibrous bands are therefore cut to improve the untethering (**b**). Left side rootlets are mapped but their stimulation elicits a consistent CMAP from the left anal sphincter at low intensity (0.5 mA). Therefore, these rootlets are preserved, and no further untethering is possible (**c**). LN, left anal sphincter; LT, left tibialis anterior; AL, left abductor hallucis. Reprinted from reference 37 (Sala et al., 2014)

can be elicited also through the stimulation of a sensory nerve, through a so-called H-reflex. Yet, the threshold to elicit a CMAP from the stimulation of the sensory roots through an H-reflex is much higher than the threshold for direct motor root stimulation, which can be as low as 0.1–0.2 mA, and this could help to discriminate between a sensory and motor root.

It should also be considered that a conduction block at the level of the grey matter of the conus, where the H-reflex is generated, may induce a loss of the muscle response regardless of the preservation of the sensory component, which ascends through the dorsal column pathway. Accordingly, the presence of a spinal SSEP recorded at the entry zone of the dorsal root (also known as "stationary potential") should be ruled out before labelling the stimulated root as nonfunctional.

Before cutting any rootlet, it is important to rule out any technical factors that may cause negative mapping, such as stimulating and recording electrode displacement, lack of stimulation, and/or anaesthesia-related factors (muscle relaxation, body temperature, halogenated gases).

Finally, it is important to never sacrifice a rootlet, which is assumed to be unfunctional, until it is proven that the same functional information, for example, anal sphincter response, is carried by another rootlet [37, 61, 87].

Cutting fibrous bands or nonfunctional rootlets significantly impact on the degree of cord untethering [26, 50, 61, 88], and the role of ION is critical to optimize the surgical results [62, 89].

Specific Neuromonitoring Scenarios

Terminal Filum Lipomas

Terminal filum lipomas represent a subtype of spinal lipomas, characterized by the fatty infiltration of the filum which causes it to thicken, eventually resulting in a terse and inelastic filum terminale. Filum lipomas almost never involve nerve roots, which remain free and maintain a normal anatomical aspect and course. Moreover, this type of lipoma never penetrates the dura mater and expands in the subcutaneous tissue [26].

Embryologic studies described different histological subtypes of filum terminale pathology: fibroadipose tissues including peripheral nerve bundles (37%), fibroadipose tissue (25%), fibrous or adipose tissue (17%), glial tissues including peripheral nerve sections (10%), and ependymal and glial tissues (10%). Durdağ's cadaveric study shows that none of the patients in whom the filum included peripheral nerve bundles showed any symptoms of neurologic deterioration, concluding that those fibres were probably not functional [90].

Fatty filum becomes a surgical entity when it manifests as clinical or radiological tethered cord syndrome. The surgical procedure consists in cutting the filum itself: it is relatively simple in experienced hands and characterized by a favourable risk/

benefits ratio. Therefore, there is an agreement to operate on patients diagnosed with filum lipomas, especially if they are symptomatic [24, 61, 26].

The filum is usually recognizable anatomically and it has still not been demonstrated that the use of ION improves the surgical outcome [91]. Filum terminale is a white and translucent, midline non-neurological structure of connective tissue and when pathologic it appears thick with a diameter more than 2 mm.

If mapping is entirely negative, the filum can be cut. However, sometimes it is still possible to elicit lower extremities muscles or the sphincter muscle response by stimulating the filum because of the presence of small rootlets adjacent to the ventral aspect of the filum, therefore not visible from the posterior approach. ION, in this case, discloses the presence of these rootlets, and by separating them from the filum, preserves them. The clinical relevance of these small rootlets is undetermined but, whenever ION is available, its use is still justified even for simple procedures such as mapping of the filum, with the overall goal of not harming the patient [61, 91, 92] (Fig. 7).

Cabrera and colleagues recently proposed a new methodology for the identification of the filum terminale with a double neurophysiological confirmation: they found that about 25% of their patients still have CAMP response despite all the precautions in order to isolate the filum terminale. In this scenario, they integrate the traditional mapping of filum terminale with a high-intensity stimulation up to 20 mA of constant current on the isolated filum terminale in a dry field for a short period of time, obtaining a bilateral-polyradicular-symmetrical response. This cauda equina nerve roots response is antidromically activated from the filum stimulation because of its anatomical continuum with the conus medullaris [93].

Mapping of the filum terminalis before sectioning is not strongly required.. Yet, in principle, if ION is available, this would spare, if any, small rootlets which may adhere to the filum. Its use should be considered an option for this, rather simple, surgical procedure.

Illustrative Case n.1

A 16-year old boy, following a growth spurt when he was 14, began to complain of a dull sensation over the perigenital area and around the anterior thighs, lower back pain worsened with physical exercise, and urinary retention (around 700 mL before feeling the urge to urinate), but without motor impairment. Symptoms progressively worsened: he underwent a first spine MRI in the supine position in July 2020, which showed an apparently normal spinal cord with no signs of myelopathy, a cervical hyperkyphosis and a conus medullaris at D12. Another lumbosacral MRI in the prone position in December 2020 showed a portion of the filum terminale in close contact with the spinal posterior wall, at the L2-L3 level, and this was considered suggestive of tethered cord syndrome (Fig. 8).

He underwent surgery to cut the filum terminale, through a L2 laminotomy.

Following stimulation of a normal motor rootlet with 0.1 mA (not shown), the filum was stimulated with intensity up to 2 mA and no CMAPs were recorded from any muscles bilaterally. Only at 2.5 mA was there some muscle activation but this

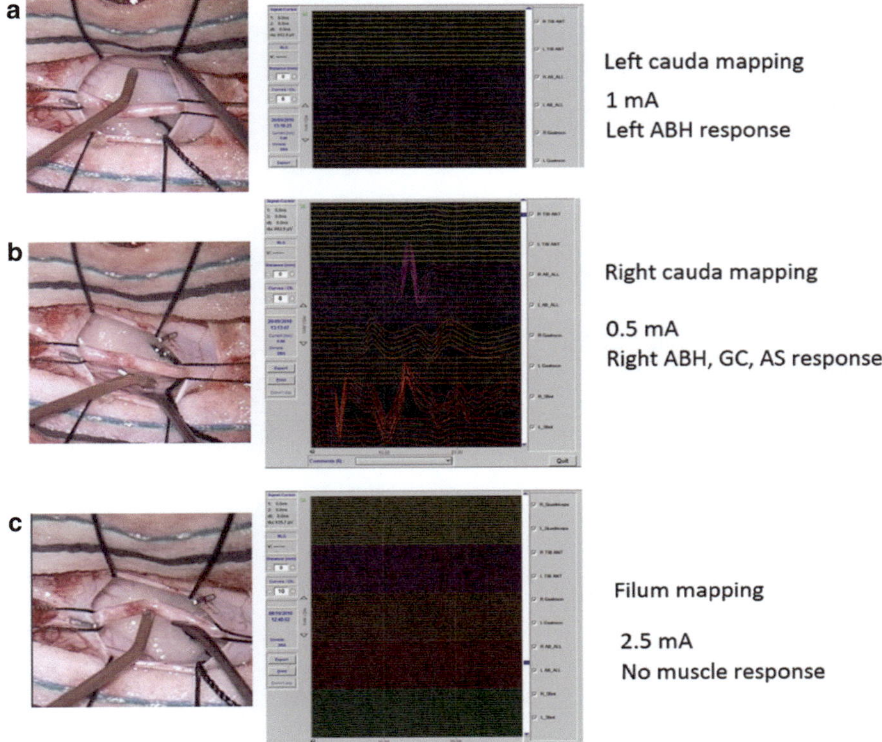

Fig. 7 Neurophysiological mapping of the filum terminale. (**a**) Direct stimulation of left cauda equina roots is performed to identify normal roots and to determine the threshold to elicit CMAPs from the lower extremity muscle. At 1 mA, a CMAP from the left abductor hallucis brevis (ABH) is obtained. (**b**) Direct stimulation of the right cauda equina roots is performed to identify normal roots on the contralateral side. At 0.5 mA, CMAPs from the right ABH, gastrocnemius (GC), and anal sphincter (AS) are obtained. This multisegmental response is likely due to nonselective stimulation of the different roots when these are packed at the level of the cauda and current spreads to adjacent roots. (**c**) Direct stimulation of the isolated filum terminaleAt 2.5 mA, no muscle response is recorded, and the filum can therefore be safely cut. If a muscle response is recorded, this warrants further investigation, and the ventral side of the filum should be inspected to identify and preserve small rootlets adjacent to the filum. Reprinted from reference 61 (Sala et al., 2013).

was deemed due to current spreading (Figs. 9 and 10). The filum was cut. The postoperative outcome was uneventful except for transitory urinary retention which required Foley catheterization, which was later discontinued after 10 days without complication. At the time of discharge, he had no sensory-motor deficits, no urinary problems, and improvement of his back pain.

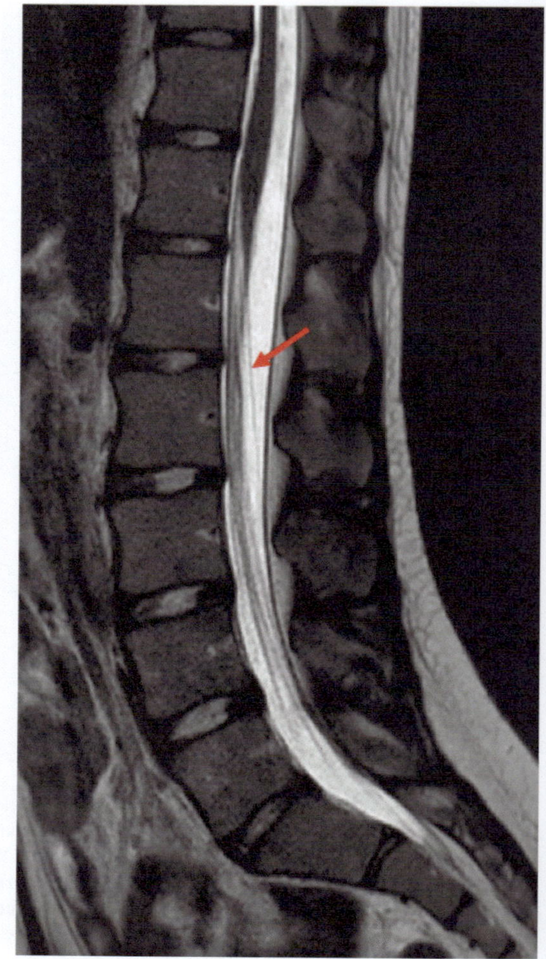

Fig. 8 Sagittal T2-weighted MRI in prone position showing the filum terminale displaced posterior to the cauda equina rootlets, in close contact with the spinal posterior wall at the L2-L3 level (red arrow). The conus is located normally at the D12 level. The patient presented with a tethered cord syndrome which improved following surgical sectioning of the filum

Conus Lipomas

In conus lipomas, a combination of monitoring and mapping techniques represents the best ION strategy. In principle, in both dorsal and transitional lipomas nerve roots leave the cord ventral to the fusion line between the lipoma and the spinal cord. Yet, it may not always be easy to determine the relationship between the dorsal rootlets and the fatty tissue. In this case, mapping along the line of adhesion between the lipoma and the dura mater can confirm the lack of any relevant neural structure before separating the two. Once the fat has been separated from the dura, one should concentrate on determining the white plane between the dorsal aspect of the cord and the ventral plane of the lipoma, aiming for total or near-total resection. At this stage of the operation, the neural structures involved are visible and there is no need

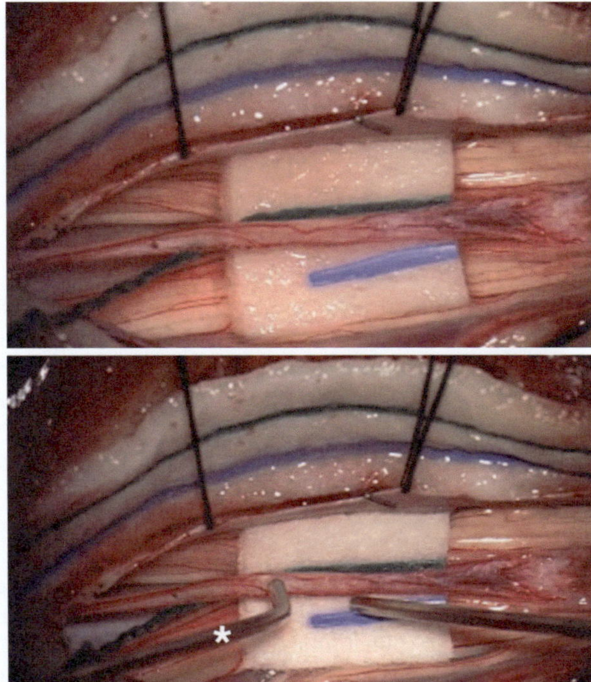

Fig. 9 Isolation and mapping of the filum terminale. Upper panel: The filum is isolated and kept separated from other roots interposing a small cottonoid. Lower panel: The filum is now stimulated with a bipolar concentric electrode (asterisk) while CSF is sucked away to keep the field dry, aiming to minimize current spreading

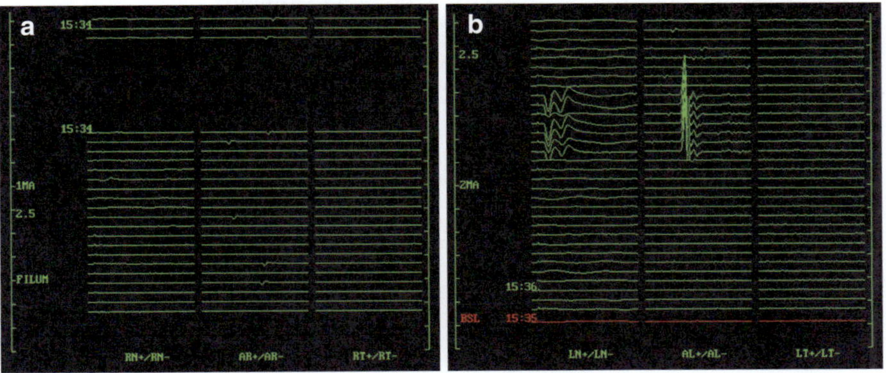

Fig. 10 Stimulation of the filum terminale: (**a**) Recordings from the right sphincter (RN), right abductor hallucis (AR) and right tibialis anterior (RT) following stimulation of the filum with a bipolar concentric electrode and increasing stimulation up to 2.5 mA. No CMAPs are recorded. (**b**) Recordings from the left sphincter (LN), left abductor hallucis (AL) and left tibialis anterior (LT) following stimulation of the filum with a bipolar concentric electrode and increasing stimulation.. No CMAPs are recorded with intensity up to 2.5 mA when some CMAPs are recorded from LN and AL due to current spreading

for mapping. Instead, monitoring of SSEPS, MEPs and BCRs warrants that no excessive traction or compression is done on the cord when attempting to progressively separate the lipoma.

In most complex lipomas, such as the chaotic ones, determining "'who is who" in the surgical field would be impossible without neurophysiological mapping. Still, due to the intermingled relationship between the lipoma and both the cauda and the conus, most often a total removal of a chaotic lipoma is not possible, even with diligent use of ION.

Illustrative Case n.2

Following a normal pregnancy and normal fetal ultrasound, a newborn baby girl presented at birth with a pedunculated fleshy structure in the sacral region with no changes in its characteristics or growth in subsequent periods (Fig. 11). The mass had an elastic consistency, it was surrounded by a cutaneous angioma and associated with a duplication of the gluteal fold.

The subsequent ultrasound evaluation with doppler showed a hyperechoic solid structure with well-defined margins, localized in the dermal layer, slightly marking the underlying adipose layer, with no flow signals detectable in its content. The MRI confirmed the suspicion of spinal dysraphism characterized by a cleft of the posterior arch of S2 with a dermal sinus that reaches the spinal canal from the subcutaneous plane. At the same level, there was an intradural lipoma of approximately 5 cm adjacent to the terminal filum. The conus ended at L2-L3 (Fig. 12).

The neurological, orthopaedic and urological evaluations were unremarkable and surgery was therefore postponed till the age of 1 year.

During surgery, SSEPs and MEPs from the lower extremity muscles, as well as anal MEPs and the BCR were monitored: MEP of the lower limbs remained stable throughout surgery (Fig. 13c), whilst there was a certain instability of the anal MEPs, and the BCR was also fluctuating throughout surgery (Fig. 13d). Surgery

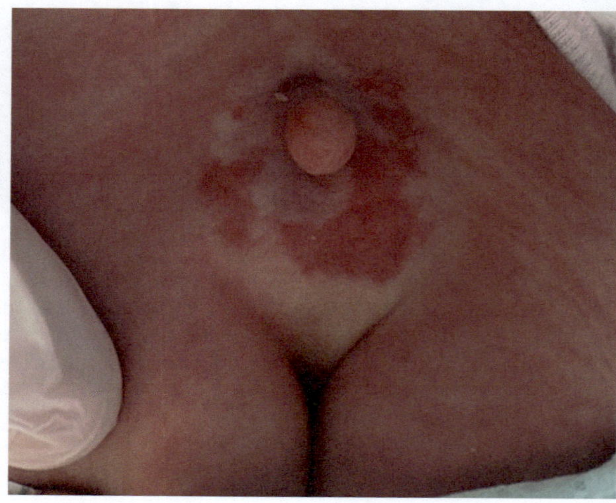

Fig. 11 Pedunculated fleshy structure in the lumbosacral region, associated with a cutaneous angioma and deviation of the gluteal fold. The association of two or more skin lesions is highly suspicious for an "occult" spinal dysraphism

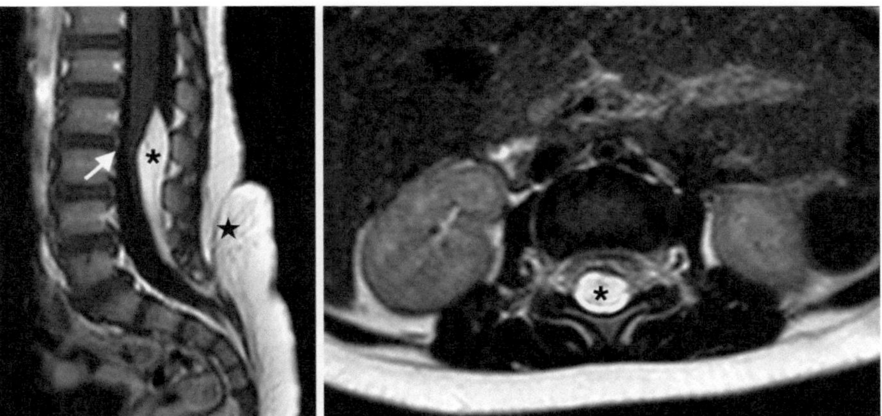

Fig. 12 Sagittal (left) and axial (right) T1-weighted MRI showing a dorsal conus lipoma (asterisk) tethering the cord at L2-L3 (arrow). A dermal sinus is also documented (star)

was transiently stopped whenever the amplitude and consistency of anal MEPs and/ or BCR worsened (Fig. 13e). Warm irrigation, transiently pausing of surgical manipulation and adjusting blood pressure whenever hypotension was noted are the corrective measures typically adopted in these cases. At the end of the surgery, the anal MEP and the BCR were slightly reduced in amplitude compared to the start of surgery, but improved following the intraoperative pause.

At the end it was possible to completely remove the lipoma and surgically neurulate the open cord. Upon awakening from anaesthesia and during the hospital stay, no neurological deficits were observed and the urinary catheter was removed a few days after surgery with no evidence of retention.

The postoperative MRI showed a total resection of the lipomatous mass. The neurological examination was completely normal at follow-up (Fig. 14).

Limited Dorsal Myeloschisis

Limited dorsal myeloschisis (LDM) is a form of spinal dysraphism characterized by two constant features: a focal "closed" midline cutaneous abnormality and a fibroneural stalk that links the skin lesion to the underlying cord. The embryogenetic hypothesis is an incomplete disjunction between cutaneous and neural ectoderms, which prevents the complete midline skin closure and allows the persistence of a physical link (fibroneural stalk) between the skin lesion and the dorsal neural tube at the non-disjunction site [94, 95].

Their features are similar to those in congenital dermal sinus (CDS), but LDM has a closed skin defect and a solid tract without a lumen; thus, in contrast to CDS, the possibility of infectious complications is low [96].

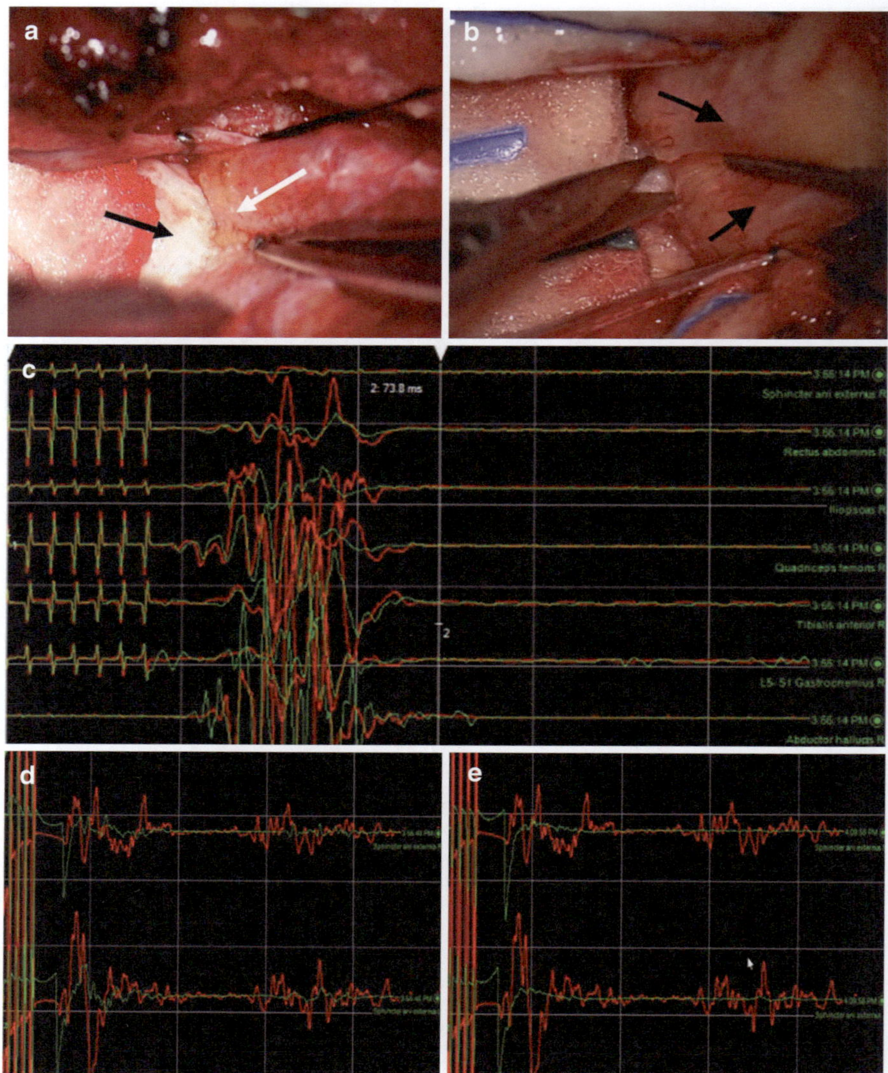

Fig. 13 Surgical removal of a dorsal lipoma. (**a**) A plane is meticulously developed between the white spinal cord (black arrow) and the lipoma (white arrow). (**b**) Only microscissors are used at this stage of the surgery while MEPs and BCR are monitored. No mapping is needed. (**c**) Lower limb MEPs are stable during surgery (red traces: baselines at the beginning of surgery; green traces: online MEPs). (**d**) Left (upper traces) and right (lower traces) BCR instability during surgery. Comparing online BCR (green traces) with baselines (red traces), both early and late components are reduced in amplitude. Further attenuation occurred towards the end of the removal of the lipoma (**e**). Surgery was temporarily halted and during closure a partial recovery of the BCR occurred (not shown). The patient required urinary catheterization for a few days but then fully recovered. At 18 months of follow-up, the patient has no clinical signs of neurogenic bladder

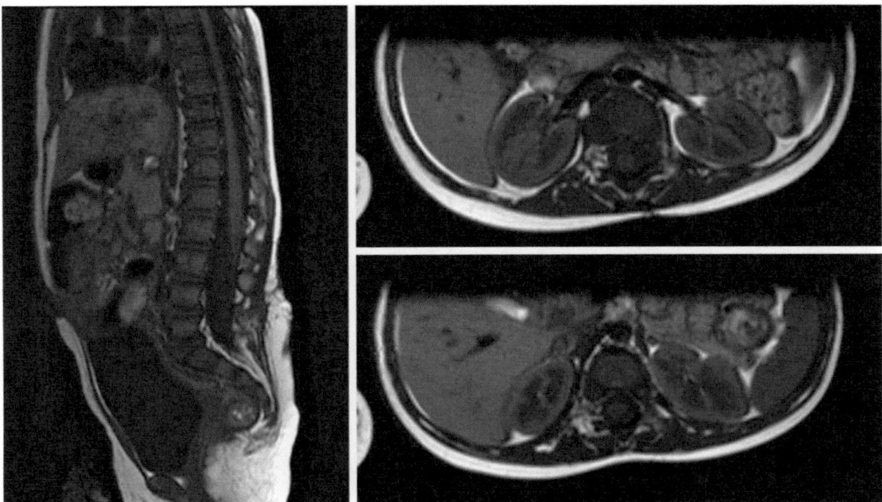

Fig. 14 Postoperative T1-weighted sagittal (left) and axial (right) MRIs showed a total resection of the lipoma

In 2010, Pang and colleagues [95] proposed a classification for LDM into non-saccular and saccular types. The non-saccular skin lesion can be divided into the variety of crater like non-skin squamous epithelium-covered midline defect (most common), or the variety with a simple cutaneous pit. The saccular LDMs can either be a skin-based protrusion with a non-skin squamous epithelial top, or a turgid sac with a skin base and a translucent epithelial top.

Any of the saccular LDMs can be associated with different internal architectures distinguishable by MRI: either a segmental myelocystocele, a stalk connecting the dome of the sac to the spinal cord (the stalk-to-dome subtype), or a basal neural nodule to which the fibroneural stalk is attached [94, 95].

The clinical relevance of LDM is related to neurologic deficits resulting from spinal cord tethering.

Illustrative Case n.3

A newborn male was born following an otherwise normal pregnancy, complicated by the finding of a sacral saccular malformation suspected for spinal dysraphism on the second trimester ultrasound. Fetal and neonatal MRI confirmed a sacral defect having a maximum calibre of about 1 cm in communication with a voluminous subcutaneous cystic structure with a maximum diameter in the axial plane of about 5 cm, and a craniocaudal span of 8 cm. The cyst consisted of two chambers of which the upper one was in continuity with the peri-medullary subarachnoid space. The spinal roots of the cauda were also stretched caudally (Fig. 15). The examination did not show intracranial pathology.

The baby underwent surgery which was performed with the support of ION. Transcranial MEPs were not performed because of safety concerns regarding

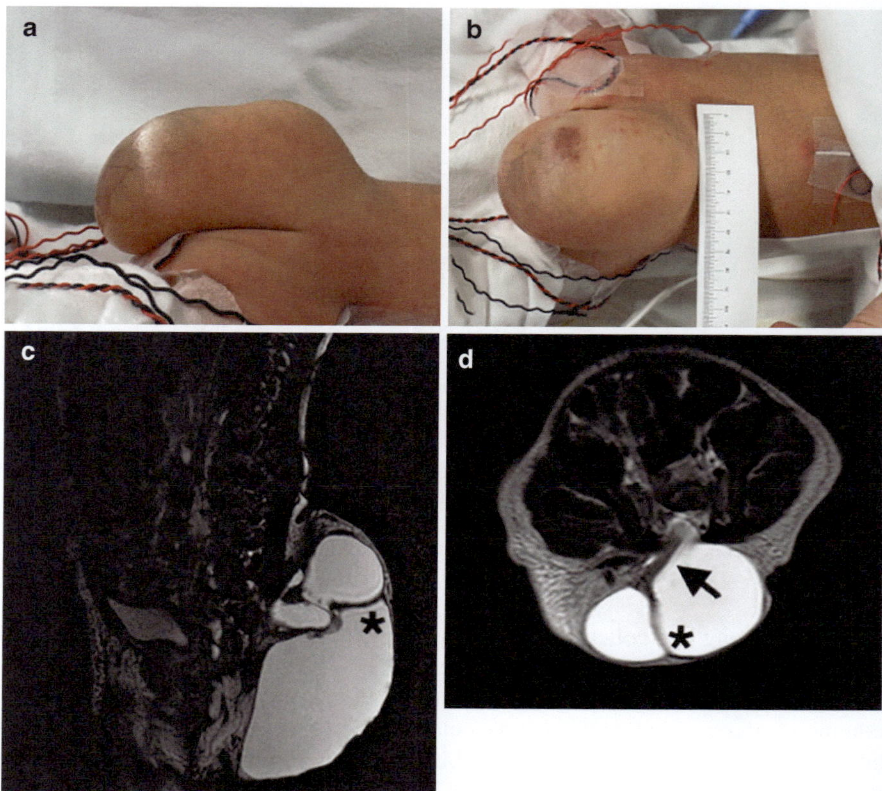

Fig. 15 Saccular limited dorsal myeloschisis. Upper panels: Lateral (**a**) and superior (**b**) view of the saccular LDM. Middle panels: T2-weighted preoperative sagittal MRI (**c**) showing a large saccular formation filled with CSF. The cystic formation has a fibrous stalk (asterisk) which divides it into two chambers. The axial view (**d**) shows that the sac is in continuity with the perimedullary subarachnoid space and the conus (arrow) appears stretched, beyond the sacral vertebral cleft, within the cystic formation and in continuity with the fibrous septation

stimulation through the open fontanel, and therefore the anaesthesiologist preferred the use of halogenated agents and avoided propofol. However, the intraoperative mapping which consisted of identifying functional and nonfunctional structures and the monitoring of the BCR were attempted and successful, despite the use of halogenated agents (Fig. 16a–e).

At the time of discharge the neuromotor examination was normal for age and the abdominal ultrasound did not show findings suspected of neurogenic bladder (such as dilation of the renal pelvis, dilation of the ureters, or bladder stagnation.).

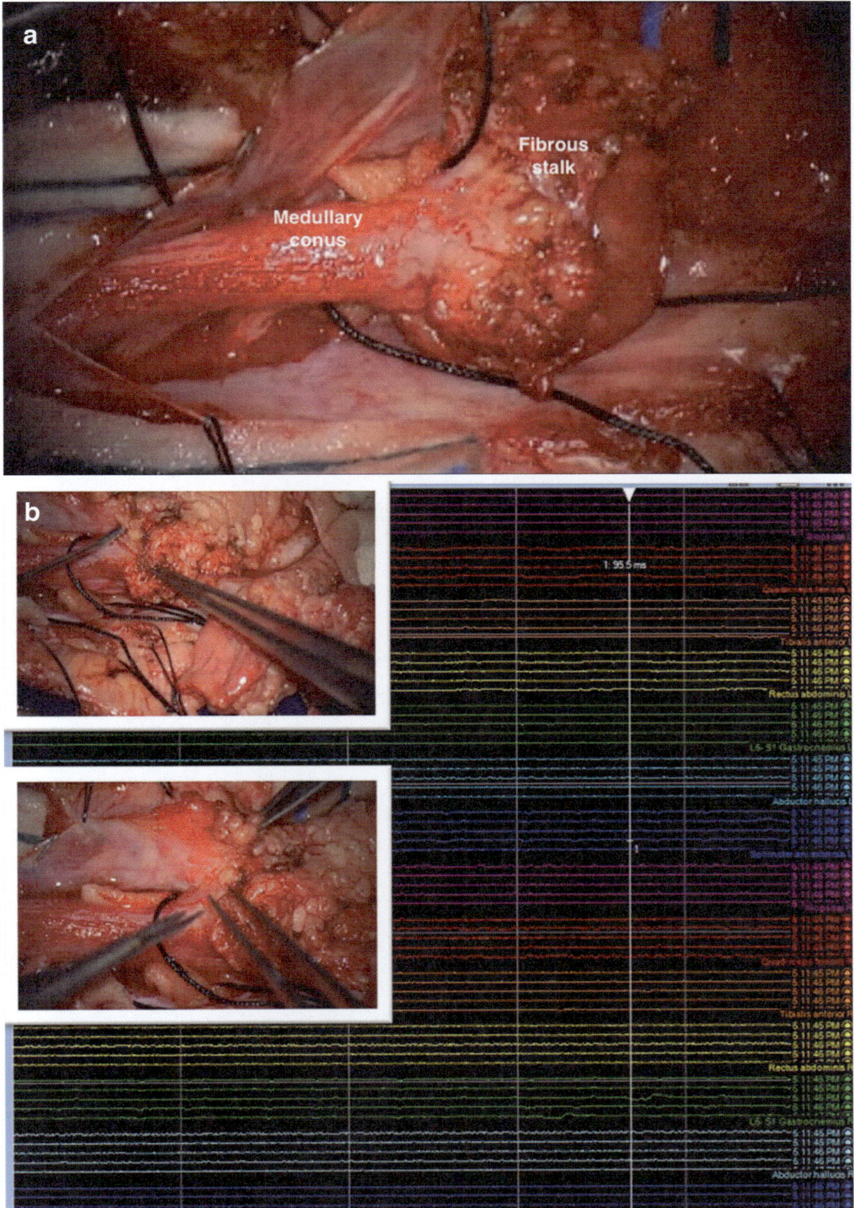

Fig. 16 (**a**) Intraoperative surgical view of the conus and the fibrous stalk. (**b**) Mapping of the junctional zone between the functional conus and the nonfunctional fibrous stalk shows no motor response from either the lower limbs MEPs or the anal sphincter, allowing a clean surgical separation of the two structures (inserts). (**c**) Mapping functional rootlets in the region of the fibrous material, with muscular response from gastrocnemius and abductor hallucis. (**d**) Mapping functional rootlets in the region of the fibrous material, with muscular response from abductor hallucis and external anal sphincter. (**e**) BCR stability (red line: baseline BCR at the beginning of surgery; green line: BCR at closure)

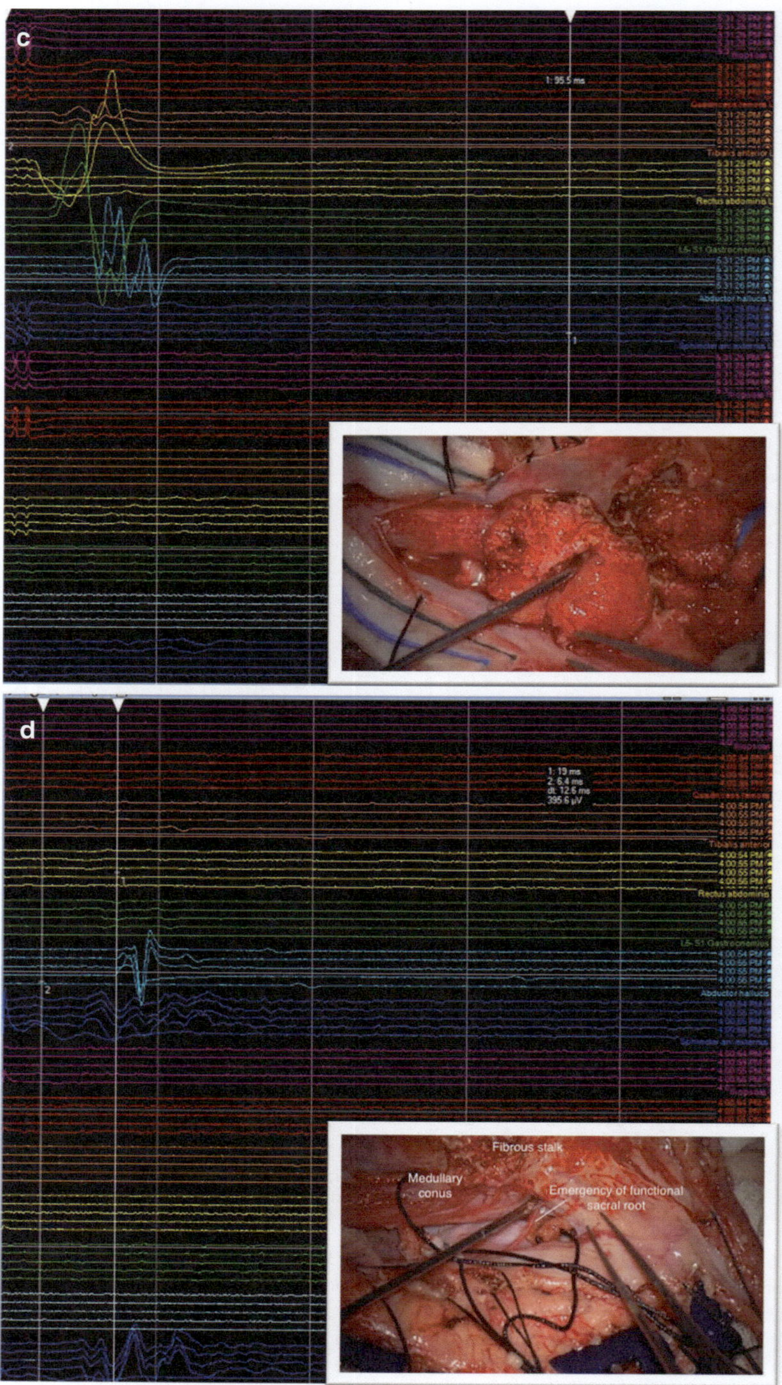

Fig. 16 (continued)

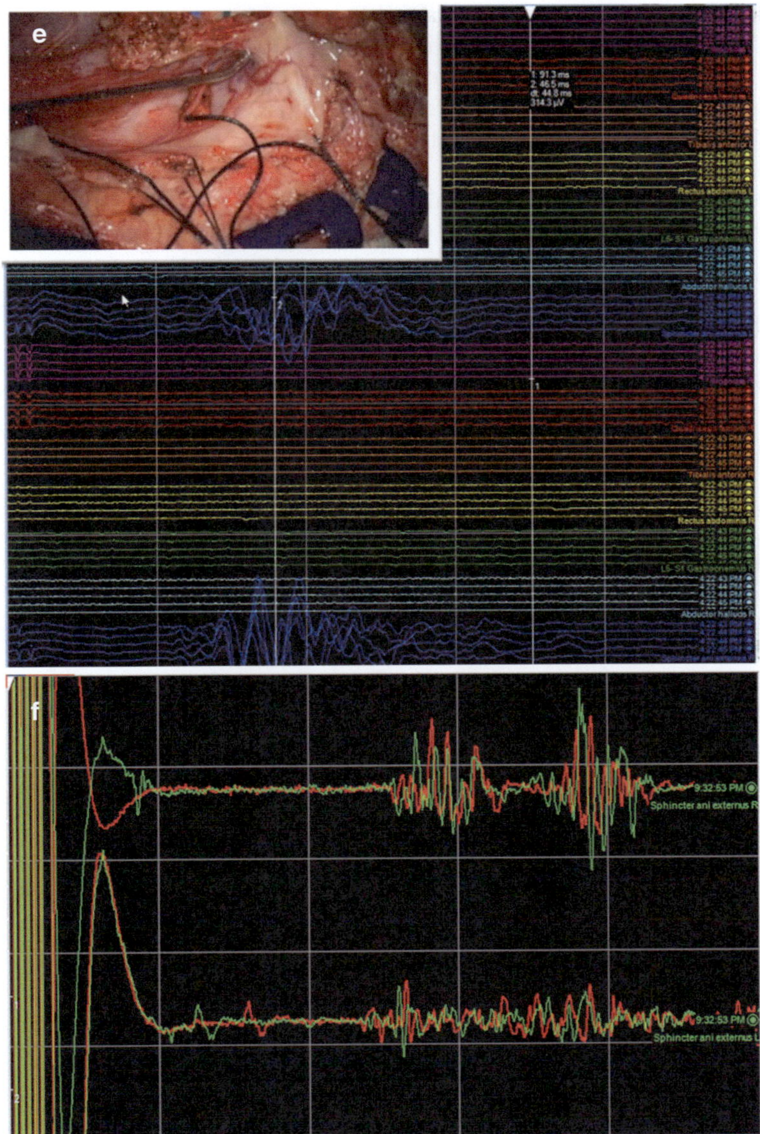

Fig. 16 (continued)

Conclusion

Tethered cord surgery remains a challenging surgical procedure, especially for certain complex occult spinal dysraphism. A deep knowledge of anatomy and embryology is a pillar to correctly address these cases but at times does not suffice as the functional, rather than anatomical, aspects are essential and cannot be disclosed in any other way than through extensive use of ION.

In addition to improving the safety of these surgical procedures, the use of mapping is also invaluable in understanding the pathophysiology of some of these disorders, which have been understood and classified also on the basis of these findings.

The use of ION cannot substitute for surgical experience but, rather, it complements the latter in providing unique functional information.

There is an ongoing debate on the value of ION in Neurosurgery. With all limitations in mind and accepting that the value of ION is not based on strong class I and II evidence according to classic EBM criteria, there is a general consensus that ION assists the surgeon not merely in predicting neurological outcome, but also in preventing or minimizing iatrogenic neurological injury. In the field of conus lipomas, we like to believe that the best long-term outcome presented by Pang et al. was also the result of their extensive use of ION.

References

1. Hoffman HJ, Hendrick EB, HR. The tethered spinal cord: its protean manifestations, diagnosis and surgical correction. Childs Brain. 1976;2:145–55.
2. Yamada S. Tethered cord syndrome. J Neurosurg Spine. 2009;10:79–81.
3. Yamada S, Zinke DE, Sanders D. Pathophysiology of 'tethered cord syndrome'. J Neurosurg. 1981;54:494–503.
4. Tani S, Yamada S, Knighton RS. Extensibility of the lumbar and sacral cord. Pathophysiology of the tethered spinal cord in cats. J Neurosurg. 1987;66(1):116–23.
5. Yamada S, Won DJ. What is the true tethered cord syndrome? Childs Nerv Syst. 2007;23(4):371–5.
6. Yamada S, Won DJ, Pezeshkpour G, Yamada BS, Yamada SM, Siddiqi J, et al. Pathophysiology of tethered cord syndrome and similar complex disorders. Neurosurg Focus. 2007;23(2):e6.
7. Pang D, Wilberger JE. Tethered cord syndrome in adults. J Neurosurg. 1982;57:32–47.
8. Weprin BE, Oakes WJ. Occult spinal dysraphism: the clinical presentation and diagnosis. Oper Tech Plast Reconstr Surg. 2000;7(2):39–52.
9. Kulkarni AV, Pierre-Kahn A, Zerah M, Chapman PH, Adelson PD, Cohen AR, et al. Conservative management of asymptomatic spinal lipomas of the conus. Neurosurgery. 2004;54:868–75.
10. Drake JM. Surgical management of the tethered spinal cord—walking the fine line. Neurosurg Focus. 2007;23(2):E4.
11. Paradiso G, Lee GYF, Sarjeant R, Hoang L, Massicotte EM, Fehlings MG. Multimodality intraoperative neurophysiologic monitoring findings during surgery for adult tethered cord syndrome: analysis of a series of 44 patients with long-term follow-up. Spine (Phila Pa 1976). 2006;31(18):2095–102.
12. Gunnarsson T, Krassioukov AV, Sarjeant R, Fehlings MG. Real-time continuous intraoperative electromyographic and somatosensory evoked potential recordings in spinal surgery: correlation of clinical and electrophysiologic findings in a prospective, consecutive series of 213 cases. Spine (Phila Pa 1976). 2004;29(6):677–84.
13. Quiñones-Hinojosa A, Gadkary CA, Gulati M, Von Koch CS, Lyon R, Weinstein PR, et al. Neurophysiological monitoring for safe surgical tethered cord syndrome release in adults. Surg Neurol. 2004;62(2):127–33.

14. Finger T, Aigner A, Depperich L, Schaumann A, Wolter S, Schulz M, et al. Secondary tethered cord syndrome in adult patients: retethering rates, long-term clinical outcome, and the effect of intraoperative neuromonitoring. Acta Neurochir. 2020;162(9):2087–96.
15. Moore KL, Persaud TVN. Lo sviluppo prenatale dell uomo. Embriologia ad orientamento medico. II. EdiSES; 2009.
16. Anastasi G. Trattato di anatomia umana. IV. Edi-Ermes; 2010.
17. Saitsu H, Yamada S, Uwabe C, Ishibashi M, Shiota K. Aberrant differentiation of the axially condensed tail bud mesenchyme in human embryos with lumbosacral myeloschisis. Anat Rec. 2007;290:251–8.
18. Pang D, Zovickian J, Moes GS. Retained medullary cord in humans: late arrest of secondary neurulation. Neurosurgery. 2011;68(6):1500–19.
19. Sarris CE, Tomei KL, Carmel PW, Gandhi CD. Lipomyelomeningocele: pathology, treatment, and outcomes. Neurosurg Focus. 2012;33(4):E3.
20. Kesler H, Dias MS, Kalapos P. Termination of the normal conus medullaris in children: a whole-spine magnetic resonance imaging study. Neurosurg Focus. 2007;23(2):E7.
21. Pinto F, Fontes R, Leonhardt MC, Amodio D, Porro F, Machado J. Anatomic study of the filum terminale and its correlations with the tethered cord syndrome. Neurosurgery. 2002;51(3):725–30.
22. Catala M. Genetic control of caudal development. Clin Genet. 2002;61:367–8.
23. Rossi A, Biancheri R, Cama A, Piatelli G, Ravegnani M, Tortori-Donati P. Imaging in spine and spinal cord malformations. Eur J Radiol. 2004;50(2):177–200.
24. Finn MA, Walker ML. Spinal lipomas: clinical spectrum, embryology, and treatment. Neurosurg Focus. 2007;23(2):e10.
25. Chapman PH. Congenital intraspinal lipomas: anatomic considerations and surgical treatment. Childs Brain. 1982;9(1):37–47.
26. Pang D, Zovickian J, Oviedo A. Long-term outcome of total and near-total resection of spinal cord lipomas and radical reconstruction of the neural placode: part I—surgical technique. Neurosurgery. 2009;65(3):511–29.
27. Pang D, Wong SZ. Surgical treatment of complex spinal cord lipomas. Childs Nerv Syst. 2013;29:1485–513.
28. Morota N, Ihara S, Ogiwara H. New classification of spinal lipomas based on embryonic stage. J Neurosurg Pediatr. 2017;19:1–12.
29. Reghunath A, Ghasi RG, Aggarwal A. Unveiling the tale of the tail: an illustration of spinal dysraphisms. Neurosurg Rev. 2021;44(1):97–114.
30. Thompson EM, Strong MJ, Warren G, Woltjer RL, Selden NR. Clinical significance of imaging and histological characteristics of filum terminale in tethered cord syndrome. J Neurosurg Pediatr. 2014;13(3):255–9.
31. Pierre-Kahn A, Zerah M, Renier D, Cinalli G, Sainte-Rose, Christian Lellouch-Tubian A, Brunelle F, et al. Congenital lumbosacral lipomas. Child's Nerv Syst. 1997;13(6):298–334.
32. Warder DE. Tethered cord syndrome and occult spinal dysraphism. Neurosurg Focus. 2001;10(1):e1.
33. Brown E, Matthes J, Bazan C, Jinkins J. Prevalence of incidental intraspinal lipoma of the lumbosacral spine as determined by MRI. Spine (Phila Pa 1976). 1994;19(7):833–6.
34. Özek MM, Cinalli G, Maixner WJ. The spina bifida. Management and outcome. Springer-Verlag Italia; 2008. 523 p.
35. Muthukumar N. Congenital spinal lipomatous malformations: part I-classification. Acta Neurochir. 2009;151:179–88.
36. Arai H, Sato K, Okuda O, Miyajima M, Hishii M, Nakanishi H, et al. Surgical experience of 120 patients with lumbosacral lipomas. Acta Neurochir. 2001;143(9):857–64.
37. Sala F, Tramontano V, Squintani G, Arcaro C, Tot E, Pinna G, et al. Neurophysiology of complex spinal cord untethering. J Clin Neurophysiol. 2014;31:326–36.
38. Rajpal S, Tubbs SR. Tethered cord due to spina bifida occulta presenting in adulthood review of 61 patients. J Neurosurg Spine. 2007;6:210–5.

39. Aufschnaiter K, Fellner F, Wurm G. Surgery in adult onset tethered cord syndrome (ATCS): review of literature on occasion of an exceptional case. Neurosurg Rev. 2008;31:371–84.

40. Selcuki M, Mete M, Barutcuoglu M, Duransoy YK, Umur AS, Selcuki D. Tethered cord syndrome in adults: experience of 56 patients. Turk Neurosurg. 2015;25:922–9.

41. Lee GYF, Paradiso G, Tator CH, Gentili F, Massicotte EM, Fehlings MG. Surgical management of tethered cord syndrome in adults: indications, techniques, and long-term outcomes in 60 patients. J Neurosurg Spine. 2006;4(2):123–31.

42. Sofuoglu OE, Abdallah A, Emel E, Ofluoglu AE, Gunes M, Guler B. Management of tethered cord syndrome in adults: experience of 23 cases. Turk Neurosurg. 2017;27:226–36.

43. Iskandar BJ, Fulmer B, Hadley M, Oakes WJ. Congenital tethered spinal cord syndrome in adults. J Neurosurg Pediatr. 1998;88:958–61.

44. Bui CJ. Tethered cord syndrome in children: a review. Neurosurg Focus. 2007;23:e2.

45. Dorward NL, Scatliff J, Hayward RD. Congenital lumbosacral lipomas: pitfalls in analysing the results of prophylactic surgery. Childs Nerv Syst. 2002;18:326–32.

46. Hoffman HJ, Taecholarn C, Bruce Hendrick E, Humphreys RP. Management of lipomyelo-meningoceles experience at the hospital for sick children, Toronto. J Neurosurg. 1985;62:1–8.

47. Alsowayan O, Alzahrani A, Alsowayan O, Farmer J-P, Capolicchio J-P, Jednak R, et al. Comprehensive analysis of the clinical and urodynamic outcomes of secondary tethered spinal cord before and after spinal cord untethering. J Pediatr Urol. 2015;1:e1–6.

48. Alsowayan O, Alzahrani A, Farmer J, Capolicchio J, Jednak R. Comprehensive analysis of the clinical and urodynamic outcomes of primary tethered spinal cord before and after spinal cord untethering. J Pediatr Urol. 2016;(February):1–5.

49. Hertzler DA. Tethered cord syndrome: a review of the literature from embryology to adult presentation. Neurosurg Focus. 2010;29(1):e1.

50. Pang D, Zovickian J, Oviedo A. Long-term outcome of total and near-total resection of spinal cord lipomas and radical reconstruction of the neural placode, part II: outcome analysis and preoperative profiling. Neurosurgery. 2010;66:253–73.

51. Sala F, Kržan MJ, Deletis V. Intraoperative neurophysiological monitoring in pediatric neuro-surgery: why, when, how? Childs Nerv Syst. 2002;18:262–87.

52. Yamada S. Filum terminale in tethered cord syndrome. J Neurosurg Pediatr. 2016;17:634.

53. Hasan MS, Tan JK, Chan CYW, Kwan MK, Karim FSA, Goh KJ. Comparison between effect of desflurane/remifentanil and propofol/remifentanil anesthesia on somatosensory evoked potential monitoring during scoliosis surgery—a randomized controlled trial. J Orthop Surg. 2018;26(3):1–7.

54. Sloan TB, Toleikis JR, Toleikis SC, Koht A. Intraoperative neurophysiological monitoring during spine surgery with total intravenous anesthesia or balanced anesthesia with 3% desflurane. J Clin Monit Comput. 2015;29(1):77–85.

55. Sloan T. Anesthesia and intraoperative neurophysiological monitoring in children. Childs Nerv Syst. 2010;26(2):227–35.

56. Sala F, Barone G, Tramontano V, Gallo P, Ghimenton C. Retained medullary cord confirmed by intraoperative neurophysiological mapping. Childs Nerv Syst. 2014;30:1287–91.

57. Fulkerson DH, Satyan KB, Wilder LM, Riviello JJ, Stayer SA, Whitehead WE, et al. Intraoperative neurophysiology of the conus medullaris and cauda equina. Childs Nerv Syst. 2010;29(4):137–44.

58. Kothbauer KF, Deletis V. Intraoperative neurophysiology of the conus medullaris and cauda equina. Childs Nerv Syst. 2010;26(2):247–53.

59. Deletis V, Vodusek D. Intraoperative recording of the bulbocavernosus reflex. Neurosurgery. 1997;40:88–92.

60. Taniguchi M, Cedzich C, Schramm J. Modification of cortical stimulation for motor evoked potentials under general anesthesia: technical description. Neurosurgery. 1993;32(2):219–26.

61. Sala F, Squintani G, Tramontano V, Arcaro C, Faccioli F, Mazza C. Intraoperative neurophysiology in tethered cord surgery: techniques and results. Childs Nerv Syst. 2013;29:1611–24.

62. Deletis V, Sala F. The role of intraoperative neurophysiology in the protection or documentation of surgically induced injury to the spinal cord. Ann N Y Acad Sci. 2006;939(1):137–44.
63. Bowman RM, Mohan A, Ito J, Seibly J, McLone D. Tethered cord release a long-term study in 114 patients. J Neurosurg Pediatr. 2009;3:181–7.
64. Scibilia A, Terranova C, Rizzo V, Raffa G, Morelli A, Esposito F, et al. Intraoperative neurophysiological mapping and monitoring in spinal tumor surgery: sirens or indispensable tools? Neurosurg Focus. 2016;41(2):E18.
65. Nuwer MR. Handbook of clinical neurophysiology. Elsevier; 2010.
66. Sala F, Manganotti P, Grossauer S, Tramontanto V, Mazza C, Gerosa M. Intraoperative neurophysiology of the motor system in children: a tailored approach. Childs Nerv Syst. 2010;26(4):473–90.
67. Husain AM, Shah D. Prognostic value of neurophysiologic intraoperative monitoring in tethered cord syndrome surgery. J Clin Neurophysiol. 2009;26(4):244–7.
68. Fulkerson DH, Satyan KB, Wilder LM, Riviello JJ, Stayer SA, Whitehead WE, et al. Intraoperative monitoring of motor evoked potentials in very young children. J Neurosurg Pediatr. 2011;7(4):331–7.
69. Gupta P. Comparison between sevoflurane and desflurane on emergence and recovery characteristics of children undergoing surgery for spinal dysraphism. Indian J Anaesth. 2015;59:482–7.
70. Singh D. Sevofluorano provides better recovery tha isofluorane in children undergoing spinal surg—abstract. J Neurosurg Anesth. 2009;21:202–6.
71. Kalkman CJ, Drummond J, Ribberink A. Effects of Propofol, etomidate, midazolam, and fentanyl on motor evoked responses to transcranial electrical or magnetic stimulation in humans. Anesthesiology. 1992;76:502–8.
72. Frei FJ, Ryhult SE, Duitmann E, Hasler CC, Luetschg J, Erb TO. Intraoperative monitoring of motor-evoked potentials in children undergoing spinal surgery. Spine (Phila Pa 1976). 2007;32(8):911–7.
73. Herta J, Yildiz E, Marhofer D, Czech T, Reinprecht A, Rössler K, et al. Feasibility of intraoperative motor evoked potential monitoring during tethered cord surgery in infants younger than 12 months. Childs Nerv Syst. 2021;38:397–405.
74. Kothbauer KF. Intraoperative monitoring for tethered cord surgery: an update. Neurosurg Focus. 2004;16(2):Article 8.
75. Journée HL, Polak HE, De Kleuver M. Conditioning stimulation techniques for enhancement of transcranially elicited evoked motor responses. Neurophysiol Clin. 2007;37(6):423–30.
76. Journée HL, Polak HE, de Kleuver M, Langeloo DD, Postma AA. Improved neuromonitoring during spinal surgery using double-train transcranial electrical stimulation. Med Biol Eng Comput. 2004;42(1):110–3.
77. Szelényi A, Kothbauer KF, Deletis V. Transcranial electric stimulation for intraoperative motor evoked potential monitoring: stimulation parameters and electrode montages. Clin Neurophysiol. 2007;118(7):1586–95.
78. Hoving EW, Haitsma E, Ophuis CMCO, Journée HL. The value of intraoperative neurophysiological monitoring in tethered cord surgery. Childs Nerv Syst. 2011;27(9):1445–52.
79. Pratheesh R, Babu KS, Rajshekhar V. Improvement in intraoperative transcranial electrical motor-evoked potentials in tethered cord surgery: an analysis of 45 cases. Acta Neurochir. 2014;156(4):723–31.
80. Tsutsui S, Iwasaki H, Yamada H, Hashizume H, Minamide A, Nakagawa Y, et al. Augmentation of motor evoked potentials using multi-train transcranial electrical stimulation in intraoperative neurophysiologic monitoring during spinal surgery. J Clin Monit Comput. 2015;29(1):35–9.
81. Sindou M, Joud A, Georgoulis G. Usefulness of external anal sphincter EMG recording for intraoperative neuromonitoring of the sacral roots—a prospective study in dorsal rhizotomy. Acta Neurochir. 2021;163(2):479–87.
82. Khealani B, Husain AM. Neurophysiologic intraoperative monitoring during surgery for tethered cord syndrome. J Clin Neurophysiol. 2009;26(2):76–81.

83. Paradiso G, Lee GYF, Hons M, Fracs MS, Cnim RS. Multi-modality neurophysiological monitoring during surgery for adult tethered cord syndrome. J Clin Neurosci. 2005;12(8):934–6.
84. Skinner SA, Vodušek DB. Intraoperative recording of the bulbocavernosus reflex. J Clin Neurophysiol. 2014;31(4):313–22.
85. Morota N. Intraoperative neurophysiological monitoring of the bulbocavernosus reflex during surgery for conus spinal lipoma: what are the warning criteria? J Neurosurg Pediatr. 2019;23(5):639–47.
86. Shinjo T, Hayashi H, Takatani T, Boku E, Nakase H, Kawaguchi M. Intraoperative feasibility of bulbocavernosus reflex monitoring during untethering surgery in infants and children. J Clin Monit Comput. 2019;33(1):155–63.
87. Pang D. Intraoperative neurophysiology of the conus medullaris and cauda equina. Childs Nerv Syst. 2010;26:411–2.
88. Pouratian N, Elias WJ, Jane JA, Phillips LH, Jane JA. Electrophysiologically guided untethering of secondary tethered spinal cord syndrome. Neurosurg Focus. 2010;29(1):E3.
89. Lall RR, Lall RR, Hauptman JS, Munoz C, Cybulski GR, Koski T, et al. Intraoperative neurophysiological monitoring in spine surgery: indications, efficacy, and role of the preoperative checklist. Neurosurg Focus. 2012;33(5):E10.
90. Durdağ E, Börcek PB, Öcal Ö, Börcek AÖ, Emmez H, Baykaner MK. Pathological evaluation of the filum terminale tissue after surgical excision. Childs Nerv Syst. 2015;31(5):759–63.
91. Srinivasan HL, Korn A, Roth J, Constantini S. Filum terminale lipomas—the role of intraoperative neuromonitoring. Childs Nerv Syst. 2020;36(12):2897–8.
92. Suess O, Mularski S, Czabanka MA, Cabraja M, Hammersen S, Kombos T. The value of intraoperative neurophysiological monitoring for microsurgical removal of conus medullaris lipomas: a 12-year retrospective cohort study. Patient Saf Surg. 2014;8(1):1–10.
93. Cabrera JP, Vigueras S, Muñoz R, López E. Double neurophysiological certification of the filum terminale during sectioning surgery in pediatric population. Surg Neurol Int. 2020;11(229):1–5.
94. Pang D, Zovickian J, Wong ST, Hou YJ, Moes GS. Limited dorsal myeloschisis: a not-so-rare form of primary neurulation defect. Childs Nerv Syst. 2013;29(9):1459–84.
95. Pang D, Zovickian J, Oviedo A, Moes GS. Limited dorsal myeloschisis: a distinctive clinico-pathological entity. Neurosurgery. 2010;67(6):1555–79.
96. Lee SM, Cheon JE, Choi YH, Kim IO, Kim WS, Cho HH, et al. Limited dorsal myeloschisis and congenital dermal sinus: comparison of clinical and MR imaging features. Am J Neuroradiol. 2017;38(1):176–82.

Urological Aspects of Spinal Dysraphism

Kwanjin Park

Spinal dysraphism includes wide variety of spinal abnormalities affecting various spinal levels. This implies various urological manifestations could be expected given the similarly looking spinal dysraphism. Additionally, the fact that substantial number of patients are not toilet-trained at the time of detection of spinal dysraphism indicates the pattern of voiding will undergo changes in the course of time. Due to abovementioned aspects, urological evaluation of spinal dysraphism is demanding even for the experienced pediatric urologists. This chapter is written for neurosurgeons who are willing to understand the urologic problems in their patients. To achieve the goal, basic physiologies and developmental changes of voiding function are described. Urological tests for patients and their implications are also included. This basic knowledge will be useful in understanding typical urodynamic patterns and practical management that will follow.

Most lesions in spinal dysraphism (SD) are found in lumbosacral area where the sacral micturition center is located, so it is not uncommon to see children with voiding dysfunction attributed to SD. Depending on the nature and the extent of lesion, patients may show various spectrum of bladder dysfunctions. This may be varied from just delay in achieving toilet training to total incontinence. A caveat that must be acknowledged is that the neural circuits affecting the bladder are long and complexly spread in the central nervous system, and the neural deficits that can be assumed from the lesions seen in current imaging and neurological examinations are not necessarily evident in that most related nervous system belongs to the

K. Park (✉)
Department of Urology, Seoul National University, College of Medicine,
Seoul, Republic of Korea

Division of Pediatric Urology, Seoul National University Children's Hospital,
Seoul, Republic of Korea
e-mail: urodori9@snu.ac.kr

273

D. Pang, K.-C. Wang (eds.), *Spinal Dysraphic Malformations*, Advances and Technical Standards in Neurosurgery 47,
https://doi.org/10.1007/978-3-031-34981-2_10

autonomic nervous system. With the visible lesion shown on the current imaging, we may predict what the patient's voiding will be like, but it is not necessarily consistent with the revealed findings. Rather it depends on how much the lesion affects the micturition pathway or the presence of unidentified upper motor neuron lesion interfering coordinated movement which is crucial for voiding. Last but not least, the neurourological development should be also taken into account in assessment. Therefore, the actual voiding pattern may look completely different even between the same spinal level of involvement of similarly looking lesions. Moreover, the urodynamics study (UDS), which is often regarded as panacea that is expected to tell everything about the patient's voiding function, may fail to simulate the patient's voiding pattern unable to define what is wrong in the bladder. Studies indicated inconsistency of interpretation between experienced examiners of urodynamics [1, 2]. Therefore, if the results of the urodynamics test could not match the clinical presentation of SD, history of current voiding, and noninvasive test of bladder function, we would say UDS alone is of little use.

Considering the characteristics of SD showing various presentations, versatile urologists in charge should be able to assume possible urodynamic patterns based on the spinal level or nature of the lesion, to assess whether the actual urodynamic pattern corresponds to their expectation, and to provide the proper management accordingly. In case of discrepancy between expected and actual urodynamic patterns, the reason should be explored and understood. In addition, the reason should be shared and discussed with neurosurgeon in charge to set an appropriate management plan. The most important consideration for urologists in the management of these symptoms is preservation of renal function by protecting the upper urinary tract (i.e., kidney function). In addition, goals of management include preserving patient quality of life by ensuring social urinary continence.

Based on our 12 years of close collaboration with neurosurgeons and performance of more than 700 cases of UDS in patients with SD, we came to understand the pathophysiology of SD better and set a strategy to see patients with SD before and after untethering. We do not propose any fixed guideline in management and follow-up but try to explain the reason of applying diagnostic tests and to show how to incorporate the results of tests into the management. This will come in handy in understanding and applying current guidelines proposed by societies and experts.

Basic Bladder Physiology and Developmental Aspects

This is the basic micturition physiology that is required to understand noninvasive and invasive urodynamic data during urologic evaluation. The two main phases of bladder function, storage and emptying of urine are controlled by a series of neurological pathways as shown in Fig. 1.

While the transition between these two functions is subject to reflex control in infants, volitional control of bladder is gradually achieved with toilet training. This type of transition of control in hollow viscus is unique in human body. At each

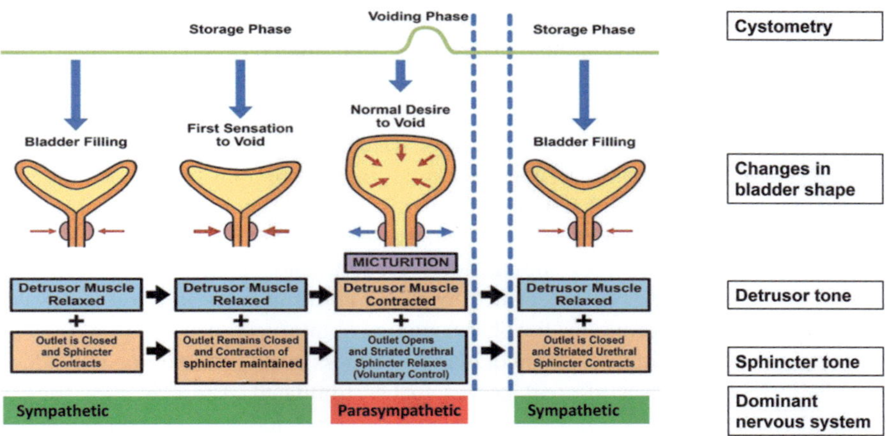

Fig. 1 The two main functional phases of bladder, storage and emptying is controlled by delicate control of several nerves, functional units of bladder. This figure shows what happens during storage and voiding phase and each cycle is divided by dotted line. The role of each relevant element during the two functional phases of bladder is also depicted

phase, the reservoir (bladder) and the outlet (urethra and urinary sphincter) are interconnected and create a complex sequence of coordinated selective excitation and inhibition governed by complex neural control system involving the brain, spinal cord, and autonomic and somatic nerves. Despite some controversies, this complex control may not be built-in at the time of birth. Conversely, several series of neural circuits which is called "simple reflex arc" are the only functional element serving the role of reflexive emptying [3]. Thus acquisition of bladder control requires meticulous control for coordinated action between abovementioned elements. This can be influenced by developmental process and varies individually. For example, babies with prematurity and low birth weight may tend to show delay in achieving proper control of bowel and bladder. Likewise, children with SD also tend to show delayed toilet training for the reason that is unclear. As the name of SD implies, inadequate structural integrity may contribute to delayed functional maturity. While relief of fecal impaction (FI) is helpful in most cases, it is unclear whether this FI is the direct result from SD attributing to delayed urinary development and needs further scrutiny.

The neurologic innervation of bladder-sphincter complex involves the central somatic and the autonomic nervous systems comprising three sets of peripheral nerves: sacral parasympathetic (pelvic nerve from S2 to S4), thoracolumbar sympathetic (hypogastric nerves and sympathetic chain from segments T10 to L2 of the spinal cord), and sacral somatic (primarily the pudendal nerve) nerves. During emptying phase when parasympathetic influence is dominant, bladder is contracted, urethra as well as urethral sphincter is relaxed facilitating micturition. On the other hand, storage phase marks activation of the sympathetic nerves leading to relaxation of the bladder body and contraction of the urethra and urethral sphincter facilitating storage. The pudendal nerves are somatic nerves from the sacral cord segments S1 to S4. They excite the voluntary external urethral sphincter, holding urine more effectively on purpose.

While the lower urinary tract is composed of the bladder, urethra, and urinary sphincter, it requires complex neural control system involving the brain, spinal cord, and autonomic and somatic nerves for normal function of abovementioned organs. These operate as a series of functioning circuits that overlay each other permitting interconnection and creation of a complex sequence of coordinated selective excitation and inhibition of the bladder, urethra, and sphincter. A variety of neurotransmitters have been identified to play significant roles in these pathways and may provide opportunities for pharmacological intervention.

During bladder filling, sensation of bladder fullness is felt by the lining of bladder (urothelium) and causes afferent nerves to be stimulated. These in turn trigger sympathetic excitatory outflow to the bladder trigone and urethra, and pudendal outflow to the voluntary external sphincter (rhabdosphincter). Sympathetic stimulation also inhibits detrusor muscle and parasympathetic ganglia around bladder. These responses in storage phase postponing micturition are collectively called the guarding reflex. This is evidenced in urodynamics as gradually increasing amplitudes of sphincteric electromyography (EMG) as well as sphincteric tone to maintain continence against increased amount of urine in neurologically normal children (Fig. 2). This guarding reflex which links bladder distention to external sphincter activity during bladder filling can activate sphincter-bladder reflex that will inhibit the parasympathetic excitatory allowing to hold more urine until reaching capacity. In addition, voluntary suppression of voiding such as vigorously repetitively crossing legs, squirting, or tucking the heel into the perineum (Vincent's curtsy) could stimulate somatic afferent pathway of the pudendal nerve leading to inhibition of detrusor contraction by sphincter-bladder inhibitory reflex. In this way, elevation of intravesical pressure is effectively suppressed with the aid of viscoelastic properties of bladder wall and the suppression of excitatory input from parasympathetic nervous system by abovementioned reflexes.

Reaching capacity, increased afferent firing from the tension receptors in the bladder leads to a shift in the efferent activity. In infants, this is elicited reflexively when bladder filling exceeds the threshold volume. However, this reflexive voiding becomes gradually under neural control of spinal or supraspinal level as the child grows. This micturition reflex consisted of the inhibition of sympathetic and somatic nervous system to release sphincter tone, and activation of sacral parasympathetic activity to contract detrusor. Micturition is a coordinated series of events involving an initial relaxation of the urethral sphincter, followed a few seconds later by the contraction of the bladder (Fig. 2), eliciting increase in bladder pressure, and resultant urinary stream. These coordinated movements are primarily orchestrated by pontine micturition center (PMC) located in medial side of dorsal tegmentum pof pons in reflexive voiding [4]. With further development, other brain regions above PMC such as cerebral cortex, cerebellum, basal ganglia, thalamus, and hypothalamus gain control over PMC allowing to control urination as needed. For example, brain lesions above PMC shows uncontrolled detrusor activity and uninhibited voiding while those below PMC show uncontrolled detrusor activity but interrupted voiding

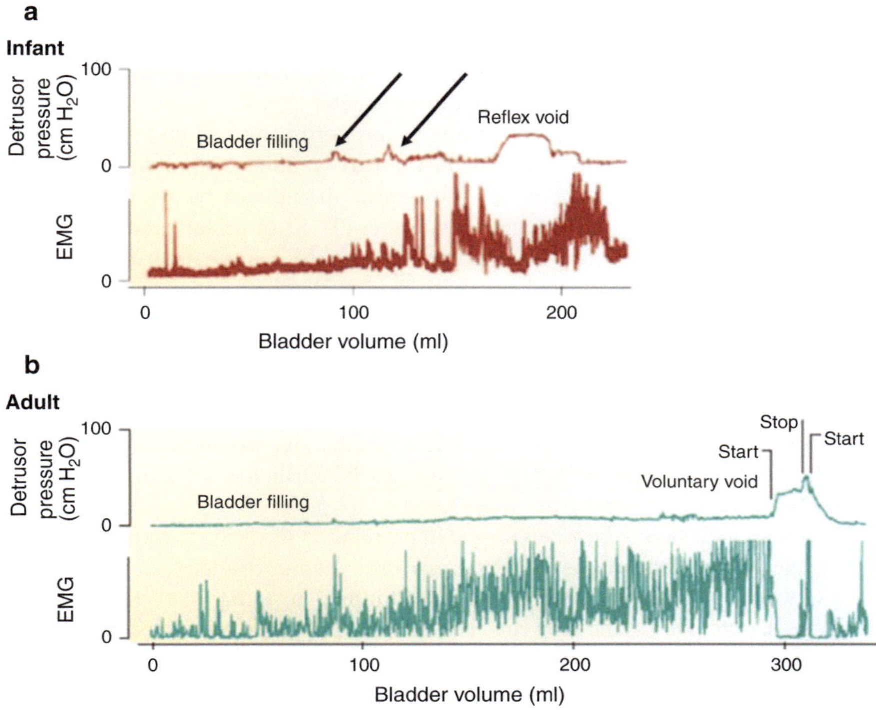

Fig. 2 Comparison of urodynamic findings between infants (**a**) and adults (**b**) to reveal the urodynamic changes during development. During bladder filling, two prominent detrusor overactivities (arrow) are seen in infants. Incomplete guarding reflex is also seen as evidenced by modest increase of electromyography activity during filling. Upon full filling of bladder, voiding commenced reflexively without volitional control. More importantly, incomplete silencing of sphincteric EMG during voiding is evident explaining the reason of detrusor sphincter discoordination (DSD) in immature voiding. Conversely, complete silencing of EMG making sure of uninterrupted voiding is seen in mature adults. The picture was originated from *Fowler CJ et al.* [5]

due to improper control of coordinated movement between detrusor contraction and sphincter (which is called detrusor sphincter dyssynergia, DSD).

Development of Bladder Function

As indicated, neonatal bladder is not always under supraspinal control, and bladder emptying is often made reflexively. This reflexive emptying is often seen as premature detrusor contractile activity before reaching estimated capacity in urodynamic study (arrows in Fig. 2). This premature contraction before reaching capacity can be called detrusor overactivity (DO) resultant from incomplete suppression of central nervous system on autonomous sacral micturition center. Also, neonates often show impaired relaxation of sphincter attributed to immature control of PMC (detrusor sphincter discoordination). It is interesting that these two urodynamic abnormalities seen in immature bladder were also known to be representative urodynamic features attributed to upper motor neuron signs which is seen in lesions located above sacral micturition center.

While most of DO and detrusor sphincter discoordination should no longer be seen in full-term neonates, they may persist in early toddler years in preterm baby or baby with delayed development. Thus these should not be regarded as the pathognomonic sign for tethered cord syndrome (TCS) in infants and there is no rush for immediate untethering for therapeutic purpose. On the other hand, "new" appearance of these signs in children who had undergone untethering could be understood as the strong evidence for secondary tethered cord syndrome (STCS) and bladder deterioration. Persistence of these two signs of immature bladder is also implicated in most nonneurogenic pediatric voiding dysfunction characterized by high bladder pressure, urinary tract infection, and high incidence of vesicoureteral reflux even in normal-looking children. Taken together, we would say that almost all of pediatric bladder dysfunction is at least partly attributed to immature neural control of bladder.

Therefore, care should be taken for the interpretation of various urodynamic tests in this age range. That means the abnormal urodynamic results seen in pediatric patients would turn out to be "temporarily abnormal," resulting in eventual normal urodynamic outcomes in the long run. This gradual improvement with development favors the decision to defer the definite treatment without compelling evidences for urgent intervention.

Normally, obtaining fecal continence precedes urinary continence. That is, nocturnal fecal continence is first seen during development, followed by daytime fecal continence and daytime urinary continence, respectively. Nocturnal urinary continence is the last obtainable event in the development of continence. Until the 5 years of age, gradual changes to voluntary control are achieved. Both urinary and fecal continence should be accomplished when children is over 5 years.

In contrast, bladder function may not fully develop in children, especially in case of immaturity. While improved control of bladder is the rule with increasing age, some factors may interfere this development. For example, developmental disorders affecting central nervous system such as general developmental delay, autism, or mental retardation may often be associated with delay in bladder control [6]. Patients with ADHD was reported to show higher prevalence of urinary as well as fecal incontinence [7]. Studies suggested that areas in brain controlling attention or short-term memory which were impaired in ADHD were in close proximity with those with bladder control explaining the relationship [8–10].

Fecal impaction is the most commonly encountered confounder on bladder control. Even those without sign and symptoms of constipation could show bladder dysfunction attributed to fecal impaction. Moreover, the amount of fecal impaction causing signs of bladder dysfunction may not be the same, highlighting the role of index of suspicion. Fecal impaction is assumed to interrupt bladder function in several ways [11]. Impacted fecal material compresses bladder eliciting DO. Also impacted fecal mass causes persistent tension to anorectal sphincters which share common neurogenic pathway letting them have cross-sensitization. This cross-sensitization is prohibitive from achieving normal urethral control leading to dysfunctional voiding. Also, persistent soiling by fecal impaction is the reason of uninterrupted invasion of uropathogenic bacteria to perineum, prone to recurrent cystitis and voiding dysfunction.

Apart from FI, high-grade vesicoureteral reflux, urinary tract infection, and urinary stone may be implicated in bladder dysfunction. Thus, if one abnormal result is found in the noninvasive urodynamics test, it is necessary to check whether the abnormal test result persists by repeating the noninvasive test rather than immediately performing the invasive test.

Urologic Tools for Investigation in Patients with Spinal Dysraphism

History

History is an important element in the evaluation. This includes urological history such as storage and emptying function, toilet training, urinary tract infection, and urinary tract anomalies. General developmental history, severity of SD (level of conus, presence of syrinx, amount, and location of lipoma) should be considered. Since the bladder and bowel at least partially share the neurological circuit and are in close proximity, the history related to bowel also provides crucial information on neurodevelopmental state of patients. In some children after untethering, high postvoid residual urine (PVR) during follow-up may require invasive urodynamics to understand the reason. However, lack of odor during diaper change or the observation of dry diaper period as opposed to continuous wetting may be the historical clues indicative of adequate emptying function. In this occasion, the invasive urodynamics could be safely postponed and treatment of fecal impaction may often lead to normalized PVR.

Nonoperative Urodynamic Studies

The primary role of nonoperative urodynamic tests is screening those who show abnormal voiding and detecting patients who should require invasive and confirmative urodynamic tests. Also, it may not be properly applied in children prior to toilet training because voiding phase can be assessed based on the sense of fullness or micturitional urge which is acquired after toilet training. However, some negative findings such as minimal postvoid residual urine may be enough to conclude adequate emptying function in case of the lack of spontaneous voiding during voiding trial after filling cystometry (pressure-flow study).

Frequency Volume Chart

In those who completed toilet training, frequency volume chart reveals the number of voiding frequency and the amount of voided volume. This gives an insight regarding patients' sensory function of bladder as well as the overall storage function of bladder. Also, this can be applied to patients undergoing clean intermittent catheterization (CIC) in order to provide information on how much urine the patients can hold at ordinary times. Usually, patients are asked to fill up the data of individual voided volume for at least 2 or 3 days to get a meaningful data. It would be better to include the amount of patient's intake (it is referred to be voiding diary) and 7 days of defecation history as a reference when considering bladder drilling in the context of behavioral treatment [12, 13]. Normal frequency volume chart usually reveals that voided volumes are within the ranges of 50–120% of estimated bladder capacity and voiding is recorded 4–8 times a day.

Uroflowmetry

In those who completed toilet training, uroflowmetry is adequate tool for evaluating emptying function. This study lets the patient void into a funnel in which a sensor will produce a flow (volume-time) curve. If it is combined with measurement of PVR, this would provide more comprehensive picture of emptying function. Good emptying function could be assumed when there will be little amount of PVR and bell-shaped uroflow curve patterns. Those with staccato or intermittent uroflowmetry were suggestive of impaired detrusor contractility or dysfunctional sphincter which interrupts urinary stream due to neurogenic or nonneurogenic causes [12, 13]. (Fig. 3).

Postvoid Residual Urine (PVR) Measurement

In case of neurologically intact spontaneous voiders, the amount of PVR urine could be an adequate estimate for the efficiency of voiding. Elevated PVR may suggest incomplete emptying function and may be caused by either insufficient detrusor contraction or inadequate opening of urethral sphincter. Serial recording and comparison of PVR during postoperative follow-up is important clue to suspect the development of TCS because TCS should be associated with DSD featuring excessive PVR due to impaired detrusor contraction by sphincter-detrusor inhibitory reflex.

For children 4–6 years of age, a single PVR greater than 30 mL or greater than 21% of bladder capacity, or repetitive PVR above 20 mL or greater than 10% of bladder capacity can be regarded as elevated. For children 7–12 years, a single PVR greater than 20 mL or 15% of bladder capacity or repetitive PVR greater than 10 mL or 6% of bladder capacity can be defined as elevated. However, single estimation of

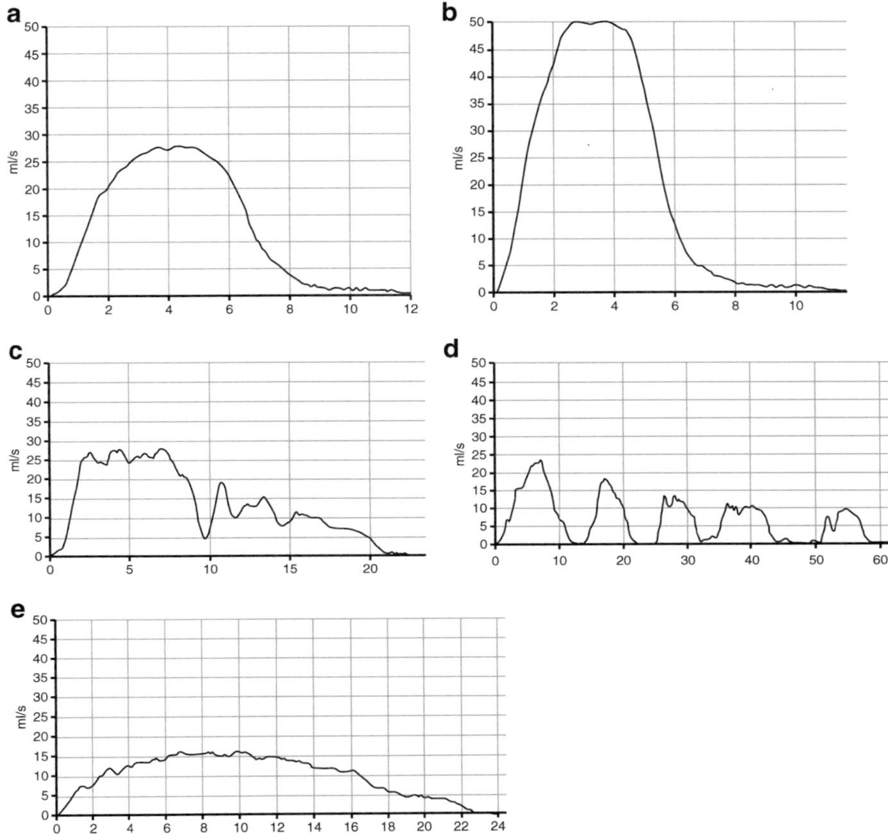

Fig. 3 Five representative types of uroflowmetry. (**a**) bell, (**b**) tower, (**c**) staccato, (**d**) intermittent, (**e**) flat. Bell and tower shape uroflowmetry is suggestive of the lack of obstruction and adequate detrusor contraction. The rest of them indicate either the presence of urethral obstruction or detrusor underactivity. Restraint of urethral stream by infravesical obstruction by either in bladder neck and urethral level shows the characteristic limited peak flow seen in c–e types

PVR is not definitive in any situation. Rather, comparing values during serial follow-up could be more reliable in deciding whether a given PVR is abnormal.

Measurement of PVR is facilitated by the introduction of automated bladder scanner sparing the need for catheterization. However, application in children has been limited and the accuracy in young children was generally unsatisfactory. Our previous study showed the questionable accuracy of individual measurement, excellent correlation was found in conglomerate of measurements [14]. This result points out that if a small amount of residual urine is seen on bladder scanner, it is actually more likely, but for a large amount of residual urine detected in the scanner, the amount may not be accurate. Despite the potential restriction, the noninvasiveness was of utmost significance that would offset all these drawbacks. Therefore, we can safely follow the patients with small PVR in bladder scanner but need to pay attention to only cases with elevated PVR making it sure that this elevation is true. While some cases for PVR elevation may be attributed to the development of TCS, other elevated PVR was found to be attributed to fecal impaction. Thus, treatment of fecal impaction may normalize the PVR, sparing the further need for invasive UDS.

Invasive Urodynamic Study

Invasive urodynamic study generally refers to tests applying urethral catheter to fill the bladder or to gauge the intravesical pressure. This includes cystometry and urethral profilometry. For evaluation of neurogenic bladder, however, cystometry is the most informative by measuring detrusor pressure and sphincteric electrical activity. Cystometry is to simulate filling and voiding phases by gradually filling bladder. The bladder and abdominal pressure are recorded by simultaneous measurement of both intravesical and intrarectal pressure, the latter representing intraabdominal pressure. By subtracting intraabdominal pressure from intravesical pressure, genuine detrusor pressure can be calculated during cystometry (Fig. 4).

Measuring perineal electromyography reveals the activity of pelvic floor muscle which gives important clues for guarding reflex and DSD.

Often fluoroscopic imaging is obtained during conventional cystometry and is called videourodynamic study. This allows to give more information such as urethral synergy, trabeculation of bladder shape, and occurrence of vesicoureteral reflux. The most significant drawback is the invasiveness related to the need for catheterization. Therefore, applying UDS is not indicated in all patients, but should be considered in case of (1) ineffective conventional treatment, (2) prior to surgery that may affect urologic function, (3) inconclusive results from noninvasive study.

According to International Continence Society (ICS), good UDS should reveal sense, detrusor contraction, compliance, capacity, and urethral function during storage phase [15]. During bladder filling, bladder is gradually filled with the rate of less than 10% of age-adjusted bladder capacity in a minute to simulate the bladder filling cycle. With the increased amount of filling, normal bladder should maintain their intravesical pressure within a limited range.

Problem list in storage phase includes abnormal capacity, gradual and persistent elevation of detrusor pressure suggestive of reduced compliance, detrusor overactivity, and sphincteric incompetence. This should be monitored and carefully recorded. Leakage during filling could be elicited by elevated detrusor pressure or incompetent sphincter which need to be accounted during cystometry. Problems in voiding phase are DSD and lack of detrusor contraction. Vesicoureteral reflux could be seen in both filling as well as voiding phases.

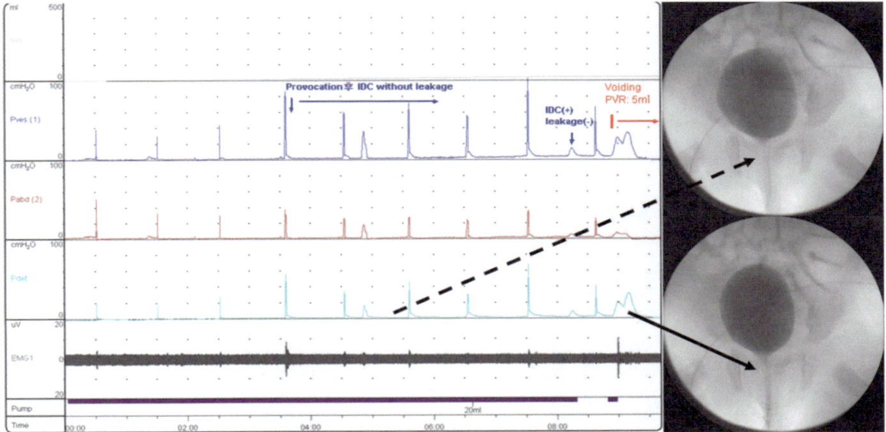

Fig. 4 Representative urodynamic study seen in those who are expected to undergo preventive untethering. Intravesical, abdominal and detrusor pressure was measured in 2,3, and fourth columns. To check in the integrity of abdominal pressure and its correspondence with vesical pressure, pressing down the bladder was done during the study. Normally no detrusor pressure elevation is seen but reflection of vesical pressure is somewhat stronger. At the end of filling spontaneous contraction of detrusor is seen (the start of arrow) and this only elevates the vesical pressure but does not elevate the abdominal pressure. Hence, elevation of detrusor pressure was shown and funneling of sphincter suggestive of synergic voiding was seen. The active change in the shapes of sphincter indicates intact neurologic control

Assessment

Having all aforementioned knowledge in bladder physiology and developmental aspect of voiding function, urological assessment of patients' status could be accurately made. Most significant urological morbidity as well as mortality inherent to TCS is renal dysfunction secondary to elevated bladder pressure and urinary tract infection. This is urodynamically revealed to be low compliance, frequent DO, reduced capacity, and high leak point pressure. This is due to DO and DSD when effective urinary drainage is virtually impossible. Urinary tract infection frequently occurs due to difficulty in clearing bacteria. Experimentally, when intravesical bladder goes over 15 cm H_2O, renal drainage to bladder was found to be hampered and eventual hydroureteronephrosis and renal parenchymal thinning appeared. High intravesical pressure is also pivotal to the development of VUR and ascending renal infection which further aggravates renal injury. Thus, presence of DO and DSD should be sought thoroughly to protect renal damages. One caveat is the detection of DSD. While DO may be found intuitively, the detection of DSD is not seen as clear as DO. Placing needle EMG in the urethral sphincter is the standard method but this is invasive and requires skill to locate the needle in the correct position. Alternatively, applying video UDS and demonstrating active sphincteric contraction in the face of elevated detrusor pressure is helpful (Fig. 5).

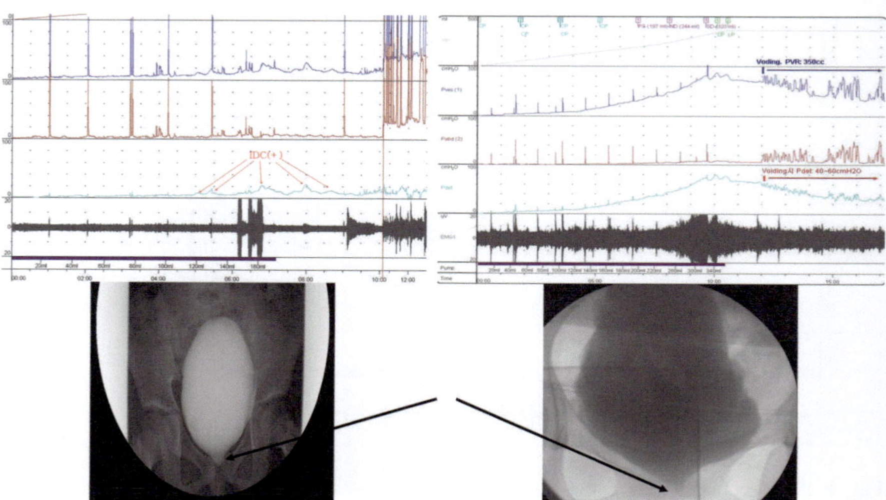

Fig. 5 Representative cases of detrusor sphincter dyssynergia seen in those receiving previous untethering. The UDS trace in the left panel shows multiple detrusor overactivities which is described as IDC (arrows). IDC referring to idiopathic detrusor contraction which is urodynamic synonym of detrusor overactivity. Also noted active sphincteric contraction in face of detrusor contraction suggestive of detrusor sphincter dyssynergia. In the right panel, both the intravesical and detrusor pressure are gradually elevated with increased filling. This is due to increased wall tension as revealed by trabeculated bladder seen below. It is assumed to be the result from chronic bladder outlet obstruction from DSD as revealed by posterior urethral dilation above abrupt sphincteric narrowing (arrow). This increased wall tension due to chronic bladder outlet obstruction leads to gradual elevation of intravesical and detrusor pressure which is also called reduced compliance

As SD is mostly found in lower lumbar or sacral spine level which corresponds to sacral micturition center, typical neurogenic bladder shows the feature of lower motor neuron disease. In most case of open SD or huge closed SD involving lumbosacral area, they typically show lack of detrusor contraction due to involvement of sacral micturition center following untethering [16]. Also, they commonly show opened bladder neck due to sphincter denervation and they will lead to persistent urine leakage. In most cases of closed SD, most of them show notable detrusor contraction, synergic urethral movement, and acceptable PVR revealed from preoperative UDS. This indicates no evidence of neurological damage in the initial presentation of closed SD. Only a few patients with closed SD may show the lack of detrusor contraction, incompetent sphincteric zone, presenting continuous dribbling due to urinary retention characteristic of lower motor neuron sign seen in open SD.

Adding more complexity, immaturity inherent to infants and toddlers should be considered in interpreting their urodynamic data. Indeed, immature bladder function may be understood as transient neurogenic bladder where abnormal neurological sign inherent to neurogenic bladder could be seen as a result of immature control of voiding reflexes.

Most patients with closed SD who showed normal synergic voiding in their preoperative UDS maintained their capability of spontaneous voiding with little PVR. During filling cystometry, bladder usually tends to maintain low vesical pressure, but incidental DO which is resultant from incomplete control of bladder is not uncommon in healthy infants. This may be elicited by immature neural control or detrusor muscle itself (myogenic origin), so DO alone could be seen in the absence of tethered cord syndrome. The typical UDS trace and corresponding cystographic findings in synergic voiders are depicted in Fig. 4. On the other hand, most untethered patients with open SD showed continuous wetting diaper (continuously dribbling urine through the urethra) due to denervated sphincter and the lack of overt urinary stream. This pattern is characteristic sign of lower motor neuron lesion involvement. Only a few showed synergic urethral movement and spontaneous voiding. PVR in these patients is usually of little amount. Most patients with closed SDs who have shown normal synergic voiding either maintained their spontaneous voiding or gradually regained their spontaneous voiding from postoperative underactive detrusor seen just after untethering. This regaining usually completed until toilet training [17].

Follow-up scheme and schedule of patients with SD may be better tailored according to the risk of urinary tract aggravation. Those with spontaneous voiding as evidenced by PVR less than 20% of age-adjusted value and streamed voiding may be spared from annual regular follow-up urodynamic study. Patients with open SD or those required CIC should receive annual follow-up UDS. In case of progressive aggravation, or encountering failure to medical treatment, UDS should be performed to clarify the reason. Our selective application of UDS and following up of most patients with spontaneous voiders with noninvasive PVR measurement may reduce the number of unnecessary invasive UDS in normal spontaneous voiders while maintaining the vigilance to patients with high risk of urological progression.

In order not to miss the cases for aggravation, understanding the implication of PVR measurement with portable ultrasound bladder scanner could be applied to determine whether urodynamic study is required. The simple and easy application of the machine makes the repetitive noninvasive measurement possible. When measured PVR in children is small, this suggests little possibility of TCS especially in those with spontaneous voiders. Rarely, TCS may be progressed in those with denervated sphincter with modest PVR. However, small PVR in bladder scanner indicates bladder is fine. This indicates that the portable bladder scanner is good for screening exempting the need for regular invasive urodynamic follow-up. Problem in interpretation may arise in cases of unacceptably high PVR, because this may be caused by either non-neurogenic or neurogenic causes. Thus, care should be taken in diagnosing neurogenic problem and determining to do urodynamic study for confirmation. The most common cause of nonneurogenic elevation of PVR is fecal impaction which is not uncommon in this age group. Careful history taking may be helpful for differential diagnosis because patients with neurogenic problem such as TCS will present elevated PVR constantly. In those with elevated PVR without neurogenic problem, this elevation appears to be more situational and more commonly seen in places unfamiliar to children such as hospital. According to the words from parents, they voided well at home. When the elevation is first identified and there is no supporting histories of urinary retention such as urinary foul odor recognized during diaper change and constant wetting of diaper which is suggestive of chronic retention of bladder may provide a historical clue of neurogenic problem. In those with elevated PVR, fecal impaction is first addressed by applying stool softener and then PVR measurement is repeated. Invasive UDS is spared for repetitive and persistent elevation of PVR despite the treatment of fecal impaction.

Achieving toilet training is an important milestone to achieve adequate bladder control. If there is no problem in continence following toilet training, there is little chance for future TCS, and TCS may be easily detected by changes in urinary symptoms. The incomplete or delayed achievement of toilet training may imply the future risk of development of TCS.

Those who could not void spontaneously are indicated for regular UDS to monitor their bladder status. According to their bladder status, regular CIC should be instituted for emptying, and anticholinergics may be added for reducing bladder tone. In those who were able to void spontaneously revealed in preoperative UDS, the lack of regaining spontaneous voiding until post-untethering 6 months may be a sign of developing retethered cord which is an unexpected consequence after the first untethering. While postoperative neuropraxia may hamper the regaining of spontaneous voiding until 6 months after the first untethering this should no longer persist than 6 months. The presence of DSD due to tethered cord syndrome could elicit sphincter-detrusor inhibitory reflex leading to lack of detrusor contraction.

In most cases for neurogenic bladder presenting DO and DSD, the bladder gets deteriorated as evidenced by high intravesical pressure, reduced compliance, and significant trabeculation. This will harbor hydroureteronephrosis, urinary incontinence, and urinary tract infection, resulting in renal damage. As there is no way to reverse DSD, control of DO by anticholinergics and diversion of urine by CIC are the mainstay of management. Despite the effort, however, some patients may experience deterioration due to failure to control DO. Aggravating bladder trabeculation will lead to decompensated bladder when no treatment is working. While surgery like augmentation cystoplasty will be the last resort, we recently reported that redo-untethering when carefully performed could be a viable option even for the candidates of augmentation cystoplasty (Fig. 6) [18]. Following the redo-untethering, not only the problem of DO and DSD but also the severe trabeculation which is the sign for decompensated bladder was normalized during follow-up [18].

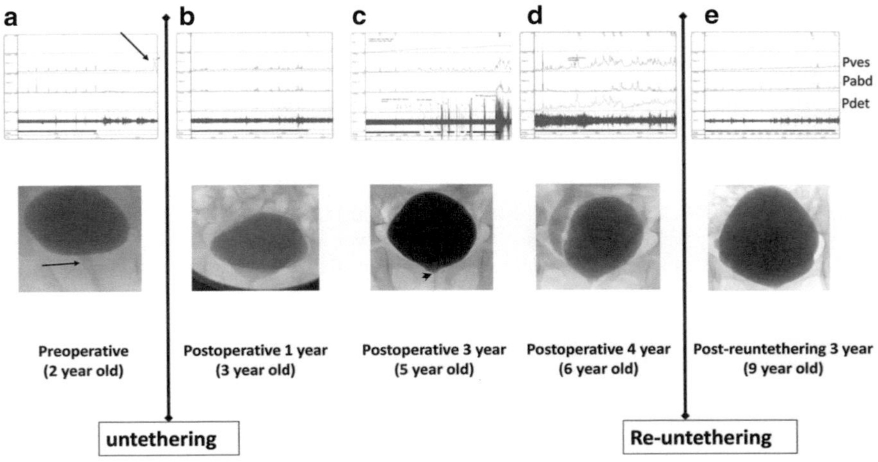

Fig. 6 Typical videourodynamic changes from before the primary untethering to after re-untethering operation in a female patient. From the *top*, each row in the urodynamic trace indicated vesical, abdominal, and detrusor pressure (*right side*). (**a**) Synergic urethral funneling movement and notable bladder contraction (*arrow*) were seen before primary untethering. (**b**) Spontaneous voiding disappeared after primary untethering, and no notable detrusor contraction was shown. Clinically, patient required intermittent catheterization to empty the bladder. (**c**) Several years later, the patient's parents complained of failure to achieve toilet training and increased urinary incontinence. In videourodynamic study, this could be explained by the emergence of detrusor overactivity and detrusor sphincter dyssynergia (*arrowhead*). (**d**)The patient's urinary incontinence was getting worse despite the conservative treatment, and the patient was suffering from repetitive and refractory urinary tract infection to conventional management. Newly appeared right dilating vesicoureteral reflux was also seen. Detrusor overactivity was getting more prominent and DSD persisted. (**e**) Following re-untethering, the patient's storage function was normalized in terms of maximal cystometric capacity, compliance, and detrusor overactivity. Moreover, the patient's sphincter remained closed due to increased compliance

Conclusion

Due to various manifestations of SD and difficulty in evaluating pediatric population, uniform evaluation protocol may not be appropriate and need to be tailored in accordance with the risk of progression. To assess the risk, understanding the pathophysiology and applying adequate combination of noninvasive and invasive tests are important. Understanding the upper motor neuron sign is crucial is diagnosing TCS.

References

1. Dudley AG, Adams MC, Brock JW 3rd, et al. Interrater reliability in interpretation of neuropathic pediatric urodynamic tracings: an expanded multicenter study. J Urol. 2018;199(5):1337–43. https://doi.org/10.1016/j.juro.2017.12.051.
2. Miller BD, Tallman CT, Boone TB, Khavari R. Low interrater reliability of videourodynamic diagnosis of detrusor external sphincter dyssynergia. Female Pelvic Med Reconstr Surg. 2021;27(5):297–9. https://doi.org/10.1097/spv.0000000000000754.
3. Andersson KE, Wein AJ. Pharmacology of the lower urinary tract: basis for current and future treatments of urinary incontinence. Pharmacol Rev. 2004;56(4):581–631. https://doi.org/10.1124/pr.56.4.4.
4. de Groat WC, Griffiths D, Yoshimura N. Neural control of the lower urinary tract. Compr Physiol. 2015;5(1):327–96. https://doi.org/10.1002/cphy.c130056.
5. Fowler CJ, Griffiths D, de Groat WC. The neural control of micturition. Nat Rev Neurosci. 2008;9(6):453–66.
6. Niemczyk J, Wagner C, von Gontard A. Incontinence in autism spectrum disorder: a systematic review. Eur Child Adolesc Psychiatry. 2018;27(12):1523–37. https://doi.org/10.1007/s00787-017-1062-3.
7. von Gontard A, Hussong J, Yang SS, Chase J, Franco I, Wright A. Neurodevelopmental disorders and incontinence in children and adolescents: attention-deficit/hyperactivity disorder, autism spectrum disorder, and intellectual disability-a consensus document of the international Children's continence society. Neurourol Urodyn. 2022;41(1):102–14. https://doi.org/10.1002/nau.24798.
8. Baeyens D, Roeyers H, Hoebeke P, Antrop I, Mauel R, Walle JV. The impact of attention deficit hyperactivity disorders on brainstem dysfunction in nocturnal enuresis. J Urol. 2006;176(2):744–8. https://doi.org/10.1016/s0022-5347(06)00295-3.
9. Baeyens D, Roeyers H, Naert S, Hoebeke P, Vande WJ. The impact of maturation of brainstem inhibition on enuresis: a startle eye blink modification study with 2-year followup. J Urol. 2007;178(6):2621–5. https://doi.org/10.1016/j.juro.2007.07.061.
10. Yu B, Kong F, Peng M, Ma H, Liu N, Guo Q. Assessment of memory/attention impairment in children with primary nocturnal enuresis: a voxel-based morphometry study. Eur J Radiol. 2012;81(12):4119–22. https://doi.org/10.1016/j.ejrad.2012.01.006.
11. Malykhina AP, Brodie KE, Wilcox DT. Genitourinary and gastrointestinal co-morbidities in children: the role of neural circuits in regulation of visceral function. J Pediatr Urol. 2017;13(2):177–82. https://doi.org/10.1016/j.jpurol.2016.04.036.
12. Austin PF, Bauer SB, Bower W, et al. The standardization of terminology of lower urinary tract function in children and adolescents: update report from the standardization Committee of the International Children's continence society. J Urol. 2014;191(6):1863–1865.e13. https://doi.org/10.1016/j.juro.2014.01.110.
13. Austin PF, Bauer SB, Bower W, et al. The standardization of terminology of lower urinary tract function in children and adolescents: update report from the standardization committee of the international Children's continence society. Neurourol Urodyn. 2016;35(4):471–81. https://doi.org/10.1002/nau.22751.
14. Do MT, Kim L, Im YJ, Park K. Can portable ultrasound bladder scanner be applied to young children less than three years old? J Pediatr Urol. 2022;18(3):344–9. https://doi.org/10.1016/j.jpurol.2022.02.001.
15. Bauer SB, Nijman RJ, Drzewiecki BA, Sillen U, Hoebeke P. International Children's continence society standardization report on urodynamic studies of the lower urinary tract in children. Neurourol Urodyn. 2015;34(7):640–7. https://doi.org/10.1002/nau.22783.
16. Tuite GF, Thompson DNP, Austin PF, Bauer SB. Evaluation and management of tethered cord syndrome in occult spinal dysraphism: recommendations from the international children's continence society. Neurourol Urodyn. 2018;37(3):890–903. https://doi.org/10.1002/nau.23382.

17. Kim L, Do MT, Jung HD, et al. Preoperative Videourodynamic study is helpful in predicting long-term postoperative voiding function in asymptomatic patients with closed spinal dysraphism. Int Neurourol J. 2022;26(1):60–8. https://doi.org/10.5213/inj.2142246.123.
18. Lee SB, Im YJ, Jung JH, et al. Clinical and urodynamic features of secondary tethered cord syndrome: how can they be found longitudinally? Neurourol Urodyn. 2022;41(1):365–74. https://doi.org/10.1002/nau.24832.